Quality and Safety in Pharmacy Practice

NOTICE

Medicine is an ever-changing science. As new research and clinical experience broaden our knowledge, changes in treatment and drug therapy are required. The authors and the publisher of this work have checked with sources believed to be reliable in their efforts to provide information that is complete and generally in accord with the standards accepted at the time of publication. However, in view of the possibility of human error or changes in medical sciences, neither the authors nor the publisher nor any other party who has been involved in the preparation or publication of this work warrants that the information contained herein is in every respect accurate or complete, and they disclaim all responsibility for any errors or omissions or for the results obtained from use of the information contained in this work. Readers are encouraged to confirm the information contained herein with other sources. For example and in particular, readers are advised to check the product information sheet included in the package of each drug they plan to administer to be certain that the information contained in this work is accurate and that changes have not been made in the recommended dose or in the contraindications for administration. This recommendation is of particular importance in connection with new or infrequently used drugs.

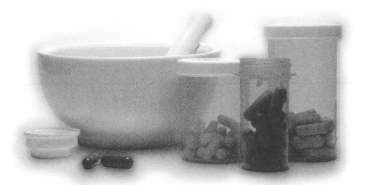

Quality and Safety in Pharmacy Practice

EDITORS

TERRI L. WARHOLAK, PHD, RPH

Assistant Professor
Department of Pharmacy Practice and Science
The University of Arizona College of Pharmacy
Tucson, Arizona

DAVID P. NAU, PHD, RPH, CPHQ

Senior Director
Research & Performance Measurement
Pharmacy Quality Alliance
Lexington, Kentucky

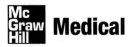 **Medical**

New York   Chicago   San Francisco   Lisbon   London   Madrid
Mexico City   Milan   New Delhi   San Juan   Seoul
Singapore   Sydney   Toronto

The **McGraw·Hill** Companies

Quality and Safety in Pharmacy Practice

1 2 3 4 5 6 7 8 9 0   DOC/DOC   14 13 12 11 10

ISBN 978-0-07-160385-0
MHID 0-07-160385-9

This book was set in Adobe Garamond Pro by Thomson Digital.
The editors were Michael Weitz and Robert Pancotti.
The production supervisor was Sherri Souffrance.
Project management was provided by Aakriti Kathuria, Thomson Digital.
The text designer was Eve Siegel; the cover designer was Mary McKeon.
Front cover photograph: Credit: Bruce Ayres/GettyImages.
RR Donnelley was printer and binder.

This book is printed on acid-free paper.

Library of Congress Cataloging-in-Publication Data

Quality and safety in pharmacy practice/editors, Terri L. Warholak,
David P. Nau.
    p. ; cm.
  Includes bibliographical references and index.
  ISBN-13: 978-0-07-160385-0 (pbk. : alk. paper)
  ISBN-10: 0-07-160385-9 (pbk. : alk. paper)
1. Pharmacy—Safety measures. 2. Medication errors—Prevention.
I. Warholak, Terri L. II. Nau, David P.
  [DNLM: 1. Pharmaceutical Services—standards—United States.
  2. Medication Errors—prevention & control—United States. 3. Quality
  Assurance, Health Care—methods—United States. 4. Safety
  Management—methods—United States. QV 737 Q11 2010]
  RS122.5.Q35 2010
  615'.10289—dc22
                              2010002972

McGraw-Hill books are available at special quantity discounts to use as premiums and sales promotions, or for use in corporate training programs. To contact a representative, please e-mail us at bulksales@mcgraw-hill.com.

DEDICATION

To Bert Ehrmann for his love and support to me during the creation of this book.

— Terri

To Martha, Jena, Paige and Maddie for their patience and love during the late nights and weekends spent on this book.

— Dave

Key Features of *Quality and Safety In Pharmacy Practice*

Everything you need to gain a complete understanding of the principles of quality improvement and their application to present and future pharmacy practice:

- Details the principles, approaches, strategies, and actions necessary to improve overall safety and effectiveness of pharmacy services

- Includes guidelines that can be implemented immediately to improve today's pharmacy practice

- Offers a complete overview of quality in general, the reasons for improving practice, and actual day-to-day changes and approaches that will positively impact the patient

- Logically divided into five parts:

  - The current and future landscape of health care quality and the business case for quality improvement and value-driven health care

  - Quality improvement concepts and tools, including statistical process control

  - Quality and safety measurement, including mechanisms for gathering consumer feedback

  - Incentives and other drivers of quality improvement

  - Application of the principles of quality improvement to pharmacy practice—complete with case examples

CHAPTER 7

Identifying Causes of Quality Problems

Terri L. Warholak and Ana Hincapie

Learning Objectives

At the end of the chapter, the reader will be able to:

1. Recognize problems associated with identifying quality issues and solutions.
2. Select an appropriate topic for analysis.
3. Support the use of root cause analysis.
4. Support the use of Healthcare Failure Modes and Effects Analysis (HFMEA^SM).

Key Definitions

- *Detectable hazard:* A very evident potential risk that will be promptly discovered before it hampers the completion of an activity (e.g., an IV bag that is leaking).
- *Effective control measure:* A barrier that eliminates or substantially reduces the likelihood of a hazardous event occurring (e.g., the pharmaceutical form of some medications prevents its use via the wrong administration route such as I tubing that only connects for IV catheter, not nasal cannula).
- *Failure mode:* Different ways that a process or subprocess can fail to provide the anticipated result.
- *Failure mode cause:* Different reasons as to why a process or subprocess would fail to provide the anticipated result.
- *Hazard analysis:* Identification and evaluation of potential hazards that are likely to produce harm in a specific process if not controlled.
- *Healthcare Failure Modes and Effects Analysis (HFMEA^SM):* A systematic approach to identify and prevent product and process problems before they occur.
- *Single point weakness:* A step in the process so critical that its failure would result in system failure or an adverse event (e.g., the prescriber order is processed for the wrong patient; this would result in the preparation, delivery, and administration of the wrong medications).

81

LEARNING OBJECTIVES provide a concise summary of what you can expect to learn from each chapter

KEY DEFINITIONS familiarize you with important words and phrases within a chapter

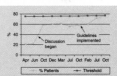

Figure 9-12. Results: percent appropriate meperidine use.

Check the change.
Post-implementation, data demonstrate that the formulary change has been successful. Pharmacy is responsible for the data collection, and data are collected from a combination of purchase and usage records, along with electronic health record (or paper) chart review. Data are collated by physician prescribing service for any outliers that are identified. With the formulary restriction and "no buy" designation, the use of meperidine has declined compared with total opioid, and the use now is in appropriate circumstances over 80% of the time (see Figures 9-12 and 9-13). Work will continue to identify outliers, upkeep the clinical information systems, and new literature.

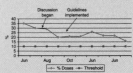

Figure 9-13. Results: percent meperidine versus total opioids.

DIAGRAMS help you visualize important data

200   Part IV ◻▸ Quality-based Interventions and Incentives

In an analysis aimed specifically at health care organizations, barriers to change are classified into three categories: input related [inputs (patients) are difficult to control and experiment with], process related (processes are complex, critical, and difficult to standardize), and output related (outputs are difficult to measure, control, and relate back to causes). These barriers stem from health care providers typically considering their work to be "sacred" and not fully incorporating patients into the system.[25]

CASE EXAMPLE 1

A consultant once worked with a pharmacy organization on a quality improvement project. The effort was promoted company-wide. In the middle of the planning stage, a staff pharmacist refused to fill a prescription for a controlled substance, because he was quite certain that the patient in question was a drug abuser. The patient complained, and the pharmacist was chastised. This case illustrates the pitfalls when goals are not congruent (i.e., the pharmacist's definition of quality patient care versus the company's definition of quality customer service). Also, it shows the importance of establishing a trust relationship between management and employees.

The policy implementation literature also has a long history of exploring obstacles to change. It is worthwhile to segment these obstacles into two categories. The first occurs when there is a lack of agreement on goals, or on what the policy/change actually should be. Policy implementation problems are often due to lack of agreement on goals because: each level of the organization has its own goals and policies, authority is never total, and interested parties try to influence policy at all levels.[26]

The second category of problems includes barriers of a more technical nature. That is, even when goal consensus exists, implementation problems may still occur in the form of technical obstacles that arise as the policy makes its way through the organization. Table 12-1 summarizes two articles from the policy literature that identify barriers to policy implementation. Each barrier is categorized as a "different goals" or "technical" problem.

Relating our discussion to the incremental quality improvement model of Six Sigma, we find that even though it is a relatively new and innovative process, barriers to its success are similar to those identified in the previous discussion. These include ambivalence of management, lack of broad participation, dependence on consensus, initiatives that are too broad or too narrow, failure to attack cultural obstacles, and, finally, lack of understanding of the principles of Six Sigma.[7]

PRACTICES THAT FACILITATE AND MAINTAIN CHANGE

The importance of addressing barriers to change cannot be overstated, as the consequences of change resistance are quite severe and include noncompliance with the new

CASE STUDIES demonstrate real world application of principles

Contents

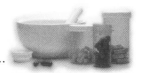

PART III   Quality Measurement

PART IV   Quality-based Interventions and Incentives

PART V   Application of Quality Improvement to the Pharmacy Practice Setting

Contributors

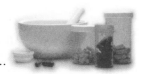

Kenneth Baker, BS Pharm, JD
Renaud Cook Drury Mesaros, PA
Phoenix, Arizona
Pharmacists Mutual Insurance Company
(Consultant, former General Counsel, and
Senior Vice President)
Algona, Iowa
Adjunct Assistant Professor
Midwestern University
Glendale, Arizona
Adjunct Assistant Professor
University of Florida
Gainesville, Florida

Susan J. Blalock, MPH, PhD
Associate Professor
Division of Pharmaceutical Outcomes
and Policy
Eshelman School of Pharmacy
University of North Carolina
Chapel Hill, North Carolina

Elizabeth A. Flynn, RPh, PhD
Associate Research Professor
Center for Pharmacy Operations
and Designs
Harrison School of Pharmacy
Auburn University
Auburn, Alabama

Ana Hincapie, MS
PhD Student
Pharmaceutical Economics,
Policy and Outcomes
The University of Arizona College
of Pharmacy
Tucson, Arizona

David A. Holdford, RPh, MS, PhD
Associate Professor
Department of Pharmacy
School of Pharmacy
Virginia Commonwealth University
Richmond, Virginia

San Keller, MS, PhD
Principal Scientist
American Institutes for Research
Health Services Research
Chapel Hill, North Carolina

Duane M. Kirking, PharmD, PhD
Professor Emeritus
College of Pharmacy
University of Michigan
Ann Arbor, Michigan

Julie Kuhle, BPharm
Pharmacy Manager
Iowa Foundation for Medical Care
West Des Moines, Iowa

Debra Legner, PharmD, MBA, MS
Pharmacist
Carlsbad Medical Center
Carlsbad, New Mexico

**Leticia R. Moczygemba,
PharmD, PhD**
Assistant Professor
Department of Pharmacy
School of Pharmacy
Virginia Commonwealth University
Richmond, Virginia

Terri Moore, PhD, MBA, RPh
Pharmacy Accreditation Reviewer
URAC
Washington, District of Columbia

David P. Nau, PhD, RPh, CPHQ
Senior Director
Research & Performance Measurement
Pharmacy Quality Alliance
Lexington, Kentucky

Ana C. Quiñones-Boex, PhD
Associate Professor of Pharmacy
    Administration
Midwestern University Chicago
    College of Pharmacy
Downers Grove, Illinois

Thomas J. Reutzel, PhD
Professor of Pharmacy Administration
Midwestern University Chicago
    College of Pharmacy
Downers Grove, Illinois

Lynne Schifreen, RN, MS, CPHQ
Quality Process Manager
Humana Pharmacy Solutions
Lees Summit, Missouri

**Virginia (Ginger) G. Scott,
PhD, MS, RPh**
Professor and Director of Continuing
    Education
Department of Pharmaceutical
    Systems and Policy
School of Pharmacy
West Virginia University
Morgantown, West Virginia

Susan J. Skledar, RPh, MPH, FASHP
Associate Professor, School of Pharmacy
    Director, Drug Use and Disease
    Management Program
University of Pittsburgh Medical Center
Department of Pharmacy
University of Pittsburgh
Pittsburgh, Pennsylvania

Mi Chi Song, PharmD
Southern Arizona
    VA Health Care System
Tucson, Arizona

Terri L. Warholak, PhD, RPh
Assistant Professor
Department of Pharmacy Practice
    and Science
The University of Arizona College
    of Pharmacy
Tucson, Arizona

**Robert J. Weber, PharmD,
MS, BCPS, FASHP**
Senior Director of Pharmaceutical Services
The Ohio State University Medical Center
Assistant Dean for Medical Center Affairs
Clinical Associate Professor—Pharmacy
    Practice and Administration
The Ohio State University College of
    Pharmacy
Columbus, Ohio

Donna West-Strum, RPh, PhD
Chair and Associate Professor
Department of Pharmacy Administration
    Research
Associate Professor
Research Institute of Pharmaceutical
    Sciences
School of Pharmacy, The University
    of Mississippi
Oxford, Mississippi

Foreword

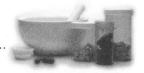

The effectiveness and safety of drug therapy and pharmaceutical services that help to insure the attainment of patient outcomes seems to be the topic of the day. Those knowledgeable of the history of pharmacy are familiar with the >100 years that the profession has put forth a continuous effort to improve the appropriate use of medicinal products by the advent of pharmaceutical services that are truly focused on maximizing the value of treatment. At any time, the issue revolves around access, cost, and quality of health care. It was not until recent years that the issue of the quality of health care including safety reached such a high point of discussion across all interested parties, including professionals, payers, regulators, and most importantly consumers. This was a result at least in part due to the release of the Institute of Medicine report, *To Err Is Human: Building a Safer Health System* (2000). The treatise articulated well the major problems in the delivery of health care in general, which indeed point to the fact that serious quality and safety issues exist throughout our health care delivery system, although many express chagrin at any reference to a "system."

The "To Err" report was followed by a second in a series of several reports on quality, titled *Crossing the Quality Chasm: A New Health System for the 21st Century* (2001). This IOM report articulates the commitment to which we all must adhere in order to improve health care to any measurable level. Health care must be not only safe and effective, but also patient-centered, timely, efficient, and equitable. The strategies needed to accomplish this goal include stronger adherence and adoption to evidence-based practice, which must be interdisciplinary, grounded in information technology, focused on management of chronic disease and increased consumer involvement/partnerships, and involve restructuring of the payment system. Additionally, the IOM published a report dealing specifically with health professions education, titled *Health Professions Education: A Bridge to Quality* (2003). This report called for dramatic changes in the education of health practitioners. Emphasis was placed on improved education in all aspects of the "quality" sciences. Interdisciplinary teams of health professionals must obtain competency in evidence-based practice, quality improvement, and informatics.

There is little doubt that the publications of the IOM reports posed many questions for each of the health professions. What measures of improvement does the profession of pharmacy propose? How does the profession propose to improve its quality efforts? How does the profession move to the next level of care that will indeed improve the safe and effective delivery of pharmaceutical services and ultimately will improve the outcomes of medication therapy? The two final reports in the IOM quality series were related to medication safety at both the research and the application level. Both reports received much public discussion; still to this day, policies and action plans are being developed and implemented based on their recommendations. *The Future of Drug Safety: Promoting and Protecting the Health of the Public* (2007) report addressed safety from the standpoint of the FDA drug approval process, including postmarketing activities to further detect safety issues as drugs are adopted for widespread use.

The *Preventing Medication Errors: Quality Chasm Series* (2007) report, which I co-chaired, was initiated by Congress to develop a national agenda for medication error reduction based on the alarming incidence of medication errors in the United States. The report focused on strategies to prevent and resolve this epidemic issue. It was noted that medication errors were prevalent in all settings of health care, including acute care, long-term care, and certainly ambulatory care. Many of my writings and publications refer to medication errors as the "silent disease" in America. I believe that the pharmacy profession is the only one of the health professions that has made the most dramatic, sweeping changes in the education of pharmacists and technical support staff to the exploration and implementation of highly significant pharmacy services based on a new paradigm of professional practice that many refer to as pharmaceutical care.

This new book is so timely and necessary to lay out the complex set of principles, approaches, strategies, and actions to improve the overall safety and effectiveness of pharmacy services with the goal of improving the quality of health care in the future. However, the book also gives guidelines that can be implemented *today* for improvement at the basic level of pharmacy services. It is essential that pharmacy students and pharmacists be educated on the principles of quality improvement. This text provides a superb overview of quality in general, the reasons for improving practice, and actual day-to-day changes and approaches that will positively impact those persons whom we serve, the patients. As a health care professional, I believe that we must strive to reduce pain and suffering of those we serve and ultimately prevent disease and the further progression of disease. Pharmaceuticals and their appropriate use can be accomplished only with quality pharmacy services. This book is our guiding tool for accomplishing this mission.

J. Lyle Bootman, PhD, ScD
Dean, College of Pharmacy
Professor of Pharmacy, Medicine and Public Health
Founding and Executive Director
Center for Health Outcomes and PharmacoEconomic Research

Preface

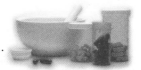

This book is the culmination of many years of academic study and real-world experience of the authors and those who have shaped our view of the world. For too long, the profession of pharmacy has functioned on the premise that quality depended solely on hiring good people who would naturally "do the right thing." We hope to shift the perspective of pharmacists and pharmacy students toward *systems thinking* wherein it is not enough merely to have good intentions. We need to understand how pharmacists interact with the system in which they work and how we can construct the system to safeguard our patients from human fallibility.

We also hope to fill the void in pharmacy curricula pertaining to quality and safety. Many pharmacists have received no formal instruction in the principles or tools of health care quality. This book provides information about the broad principles of quality improvement (QI) along with insights on their application to the practice of pharmacy. It also shows practical tools for QI that the reader can adapt to his or her specific needs.

Chapters 1–4 describe the current and future landscape for health care quality and provide a framework for examining standards of medication use. These chapters also establish the business case for QI and value-driven health care. There are clear consequences for ignoring the safety and quality deficits in our current medication-use system and we hope to establish the need for QI in the everyday practice of pharmacy.

Chapters 5–8 lay the foundation for understanding the concepts and tools of QI. The foundation is built on the theoretical frameworks proposed by quality gurus such as W. Edwards Deming, Walter Shewart, and Avedis Donabedian. We believe that it is important for pharmacists to understand how to think about quality so they can truly build the culture that is necessary for optimizing the safety and quality of our pharmacies and other health care organizations. In addition, these chapters outline key tools that are crucial to identification of problems, assessment of problems, refinement of systems, and continuous evaluation of quality.

Chapters 9–11 further examine methods for measuring safety and quality, including mechanisms for gathering consumer feedback on pharmacy quality. As with the other chapters, the authors seek to apply well-established measurement frameworks to the contemporary practice of pharmacy. The chapter on consumer feedback describes the development, testing, and potential uses of a survey that was sponsored by the Pharmacy Quality Alliance; the survey is modeled after the oft-used CAHPS measures throughout other sectors of health care. Finally, in Chapter 11, Kenneth

Baker provides insights on how to integrate QI concepts and tools into a robust risk-management program.

Chapters 12–15 offer guidance on implementing changes that improve safety and quality. This part of the book includes discussion of how financial incentives and public reports on pharmacy quality may stimulate greater adoption of QI programs, and how effective teamwork and leadership can make these programs more effective. Chapters 16 and 17 then provide case studies and examples for implementing highly effective QI programs.

We believe that this book will be useful to practicing pharmacists as well as to pharmacy students. To assist pharmacy educators, we have developed a companion set of lectures and exercises that mirror the content of this book. This academic toolkit is known as *Educating Pharmacy Students and Pharmacists to Improve Quality (EPIQ)* and is available from the Pharmacy Quality Alliance, Inc (www.pqaalliance.org).

Acknowledgments

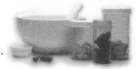

We wish to thank our chapter authors for giving their time and expertise so that this book could be created, and special thanks to David Holdford and Donna West for helping to create the Educating Pharmacy Students and Pharmacists to Improve Quality (EPIQ) program for pharmacy educators, which serves as a companion to this book. We also appreciate the support of Laura Cranston of PQA for the creation of EPIQ and her dedication to improving the quality of pharmacy services. Finally, the book never would have been finished without the guidance and encouragement of Michael Weitz and Robert Pancotti.

Part I
Status of Quality Improvement and Reporting in the U.S. Health Care System

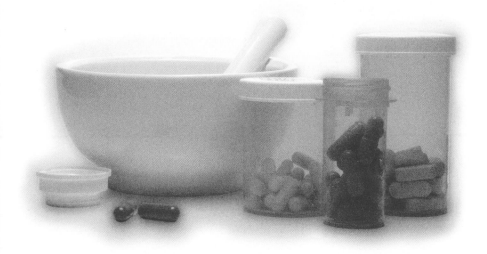

Part 1
Status of Quality Improvement and Reporting in the U.S. Health Care System

CHAPTER 1

Quality and the Future of Health Care

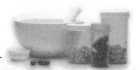

David P. Nau

Learning Objectives

At the end of the chapter, the reader will be able to:

1. Summarize major recommendations of the Institute of Medicine (IOM) regarding health care quality.
2. Define what is meant by quality in general and health care quality in particular.
3. Describe what is meant by "value-driven health care."
4. Argue the case for multiple strategies for improving health care.
5. Explain why quality must be measured.

> It was the best of times; it was the worst of times.
>
> Charles Dickens, *A Tale of Two Cities*

It is a time of great transition in health care. Rapidly increasing costs for health care services, along with recognition of suboptimal quality, have forced our government and the private sector to re-examine the U.S. health care system. One could view the current challenges in health care as being the "worst of times" but one could also envision the "best of times" by identifying many opportunities for enhancing quality and value. I hope that the profession of pharmacy will eventually look back on the first decades of the 21st century as the time when pharmacists delineated their role as promoters of quality and value.

The importance of pharmaceuticals to the treatment of chronic disease received increased attention since the implementation of the Medicare Part D drug benefit. The utilization of prescription medications by the elderly increased by 12.8% after the implementation of Part D, and the Congressional Budget Office has projected that Medicare cumulative outlays on Part D medications will reach nearly $800 billion by 2015.[1] Unfortunately, there is evidence that many patients experience *preventable* adverse medication-related events or fail to receive appropriate drug therapy due to the shortcomings of our complex and disjointed medication-use system in the United States.[2–4] Researchers have estimated that for every dollar we spend on pharmaceuticals, we spend another dollar on treating the problems that stem from suboptimal medication use and therefore waste billions of dollars in health care resources every year.[5] The economic value of the health care system is far from ideal.

Improving the value of the health care system will require improved quality and/ or better cost control (and ideally both). The Secretary of Health and Human Services is repositioning the federal government to be a value-based purchaser of health care services. Private-sector payers have already increased their scrutiny of quality and costs and created incentives for providers to boost performance. Realigning the incentives within the private and public sectors to drive improvements in quality and reductions in inefficiency is also known as value-driven health care.

The Institute of Medicine (IOM) has also pointed out the shortcomings of the U.S. health care system and called for a redesign for our antiquated processes of care including a renewed look at processes for prescribing, dispensing, and monitoring the use of medications.[6] The National Quality Forum (NQF) has also given increased attention to the quality of medication-use systems through development of *A National Framework and Preferred Practices for Therapeutic Drug Management Quality and Reporting.*[7] Both the NQF and IOM have called for better coordination of care across health care institutions and health professions, including a revised role for pharmacists in optimizing the use of medications. The demand for better quality and value in health care presents a significant opportunity for pharmacists.

Over the past 50 years, the profession of pharmacy has been undergoing an evolution from compounders and dispensers of medications to providers of medication therapy management (MTM). This evolution has been spurred by various forces, both social and technological. New drug discoveries, modern manufacturing methods, and efficient distribution systems have diminished the need for pharmacists to compound medications, to the point where the art of compounding survives only as a niche business for a small number of pharmacists. The increasing size of the drug armamentarium, along with an increased recognition of the need to tailor drug regimens based on various physiological, genetic, and cultural parameters, has heightened the demand for experts in MTM. Colleges of Pharmacy have adapted to this changing environment by converting all pharmacy education programs to the PharmD degree wherein all students are clinically trained to be experts in drug therapy. The increased demand for efficient and effective medication management, coupled with the growth in clinically trained pharmacists, creates an opportunity for the health care system to integrate pharmacists into the care of patients with chronic diseases.

Although clinical pharmacist services in academic medical centers have been well established for several decades, the ambulatory sector for pharmacy has been a very different world. Despite a number of small studies that have demonstrated the ability of community pharmacists to improve the quality of drug therapy and enhance clinical outcomes, there has been little demand for MTM by community pharmacists. The community pharmacy is still often viewed as a distribution center for medications with no professional services beyond the identification of potential drug—drug interactions or excessive doses. However, the opportunity for heightening the patient-care role of pharmacists has never been better.

When creating the Medicare drug benefit, the Centers for Medicare & Medicaid Services (CMS) included requirements for drug plans to provide MTM programs. Although the requirement for MTM was initially heralded as a watershed moment for community pharmacists, the profession soon realized that the nonspecific language in the requirement allowed drug plans to define MTM for themselves. A survey of Medicare plans that offer prescription drug coverage showed that the majority of plans did *not* include community pharmacists within their model for MTM at the onset of Part D.[8] Additionally, the restrictive eligibility criteria for MTM programs exclude the majority of Medicare enrollees from MTM.[9]

It is understandable that the CMS did not provide more detail in their initial requirements for MTM. There was considerable pressure to get the drug benefit implemented quickly, and there was little evidence to show that one approach to MTM was considerably better than another. Recent actions by the CMS suggest that they will be giving greater scrutiny to the quality and safety of medication use in prescription drug plans, and will be evaluating how different methods of MTM impact the overall quality of care. This may create an opportunity for community pharmacists to play an important role within a value-driven health care system; however, capitalizing on this opportunity will require increased transparency of the quality and costs of pharmacy services in order to establish the value of pharmacy within the broader health care system.

MEASURING QUALITY IN PHARMACY SERVICES

Two cornerstones of value-driven health care are transparency of quality and transparency of costs. Although there has been considerable attention to the costs of pharmaceuticals, there has been little effort to systematically measure the quality of pharmacy services or the cost-effectiveness of these services. A few studies have sought to measure the quality and cost-effectiveness of pharmacy services, but there has been no widely adopted set of measures of pharmacy quality. Thus, the profession of pharmacy has trailed physicians, hospitals, and long-term care facilities in the quality revolution.

While serving as CMS Administrator, Mark McClellan stimulated the creation of the Pharmacy Quality Alliance (PQA) with the goal that this alliance would identify the most appropriate ways to measure the quality of pharmacy services for Medicare Part D enrollees as well as other patients. The PQA was envisioned as a counterpart to the Ambulatory Quality Alliance (AQA) and Hospital Quality Alliance (HQA) and recently joined the Quality Alliance Steering Committee. Nearly 60 organizations comprise the membership of the PQA and include federal agencies [CMS and Agency for Healthcare Research and Quality (AHRQ)], America's Health Insurance Plans (AHIP), and numerous health/drug plans, pharmacy associations, pharmacy benefit managers, quality-improvement organizations, and pharmaceutical research and manufacturing companies. More information on PQA is available at www.pqaalliance.org.

Given the dearth of quality measures for ambulatory pharmacy services, the PQA spent much of its time during 2006 and 2007 identifying potential measures of pharmacy quality and pilot testing these measures with organizations experienced in quality measurement. PQA partnered with NCQA to develop specifications for over 30 measures that could potentially be derived from drug claims data. At the conclusion of pilot testing, 15 of these measures demonstrated favorable attributes for performance measurement and were submitted to the NQF for endorsement consideration in 2008. PQA also partnered with the American Institute for Research to develop a questionnaire that could gather the consumer perspective on the quality of pharmacy services. The English and Spanish versions have been submitted to the AHRQ for consideration of including the questionnaire within the family of measures known as Consumer Assessment of Healthcare Providers and Systems (CAHPS).

Although several measures of pharmacy quality have now been developed and tested, the key issues for the future are how best to utilize the measures in value-based purchasing of health care services, and how to stimulate the improvement of quality in medication use. In the summer of 2008, PQA initiated a series of demonstration projects to begin testing different models for implementing quality-focused performance reports for community pharmacies and to explore how pharmacists might collaborate with other health care providers and health plans to improve the quality of medication utilization for high-risk patients.

PQA DEMONSTRATION PROJECTS

In the summer of 2008, PQA initiated a demonstration project in five states to test the feasibility and potential usefulness of creating performance reports for community pharmacies. This 1-year demonstration project gathered feedback about the performance report system from hundreds of community pharmacies, as well as their partners, and set the stage for a second phase of demonstration projects that will determine the capability of community pharmacists to enhance the quality and safety of medication use. The Phase I demonstration sites and partners are listed in Table 1-1.

The subsequent demonstrations that are to be facilitated by PQA should help to answer many important questions about the integration of pharmacy services into the broader system of value-driven health care. These questions include: (1) to what extent can pharmacists improve the quality and safety of medication utilization; (2) can financial incentives stimulate the improvement of pharmacy performance and how much incentive is necessary to boost performance by a clinically meaningful amount; and (3) is there a significant return on investment to the health care system for providing targeted incentives to pharmacies and is there a reasonable return on investment to pharmacy owners for investing in better quality and safety?

Financial incentives may include more than just "payment for cognitive services" by pharmacists. The ideal compensation system would stimulate improved quality by providing higher payment to providers that achieve higher levels of quality. Many private payers as well as the federal government are experimenting with various types of financial incentives for physicians, hospitals, and home health providers to boost the quality and value of health care. Thus, it is important that we examine how similar incentives might be structured for the pharmacy sector to elevate the quality and safety of medication use. Details on financial incentives are provided in Chapter 15.

TABLE 1-1. PQA Demonstration Project Partners

State	Lead Organization	Partners
Indiana	Purdue	Regenstrief Institute, Indiana Health Information Exchange, numerous retail pharmacies
Iowa	University of Iowa	Iowa Foundation for Medical Care, Iowa Medicaid, Wellmark, numerous retail pharmacies
North Carolina	Outcomes Pharmaceutical Health Care	Kerr Drug
Pennsylvania	Highmark	Rite Aid, CE City
Wisconsin	Pharmacy Society of Wisconsin	University of Wisconsin, numerous health plans, WI Pharmacy Quality Collaborative

INCREASING TRANSPARENCY

The availability of information on health care quality is rapidly expanding. Within the last decade, numerous websites have been developed by the CMS as well as the private sector to provide comparative information on health care providers and insurers. The CMS-sponsored sites include: *Hospital Compare* (www.hospitalcompare.hhs.gov), *Home Health Compare* (www.medicare.gov/HHcompare), and *Nursing Home Compare* (www.medicare.gov/NHcompare). The Joint Commission also hosts a website with quality-related information on hospitals, nursing homes, home health agencies, and other facilities accredited by the Joint Commission (www.qualitycheck.org). All of these sites allow consumers or payers to view each institution's performance on numerous quality measures. General information on the quality of health plans can be found on NCQA's website, and in-depth comparative information can be purchased through membership in *Quality Compass* (www.qualitycompass.org). In some states, the public can also find quality reports on physicians and clinics. For example, the Wisconsin Collaborative for Healthcare Quality (WCHQ) allows a consumer to find information for all clinics within a specific zip code or city in Wisconsin (www.wchq.org).

Community pharmacies have only recently begun to experience public reports. Many of these reports focus only on customer satisfaction and may only provide aggregate information for an entire chain. For example, JD Power conducts a web-based survey of consumers and provides rankings of chains, supermarkets, and mass merchandisers (www.jdpower.com/healthcare). In anticipation of consumer demand for more robust reports on individual community pharmacies, the PQA has developed a prototype website that would allow much of the same functionality of the WCHQ website.

Once active, this website will allow consumers to find information on the quality of pharmacies in their community. Thus, the realm of community pharmacy is expected to soon come under the same level of transparency as other health care providers.

KEY POINTS

◉ Health care reform efforts in the federal and state governments as well as the private sector are driving the demand for more evidence of the quality and value of various providers and services.

◉ The PQA was created in 2006 to facilitate the development of quality measures for community pharmacies and drug plans. It has conducted demonstration projects in five states and more are planned to ascertain the feasibility of creating pharmacy-specific quality reports and the ability of pharmacies to drive improvements in quality.

◉ The public reporting of information about the quality of health care providers has grown rapidly in the last decade. Although community pharmacies have been immune from this trend, it is expected that pharmacy performance reports will soon be available to the public.

REFERENCES

1. Lichtenberg FR, Sun SX. The impact of Medicare Part D on prescription drug use by the elderly. *Health Aff.* 2007;26(6):1735–1744; Congressional Budget Office. *Projection of Spending for the Medicare Part D Benefit;* 9 February 2005.
2. Nau DP, Kirking DM. Why is medication use less than appropriate? In: Fulda TR, Wertheimer AI, eds. *Pharmaceutical Public Policy.* New York: Haworth Press; 2007: 477–498.
3. Aparasu R, Mort J. Inappropriate prescribing for the elderly: Beers criteria-based review. *Ann Pharmacother.* 2000;34:338–346.
4. Budnitz DS, Pollock DA, Weidenbach KN, et al. National Surveillance of Emergency Department Visits for Outpatient Adverse Drug Events. *JAMA.* 2006;296:1858–1866.
5. Johnson JA, Bootman JL. Drug-related morbidity and mortality: a cost-of-illness model. *Ann Intern Med.* 1995;155:1949–1956.
6. Institute of Medicine. *Crossing the Quality Chasm.* Washington, DC: National Academy Press; 2001.
7. National Quality Forum. *A National Framework and Preferred Practices for Therapeutic Drug Management Quality Measurement and Reporting.* http://www.qualityforum.org/projects/ongoing/therapeutic/index.asp. Accessed January 8, 2008.
8. Touchette DR, Burns AL, Bough MA, Blackburn JC. Survey of medication therapy management programs under Medicare Part D. *J Am Pharm Assoc.* 2006;46:683–691.
9. Centers for Medicare & Medicaid Services. *CY07 MTM Fact Sheet.* http://www.cms.hhs.gov/PrescriptionDrugCovContra/Downloads/MTMFactSheet.pdf. Accessed January 8, 2008.

CHAPTER 2

Understanding Problems in the Use of Medications

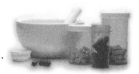

David P. Nau and Duane M. Kirking

Learning Objectives

At the end of the chapter, the reader will be able to:

1. Develop a general understanding of how problems occur in the use of medications.
2. Identify and describe eight types of drug-related problems.
3. Discuss relationships between drug-related problems and drug-related morbidity.

Medications are one of the key tools in the therapeutic management of disease. However, they are not always used in an ideal, or appropriate, manner.[1,2] When medications are not used appropriately, patients may experience adverse events or fail to achieve their therapeutic goals. In turn, this results in suboptimal quality of life and wasted resources for our society.

Hepler and Strand have used the term "drug-related morbidity" to describe the phenomenon of therapeutic malfunction – the failure of a therapeutic agent to produce the intended therapeutic outcome.[3] This concept encompasses both treatment failure and the production of new medical problems. Considering that drug-related morbidity accounts for at least 7% of hospital admissions and billions of dollars in unnecessary health care expenditures, drug-related morbidity is an important public health issue.[4–6]

Drug-related morbidity is often preceded by a drug-related problem (DRP).[7] A DRP is an event or circumstance involving drug treatment that actually or potentially interferes with the patient experiencing an optimum outcome of medical care. Strand et al. delineated eight categories of DRPs:

1. *Untreated indications*: the patient is in need of a drug that was not prescribed.
2. *Improper drug selection*: the wrong drug is being used.
3. *Subtherapeutic dosage*: too little of an appropriate drug is being used.
4. *Overdosage*: the patient receives too much of an appropriate drug.
5. *Failure to receive drug*: the patient does not obtain/use the drug that was prescribed.

6. *Adverse drug reaction*: an unintended and potentially harmful effect of a drug.
7. *Drug interactions*: undesirable consequences of drug–drug or drug–food interactions.
8. *Drug use without indication*: the patient is taking a drug for which he or she has no medical need.[7]

DRPs may arise due to inappropriate prescribing, inappropriate dispensing/administration of the drug, inappropriate behavior by the patient, inappropriate monitoring of the patient, or patient idiosyncrasy. Although idiosyncrasy is inherently unpreventable, most of the other causes of DRPs can be prevented. The following section of this chapter will provide a framework for examining the causes of suboptimal medication use.

A FRAMEWORK FOR EXAMINING THE QUALITY OF MEDICATION USE

Hepler and Grainger-Rousseau's conceptualization of a pharmaceutical care system offers a good framework for examining the quality of medication use.[8] The pharmaceutical care system is similar to the drug-use process described by Knapp et al.[9] but adds the functions of drug monitoring and management to denote the importance of ongoing attention to the patient and drug regimen. Hepler and Grainger-Rousseau suggest that there are three key elements to the proper functioning of a pharmaceutical care system: (1) initiating therapy; (2) monitoring therapy; and (3) managing (i.e., correcting) therapy.

Appropriate initiation of therapy requires the recognition and assessment of the patient's signs and symptoms to generate an appropriate diagnosis and therapeutic plan. It also entails the prescribing of a drug that, based on the knowledge of the prescriber and information available to the prescriber, would be the most appropriate product for the individual patient. Furthermore, the patient must obtain the prescribed medication (most often from a pharmacy that presumably has dispensed the appropriate medication along with appropriate advice to the patient) and the patient must begin using it. Given the numerous steps and people involved in the initiation of drug therapy, it is easy to identify many potential reasons for failures in this process.

Problems with Initiation of Therapy

If patients do not recognize a potential health problem that could be treated with a medication, or do nothing about a recognized problem, then the initiation of drug therapy will not occur. Patients may not recognize a problem because the problem may be asymptomatic or because they lack an understanding of the significance or meaning of symptoms. They may also choose not to seek the advice of a health professional due to fears of what they may be told, or because of a distrust of providers. They may also lack access to health care due to an inability to pay for services or geographic barriers.

Once a patient accesses the health care system, an evaluation of his or her signs or symptoms should be conducted. However, if the patient is unable to communicate clearly with the provider, an accurate assessment of the problem becomes difficult. The provider may also lack the necessary skills or equipment to accurately diagnose the problem, or may not give adequate attention to the patient's problem. If the problem is not correctly diagnosed, it is unlikely that appropriate drug therapy will be prescribed.

Once the diagnosis is made, the clinician then needs to decide whether a drug is warranted for treating the patient. If so, the selection of the drug (along with an appropriate dose, route, duration, and instructions) can be challenging. Given the thousands of drug products that are available, and the characteristics of the patient (e.g., age, weight, renal function, and cognitive function), the clinician is tasked with selecting the most appropriate therapy for the disease in this patient at this time. The task is made more complex for the physician by having to deal with multiple payers who may each specify a different preferred drug for a given condition, as well as by advertisements that lead patients to request specific products, or by conflicting data from clinical trials. Most often, the clinician is working from his or her memory of the numerous products indicated for a particular disease, and uses simple decision rules to reduce the complexity and uncertainty inherent in product selection (e.g., "If the patient is a child with uncomplicated otitis media, and no other health problems, I prescribe amoxicillin"). Numerous studies have been conducted of how physicians select drug products and the detailed findings of these studies are beyond the space available in this chapter.[10–14]

Once the prescription for drug therapy is generated, the ambulatory patient generally obtains the medication from a pharmacy. The pharmacist is charged with confirming the appropriateness of the medication for the patient and then dispensing the product, along with instructions on proper use, to the patient or caregiver. The process by which the pharmacist evaluates the appropriateness of the prescribed therapy is sometimes called "prospective drug-utilization review" (PDUR).[15] Although the pharmacist should be readily able to detect any obvious problems with the prescription (e.g., a 10-fold overdose of chloral hydrate for an infant), this does not always happen. An individual pharmacist may lack the knowledge of appropriate drug therapy, or may not be paying close attention to the prescription in the hurried environment of many community pharmacies. Computerized PDUR systems have been developed to assist in identifying potential problems with prescriptions; however, the alerts generated by these systems may not always provide clear guidance on the action to be taken by the pharmacist, and a high volume of low-risk alerts may lead to high-risk alerts being overlooked.[16,17] Another challenge for the pharmacist is the lack of information regarding the patient's medical condition. The patient's diagnosis and other pertinent clinical information are not often immediately available to the pharmacist, and thus the task of PDUR becomes more challenging.

If the pharmacist has deemed the prescribed therapy to be appropriate, then the correct drug and information need to be provided to the patient or the patient's caregiver. Within hospitals, the product is usually provided by the pharmacy to a nurse who then administers the drug to the patient. However, hospitals may also have medications stocked within a nursing unit and the pharmacist may be bypassed altogether. This limits the opportunity to double-check the order prior to the drug's administration. Regardless of setting, there are numerous steps involved with the dispensing and/or administration of a drug product and often several personnel are involved in processing the drug order before the product reaches the patient. This creates many opportunities for error.

Dispensing-related medication errors often result from a combination of human factors and systems failures. Some of the most frequently cited factors include: (1) the lack of a consistent dispensing process, or unclear roles within the process; (2) a workload that exceeds the capacity of the personnel and dispensing process; (3) excessive distractions in the dispensing process; (4) unclear handwritten prescriptions; (5) similar drug names that can easily be confused; (6) products or packaging that look identical; (7) lack of training for personnel; and (8) failure to communicate with patients.

Pharmacist–patient communication is important for at least three reasons. First, it provides the pharmacist with information to assess the appropriateness of the prescribed regimen. Second, talking to the patient about the prescribed medication can reveal potential medication errors before the patient receives the medication (e.g., the pharmacist had interpreted the handwritten prescription as being for a cardiovascular drug, but the patient says that she was prescribed the drug for breast cancer). Lastly, the pharmacist can provide the patient with information regarding the appropriate use of the medication and can confirm that the patient understands the information.

Unfortunately, verbal communication between pharmacist and patient does not always occur. There are several reasons for this. Some pharmacists perceive that patients do not want to talk to them, and thus they do not attempt to initiate a dialogue. However, research has indicated that many patients want more information about their medications.[18] Even when pharmacists do attempt to communicate drug-related information, the patient or caregiver may have difficulty engaging in a productive dialogue if they feel ill or are distracted by a sick child. There is also a financial disincentive for pharmacy personnel to spend time talking with patients, since payment to the pharmacy is based on sale of the product regardless of whether the pharmacist and patient converse about the medications. Thus, spending time in conversation with patients detracts from dispensing more prescriptions and maximizing revenue. Additionally, patients may expect to receive their medications within a few minutes of presenting the prescription and the pharmacist may feel compelled to minimize the processing time for prescriptions by not talking with patients. Finally, some pharmacists feel apprehensive about talking with patients and may avoid conversations altogether.[19]

Perhaps the most important participant in a pharmaceutical care system is the patient. The patient ultimately decides if, and how, he or she will take the medication. Patients may choose not to fill the prescription or may alter the regimen in ways that are not conducive to optimal outcomes. This may stem from concerns over side effects or addiction, a perceived lack of effectiveness of the drug, or an inability to pay for the medications. Additionally, it may be difficult for some patients to manage a complex drug regimen that involves many medications or complicated directions. Thus, patients may unintentionally miss doses because of the burden involved.

Problems in Monitoring and Managing Drug Therapy

The monitoring and management of drug therapy are crucial elements of the pharmaceutical care system, since they facilitate the identification of problems with the initial therapeutic plan or problems with the patient's use of the medications. However, these are also the elements of pharmaceutical care that are most often neglected. The ongoing management of drug therapy may not happen if clinicians or patients fail to monitor the progress toward the therapeutic goals or if they fail to act despite the monitoring data clearly showing the need for change in the plan.

Phillips et al. have used the term "clinical inertia" to describe the "failure of health care providers to initiate or intensify therapy when indicated."[20] Clinical inertia is due to at least three problems: overestimation of care provided, use of soft reasons to avoid intensification of therapy, and practice organization not being designed for achieving therapeutic goals. Several studies have noted that physicians overestimate their care provided for chronic illnesses, including overestimation of the extent to which they screened for, and monitored, diseases such as diabetes and coronary heart disease.[21,22]

Even when monitoring data indicate that the therapeutic goal is not being achieved, physicians may use "soft" reasons to justify their decisions not to intensify therapy. For example, if the physician perceives the control of the disease has improved, then he or she may be reluctant to intensify therapy despite the therapeutic target not being achieved.[23] Physicians may also choose not to intensify therapy if they perceive that the patient would not adhere to the intensified therapy.[23] These barriers may stem from concerns over side effects or a belief that the therapeutic targets proposed in clinical guidelines may not be appropriate for a specific patient, or a lack of physician training to "treat to goal."[20]

Many physicians were not trained to intensify drug therapy until therapeutic targets are achieved.[20] Additionally, many practice sites are not organized to systematically identify patients who are not achieving the therapeutic goal and to prompt action for further monitoring or intensification of therapy. Many practices are organized to focus on the patient's current medical complaint without attention to the ongoing control of chronic disease. For example, a 65-year-old woman with diabetes may present to the physician's practice to discuss menopausal symptoms. The physician may discuss menopause but then fail to identify that the patient has not had an assessment of glycemic control for the past 2 years. Although office-based quality improvement initiatives have been developed in recent years to counter this problem, the majority of physician practices are still not engaging in quality improvement efforts toward this aim.[20,24]

Many quality improvement efforts have recognized the important role that non-physician providers can play in a pharmaceutical care system. Nurses and pharmacists can play a significant role in educating and monitoring patients with chronic illnesses, and identifying those patients in need of therapy modification. Since pharmacists often encounter patients monthly for drug refills, they are in an excellent position to collect objective monitoring information (e.g., blood pressure and hemoglobin A1c) and solicit subjective feedback from patients regarding their experience with the drugs (e.g., side effects and symptom resolution) to identify those patients in need of further evaluation by a physician. A recent multistate project demonstrated that community pharmacists who provided enhanced services to diabetes patients helped the patients achieve better health and reduced total health care expenditures.[25] Several other recent studies have shown that pharmacists' consultations may also have a positive impact on patients' health.[26–28] Unfortunately, only a small percentage of patients with chronic diseases receive medication therapy management services.[29]

Problems with Information Flow

A cross-cutting theme regarding the suboptimal use of medications is the poor flow of information throughout the pharmaceutical care system. In order for clinicians to make informed decisions regarding the initiation or modification of drug therapy, they need to have timely access to objective and subjective data regarding the patient. In order for pharmacists to evaluate the appropriateness of a prescribed drug, they need to have information such as the patient's diagnosis, weight, and other medications. The patient also needs to know the therapeutic goals, how to appropriately use the medication, how to self-monitor for side effects and therapeutic effectiveness, and how and when to contact various clinicians.

It is important to recognize that information flow, by itself, does not always lead to better decisions or greater achievement of therapeutic goals. Electronic prescribing systems have the potential to decrease several types of medication errors; however, they may also create other types of errors.[30] Furthermore, providing pharmacists with more information about the patient does not necessarily lead to better care by pharmacists.[31] This is particularly true if the pharmacy's operations are not designed to facilitate interaction between patients and pharmacists. Nonetheless, increasing the electronic connectivity between providers and with patients reduces barriers that impede the appropriate initiation, monitoring, and management of drug therapy.

HOW OFTEN DO PROBLEMS OCCUR IN THE USE OF MEDICATIONS?

Hundreds of studies have been conducted over the past several decades that document a myriad of problems with the use of medications. We selected examples of studies from each of the eight categories of DRPs as defined by Strand and colleagues,[7] as well as from the literature on medication errors. It is important to note that the evidence presented in the category of *adverse drug events* (ADEs) is not limited to reports of idiosyncratic drug reactions, and includes reports of both preventable and nonpreventable ADEs.

Adverse Drug Events

A recent study using the National Ambulatory Medical Care Survey estimated that there were 4.3 million ambulatory visits in the United States during 2001 for the treatment of an ADE.[32] This equates to 15 visits per 1000 population with nearly half of these visits being to a hospital emergency department. The authors of this national study also found that the elderly and women were most likely to receive care for an ADE.

In 1995, Bates et al. found that ADEs occurred in 6.5% of all adult, nonobstetrical, hospital admissions.[33] They estimated that 28% of the ADEs were preventable. A study of pediatric patients found that ADEs and potential ADEs occurred in 2.3%

and 10%, respectively, of admitted patients.[34] Yet another study found that ADEs occurred in more than 12% of patients within 3 weeks of discharge from a hospital.[35] The majority of these ADEs were judged to be preventable or ameliorable. Other studies of ADEs have shown similar results.[36] Changes to the inpatient medication-use system such as computerized physician order entry, clinical decision-support programs, and pharmacist involvement with the medical team have been shown to decrease the risk of medication errors and ADEs.[37–41]

Untreated Indications

The patient may have a need for drug therapy (a drug indication), but is not receiving a drug for that indication. It has been estimated that less than half of persons who qualify for lipid-modifying therapy are receiving it.[42] The treatment of hypertension is only slightly better with 59% of persons with hypertension receiving drug therapy.[43] Although it is possible that some persons with dyslipidemia and hypertension could achieve control of their disease without a medication, only 20% of patients with coronary heart disease achieve their goal for LDL cholesterol and 34% of hypertensive patients achieve their blood pressure goal.[42,43] However, the proportion of diabetic patients receiving drug therapy for dyslipidemia increased from 28% in the early 1990s to 56% by 2000.[44] Increases were also seen in the use of drug therapy for hypertension and glycemic control in the same population. Thus, there has been improvement in the treatment of chronic disease in recent years, although many people still do not receive drug therapy when needed.

Inappropriate Prescribing

Examples of inappropriate prescribing include: (1) selecting a drug that will not be effective for treating the patient's condition (i.e., wrong drug); (2) selecting a dose that is too low to be effective; (3) selecting a dose that is too high and potentially harmful; or (4) selecting a drug that is inappropriate based on the patient's comorbidities or concurrent drug use (drug–disease or drug–drug interactions). Researchers of inappropriate prescribing often combine some of the aforementioned categories when reporting the results of their studies.

A recent trend is to examine the use of potentially inappropriate medication (PIM) in the elderly based on criteria developed by Beers et al.[45,46] The Beers criteria focus on drugs that may be inappropriate for use in the elderly due to their propensity to cause ADEs in this population. The elderly are an important population for medication-use studies, since they may be more vulnerable to adverse drug-related events and often use many medications.

Lau et al. used the Beers criteria to identify PIM use among elderly nursing home residents.[47] They found that over 50% of residents experienced inappropriate prescribing of medications. Specifically, 40% of residents experienced inappropriate drug selection, 11% had excess dosage, and 13% had a drug–disease interaction. In a follow-up report, Lau et al. determined that residents who experienced inappropriate prescribing had greater odds of hospitalization in the month following exposure to PIM.[48]

Curtis et al. examined the frequency of PIM in noninstitutionalized elderly patients using prescription claims from 1999.[49] They found that 21% of older adults received at least one drug included on the revised Beers list and 15% received at least two drugs of concern. Rigler et al. compared the frequency of PIM in three cohorts with the Kansas Medicaid program (nursing home residents, recipients of home and community-based services for the frail elderly, and ambulatory patients).[50] They found that PIM occurred in 38%, 48%, and 21%, respectively, of nursing home residents, frail elderly, and ambulatory patients.

One limitation of the numerous studies of PIM in the elderly is that they frequently assess the use of individual medications that are considered inappropriate regardless of the patient's diagnoses or concurrent use of other drugs. To overcome this limitation, Zhan et al. examined the frequency of 6 drug–drug combinations and 50 drug–disease combinations that place the elderly at risk for ADEs.[51] Using data from two national surveys regarding ambulatory visits, they estimated that 0.74% of visits involving two or more prescriptions had at least one inappropriate drug–drug combination, and 2.58% of visits involving at least one prescription had an inappropriate drug–disease combination. Thus, when more stringent criteria are used to assess PIM in the elderly, the rate of inappropriate prescribing appears much lower.

It is not just the elderly who may have inappropriate drugs prescribed. Some hospitalized patients receive antibiotics that are not appropriate for the identified or suspected pathogen.[52] Patients with mental health disorders may also receive drugs that are not appropriate for their diagnoses.[53] For example, some patients with depression receive only tranquilizers, perhaps because a physician failed to recognize that the patient's sleep disorder stemmed from depression.[54]

Even when appropriate drugs are selected, the prescribed dose may be insufficient to achieve the desired therapeutic benefit. A study of the California Medicaid population revealed that two thirds of patients using antidepressants were receiving a subtherapeutic dose.[55] The majority of patients with diabetes receive drug therapy that is inadequate to achieve glycemic control.[56–58] Specialists are marginally better than primary care physicians at intensifying therapy in response to elevated blood glucose levels, but the majority of diabetes patients still do not receive intensification of drug therapy when warranted.[57] Pain control medications are also underdosed frequently, particularly in terminally ill patients.[59–63]

Doses that are too high may also be prescribed. One reason for excessive doses is the failure of the prescriber to account for a patient's renal impairment.[61] This is particularly important for drugs with a narrow therapeutic index that are excreted in the urine (e.g., aminoglycosides and digoxin). Many U.S. hospitals have developed pharmacokinetic dosing services to ensure that renally impaired patients receive appropriate doses of medications.[62] Small children, particularly infants, require weight-based dosing of many drugs to ensure that they do not receive overdoses. However, medication overdoses, particularly related to oncology medications, continue to occur in hospitalized children.[63] The drug class most commonly associated with overdoses in nonhospitalized children is analgesics, particularly acetaminophen.[64] Overall, approximately 7.5%

of all overdoses treated in emergency centers in the United States are due to errors in prescribing, dispensing, or monitoring drug therapy.[64]

Failure to Receive Drug

Even if the patient is prescribed a drug when appropriate, and an appropriate medication and dose are selected, the patient may not receive the drug. A survey of Medicare beneficiaries in 2003 found that 4 in 10 seniors did not take all of the medications prescribed for them in the last year.[65] The reasons most frequently given for not taking all of their medications were: (1) the costs were too high; (2) they did not think the drugs were helping them; and (3) the drug made them feel worse. Approximately 26% of subjects did not fill a prescription or cut their dose of a drug because of cost concerns, while 25% stopped taking a drug because it made them feel worse or they perceived the drug was not helping. Subjects who had prescription drug benefits were less likely to go without medication due to the cost of medications.

The reasons for suboptimal adherence to medications may depend partly on the type of drug therapy regimen and may be multifactorial. A study of lipid-lowering therapy identified that only 26% of elderly patients maintained a high level of use of statin drugs over 5 years, with the greatest decline in adherence occurring in the first 6 months of therapy.[66] A similar study noted that only 31% of patients were adherent at 3 years after initiation of therapy, with the greatest decline happening in the first 3 months.[67] This study also noted that the short-term effectiveness of the drug therapy was associated with higher adherence in subsequent months. Thus, patients may be more likely to discontinue therapy with statin drugs when they see no improvement in their cholesterol levels and do not feel better. The perceived lack of effectiveness, when coupled with the high cost of statin drugs, may be leading to the high discontinuation rates of these drugs.

Side effects may also contribute to poor adherence with some drug regimens. In particular, antidepressants may produce undesirable side effects such as lethargy and sexual dysfunction with about one third of depressed patients discontinuing therapy prematurely.[68] Side effects are also noted frequently as a contributing factor in poor adherence to highly active antiretroviral therapy (HAART).[69] However, side effects alone do not explain much of the variance in medication nonadherence, and they are most likely weighed against the perceived benefits of the medication when patients decide whether to continue taking a medication.[70–73] Many patients taking antidepressant or antiretroviral drugs discontinue their regimens when their "concerns" about the medications exceed the perceived "necessity" of the medications.[72,73]

Drug Use Without Indication

In this category, the patient is taking a drug for which he or she has no medical need. According to the 2007 National Survey on Drug Use and Health, an estimated 5.2 million Americans are using prescription pain-reliever drugs for nonmedical purposes.[74] This represents 2.1% of the U.S. population over the age of 12 years. However, an estimated 3.4% of 12- to 17-year-olds reported past-month prescription drug abuse. The rate of prescription drug abuse among American youth has increased considerably since 1990.[74]

Some "nonindicated" drug use stems from over-prescribing of drugs by physicians. For example, the majority of patients who are diagnosed with an upper respiratory infection receive antibiotics despite the lack of effectiveness of antibiotics for these conditions.[75,76] It is estimated that 17–20% of the patients who receive antibiotics lack an indication for the drug.[77,78] The high rate of nonindicated antibiotic utilization may be partly driven by patients' misunderstandings about antibiotic effectiveness for viral infections, physician desires to satisfy patients' demands, and marketing campaigns for new antibiotics.[79]

Medication Dispensing/Administration Errors

Although many of the DRPs listed in the preceding sections could result from errors in diagnosis, prescribing, consumption, or monitoring of patients, it is also important to examine errors in the dispensing or administration of medications. There has been considerable variation in the rates of dispensing errors across numerous studies in ambulatory settings. However, a recent, well-conducted study provided a national benchmark rate of 17 errors out of every 1000 prescriptions dispensed (1.7%).[80] Approximately 6.5% of the errors were judged as having the potential for clinically significant consequences for the patient. Given that more than 3 billion prescriptions are dispensed in the United States each year, an estimated 51 million dispensing errors occur annually.

Medication errors also occur within institutional settings. In 2002, a study of 36 hospitals and skilled nursing facilities found that 19% of doses were in error with 7% of errors being potentially harmful.[81] The most common types of errors involved giving the drug at the wrong time or omitting a scheduled dose. Given the frail health of many persons in hospitals and nursing homes, these medication administration errors can be particularly devastating.

Although the aforementioned studies derived their estimates of errors via observation of pharmacists or nurses, the public's perception of errors is also important. In 2002, the Commonwealth Fund conducted a nationwide survey regarding consumer perceptions of health care quality.[82] Approximately 22% of respondents reported that they, or a family member, had experienced a medical error, and 16% had (at some point in their lives) received the wrong medication or wrong dose of medication. A more recent survey of an insured population found that about 18% of respondents had experienced an error by an ambulatory pharmacy at some point in their lives, with 6.8% of subjects experiencing an error within the last year.[83] Despite the personal experiences of the public with medical error, and media attention to this issue, only 6% of the public and 5% of physicians viewed medical errors as one of the nation's most important health issues.[84] Concerns about errors ranked far below concerns about the costs of medical care and prescription drugs.

CONCLUSION

The medication-use system is amazingly complex. While we may commonly equate medication use with consumption by the patient, the management of medication use involves physicians, pharmacists, nurses, and other health professionals as well as those involved in the organization and financing of health care. In addition, these persons work in a mélange of physical settings, adding to the complexity. To make such a complex system operate well, there must be sharing of information and other elements of collaboration across providers who may be in separate physical locations.

The thousands of different medications that make up our armamentarium and the unique characteristics of individual patients make the selection of medication regimens complicated even in the best system of care. Coupled with this complexity is uncertainty as to how individual patients may respond to a drug and uncertainty generated by conflicting clinical trial results. While the complexity and uncertainty of health care create challenges in initiating and managing drug therapy for an individual patient, the same factors complicate our efforts to build a better medication-use system.

Uncertainty as to the frequency and nature of DRPs, and uncertainty about the effectiveness of various system-level interventions, complicates our efforts to modify an already complex medication-use system. The complexity of research on DRPs heightens this uncertainty. For example, definitive assessment of the preventability of ADEs is not always possible. Furthermore, the extent and nature of drug-related morbidity in the elderly have been obfuscated by the proliferation of studies that examine "PIMs" with varying criteria. Thus, it is not clear how many elderly patients are experiencing actual drug-related morbidity versus "potential" DRPs.

Also contributing to the uncertainty is the difficulty in detecting and measuring some types of DRPs. For example, the untreated indication is harder to detect than a drug–drug interaction. More broadly, errors of omission (not doing what is needed) may be more difficult to identify than errors of commission (doing something wrong), since there may be no sentinel event, and no easily accessed data, in the case of omissions. Thus, the frequency of untreated indications is less well known than the frequency of drug–drug interactions, and the prevention of untreated indications may be more challenging.

If complexity and uncertainty are the root causes of many DRPs, then quality improvement efforts for the medication-use system should focus on methods to reduce complexity and uncertainty. Information systems that facilitate evidence-based decision-making and that improve both the nature and content of communication between all the participants in health care will go a long way toward reducing DRPs. Teamwork, systems thinking, and continuous learning from successes and failures are also essential components to building a safe and effective medication-use system. At the same time, the importance of the individual must not be overlooked. The strong covenantal relationship between provider and patient can establish an environment that facilitates a truly helpful dialogue. Once we develop a better understanding of how to improve the quality of the medication-use system, we can design payment systems and health care policies that facilitate the appropriate use of medications.

KEY POINTS

- Drug-related morbidity is the phenomenon of therapeutic malfunction – the failure of a therapeutic agent to produce the intended therapeutic outcome. This concept encompasses both treatment failure and the production of new medical problems.

- Hepler and Grainger-Rousseau suggested that there are three main elements to the proper functioning of a pharmaceutical care system: (a) initiating therapy; (b) monitoring therapy; and (c) managing (i.e., correcting) therapy.
- Quality improvement efforts for the medication-use system should focus on methods to reduce complexity and uncertainty.

REFERENCES

1. Manasse HR. Medication use in an imperfect world: drug misadventuring as an issue of public policy, part 1. *Am J Hosp Pharm*. 1989;46:929–944.
2. Manasse HR. Medication use in an imperfect world: drug misadventuring as an issue of public policy, part 2. *Am J Hosp Pharm*. 1989;46:1141–1152.
3. Hepler CD, Strand LM. Opportunities and responsibilities in pharmaceutical care. *Am J Hosp Pharm*. 1990;47:533–543.
4. Johnson JA, Bootman JL. Drug-related morbidity and mortality: a cost-of-illness model. *Arch Intern Med*. 1995;155:1949–1956.
5. Bootman JL, Harrison DL, Cox E. The health care cost of drug-related morbidity and mortality in nursing facilities. *Arch Intern Med*. 1997;157:2089–2096.
6. Winterstein AG, Sauer BC, Hepler CD, Poole C. Preventable drug-related hospital admissions. *Ann Pharmacother*. 2002;36:1238–1248.
7. Strand LM, Morley PC, Cipolle RJ, Ramsey R, Lamsam GD. Drug-related problems: their structure and function. *DICP Ann Pharmacother*. 1990;24:1093–1097.
8. Hepler CD, Grainger-Rousseau T-J. Pharmaceutical care versus traditional drug treatment. Is there a difference? *Drugs*. 1995;49:1–10.
9. Knapp DA, Knapp DE, Brandon BM, West S. Development and application of criteria in drug use review programs. *Am J Hosp Pharm*. 1974;31:648–658.
10. Denig P, Haaijer-Ruskamp FM, Zijsling DH. How physicians choose drugs. *Soc Sci Med*. 1988;27:1381–1386.
11. Denig P. Scope and nature of prescribing decisions made by general practitioners. *Qual Saf Health Care*. 2002;11:137–143.
12. Groves KEM, Flanagan PS, MacKinnon NJ. Why physicians start or stop prescribing a drug: literature review and formulary implications. *Formulary*. 2002;37:186–194.
13. Schwartz RK, Soumerai SB, Avorn J. Physician motivations for nonscientific drug prescribing. *Soc Sci Med*. 1989;28:577–582.
14. Segal R, Wang F. Influencing physician prescribing. *Pharm Pract Manage Q*. 1999;19:30–50.
15. Chrischilles EA, Fulda TR, Byrns PJ, et al. The Role of Pharmacy Computer Systems in Preventing Medication Errors. *J Am Pharm Assoc*. 2002;42:439–488.
16. Chrischilles EA, Fulda TR, Byrns PJ, et al. The role of pharmacy computer systems in preventing medication errors. *J Am Pharm Assoc*. 2002;42:439–448.
17. The US Pharmacopeia Drug Utilization Review Advisory Panel. Drug utilization review: mechanisms to improve its effectiveness and broaden its scope. *J Am Pharm Assoc*. 2000;40:538–545.
18. Kimberlin C, Brushwood D, Allen W, et al. Cancer patient and caregiver experiences: communication and pain management issues. *J Pain Symptom Manage*. 2004;28:566–578.

19. Anderson-Harper HM, Berger BA, Noel R. Pharmacists' predisposition to communicate, desire to counsel and job satisfaction. *Am J Pharm Educ.* 1992;56:252–258.
20. Phillips LS, Branch WT, Cook CB, et al. Clinical inertia. *Ann Intern Med.* 2001;135: 825–834.
21. McBride P, Schrott HG, Plane MB, et al. Primary care practice adherence to National Cholesterol Education Program guidelines for patients with coronary heart disease. *Arch Intern Med.* 1998;158:1238–1244.
22. Drass J, Kell S, Osborn M, et al. Diabetes care for Medicare beneficiaries. Attitudes and behaviors of primary care physicians. *Diab Care.* 1998;21:1282–1287.
23. El-Kebbi IM, Ziemer DC, Gallina DL, et al. Diabetes in urban African-Americans. XV. Identification of barriers to provider adherence to management protocols. *Diab Care.* 1999;22:1617–1620.
24. Institute of Medicine. *Crossing the Quality Chasm.* Washington, DC: National Academy Press; 2001.
25. Fera T, Bluml BM, Ellis WM. Diabetes ten city challenge: final economic and clinical results. *J Am Pharm Assoc.* 2009;49:383–391.
26. Pindolia VK, Stebelsky L, Romain RM, Luoma L, Nowak SN, Gillanders F. Mitigation of medication mishaps via medication therapy management. *Ann Pharmacother.* 2009;43:611–620.
27. Welch EK, Delate T, Chester EA, Stubbings T. Assessment of the impact of medication therapy management delivered to home-based Medicare beneficiaries. *Ann Pharmacother.* 2009;43:603–610.
28. Robinson JD, Segal R, Lopez LM, Doty RE. Impact of a Pharmaceutical Care Intervention on Blood Pressure Control in a Chain Pharmacy Practice. *Ann Pharmacother.* 2010;44:88–96.
29. Medicare Part D Medication Therapy Management (MTM) Program Fact Sheet 2008. http://www.cms.hhs.gov/PrescriptionDrugCovContra/Downloads/MTMFactSheet.pdf. Accessed July 19, 2009.
30. Institute for Safe Medication Practices. *Remote Electronic Prescribing can lead to Wrong Patient Errors.* http://www.ismp.org/Newsletters/nursing/Issues/NurseAdviseERR200812. pdf. Accessed August 17, 2009.
31. Weinberger M, Murray MD, Marrero DG, et al. Effectiveness of pharmacist care for patients with reactive airways disease. *JAMA.* 2002;288:1594–1602.
32. Zhan C, Arispe I, Kelley E, et al. Ambulatory care visits for treating adverse drug effects in the United States, 1995–2001. Jt Comm J Qual Patient Saf. 2005;31:372–378.
33. Bates DW, Cullen D, Laird N, et al. Incidence of adverse drug events and potential adverse drug events: implications for prevention. *JAMA.* 1995;274:29–34.
34. Kaushal R, Bates DW, Landrigan C, et al. Medication errors and adverse drug events in pediatric inpatients. *JAMA.* 2001;285:2114–2120.
35. Forster AJ, Murff HJ, Peterson JF, Gandhi TK, Bates DW. The incidence and severity of adverse events affecting patients after discharge from the hospital. *Ann Intern Med.* 2003;138:161–167.
36. Lazarou J, Pomeranz BH, Corey PN. Incidence of adverse drug reactions in hospitalized patients: a meta-analysis of prospective studies. *JAMA.* 1998;279:1200–1205.
37. Leape LL, Bates DW, Cullen DJ, et al. Systems analysis of adverse drug events. *JAMA.* 1995;274:35–43.

38. Bates DW, Leape LL, Cullen DJ, et al. Effect of computerized physician order entry and a team intervention on prevention of serious medication errors. *JAMA*. 1998;280:1311–1316.

39. Evans RS, Pestotnik SL, Classen DC, et al. A computer-assisted management program for antibiotics and other antiinfective agents. *N Engl J Med*. 1998;338:232–238.

40. Leape LL, Cullen DJ, Clapp MD, et al. Pharmacist participation on physician rounds and adverse drug events in the intensive care unit. *JAMA*. 1999;282:267–270.

41. Kucukarslan SN, Peters M, Mlynarek M, et al. Pharmacists on rounding teams reduce preventable adverse drug events in hospital general medicine units. *Arch Intern Med*. 2003;163:2014–2018.

42. National Cholesterol Education Program. *Third Report of the Expert Panel on Detection, Evaluation, and Treatment of High Blood Cholesterol in Adults*. NIH Publication No. 02-5215. Bethesda, MD: National Heart, Lung and Blood Institute; 2002:284 pp.

43. Chobanian AV, Bakris GL, Black HR, et al. Seventh report of the Joint National Committee on prevention, detection, evaluation, and treatment of high blood pressure. *Hypertension*. 2003;42:1206–1252.

44. Saydah SH, Fadkin J, Cowie CC. Poor control of risk factors for vascular disease among adults with previously diagnosed diabetes. *JAMA*. 2004;291:335–342.

45. Beers MH, Ouslander JG, Rollingher I, et al. Explicit criteria for determining inappropriate medication use in nursing home residents. *Arch Intern Med*. 1991;151:1825–1832.

46. Fick DM, Cooper JW, Wade WE, et al. Updating the Beers criteria for potentially inappropriate medication use in older adults: results of a US consensus panel of experts. *Arch Intern Med*. 2003;163:2716–2724.

47. Lau DT, Kasper JD, Potter DEB, Lyles A. Potentially inappropriate medication prescriptions among elderly nursing home residents: their scope and associated resident and facility characteristics. *Health Serv Res*. 2004;39:1257–1276.

48. Lau DT, Kasper JD, Potter DEB, Lyles A, Bennett RG. Hospitalization and death associated with potentially inappropriate medication prescriptions among elderly nursing home residents. *Arch Intern Med*. 2005;165:68–74.

49. Curtis LH, Ostbye T, Sendersky V, et al. Inappropriate prescribing for elderly Americans in a large outpatient population. *Arch Intern Med*. 2004;164:1621–1625.

50. Rigler SK, Jachna CM, Perera S, Shireman TI, Eng ML. Patterns of potentially inappropriate medication use across three cohorts of older Medicaid recipients. *Ann Pharmacother*. 2005;39:1175–1181.

51. Zhan C, Correa-de-Araujo R, Bierman AS, et al. Suboptimal prescribing in elderly outpatients: potentially harmful drug–drug and drug–disease combinations. *JAGS*. 2005;53:262–267.

52. Hecker MT, Aron DC, Patel NP, et al. Unnecessary use of antimicrobials in hospitalized patients. *Arch Intern Med*. 2003;163:972–978.

53. Edgell ET, Summers KH, Hylan TR, Ober J, Bootman JL. A framework for drug utilization evaluation in depression: insights from outcomes research. *Med Care*. 1999;37: AS67–AS76.

54. Wells KB, Katon W, Rogers WH. Use of minor tranquilizers and antidepressant medications by depressed outpatients: results from the Medical Outcomes Study. *Am J Psychiatry*. 1994;151:694–700.

55. McCombs JS, Nichol MB, Stimmel GL. The cost of antidepressant drug therapy failure: a study of antidepressant use patterns in a Medicaid population. *J Clin Psychiatry*. 1990;51:60–69.

56. Grant RW, Cagliero E, Dubey AK, et al. Clinical inertia in the management of type 2 diabetes metabolic risk factors. *Diab Med*. 2004;21:150–155.

57. Shah BR, Zinman B, Hux JE, van Walraven C, Laupacis A. Clinical inertia in response to inadequate glycemic control: do specialists differ from primary care physicians? *Diab Care*. 2005;28:600–606.

58. Wetzler HP, Snyder JW. Linking pharmacy and laboratory data to assess the appropriateness of care in patients with diabetes. *Diab Care*. 2000;23:1637–1641.

59. Cleeland CS, Gonin R, Hatfield AK, et al. Pain and its treatment in outpatients with metastatic cancer. *N Engl J Med*. 1994;330:592–596.

60. Larue F, Colleau SM, Brasseur L, Cleeland CS. Multicentre study of cancer pain and its treatment in France. *BMJ*. 1995;310:1034–1037.

61. Olyeai A, de Matos A, Bennet W. Prescribing drugs in renal disease. In: Brenner B. *The Kidney*. 6th ed. Philadelphia, PA: WB Saunders Co; 2000:2606–2653.

62. Pedersen CA, Schneider PJ, Scheckelhoff DJ. ASHP national survey of pharmacy practice in hospital settings: monitoring and patient education – 2003. *Am J Health Syst Pharm*. 2004;61:457–471.

63. Liem RI, Higman MA, Chen AR, Arceci FJ. Misinterpretation of a Calvert-derived formula leading to carboplatin overdose in two children. *J Pediatr Hematol Oncol*. 2003;25: 818–821.

64. Litovitz TL, Klein-Schwartz W, Rogers GC Jr, et al. 2001 annual report of the American Association of Poison Control Centers Toxic Exposure Surveillance System. *Am J Emerg Med*. 2002;20:391–452.

65. Safran DG, Neuman P, Schoen C, et al. Prescription drug coverage and seniors: findings from a 2003 national survey. *Health Aff*. 2005;W5:152–166.

66. Benner JS, Glynn RJ, Mogun H, et al. Long-term persistence in use of statin therapy in elderly patients. *JAMA*. 2002;288:455–461.

67. Benner JS, Pollack MF, Smith TW, et al. Association between short-term effectiveness of statins and long-term adherence to lipid-lowering therapy. *Am J Health Syst Pharm*. 2005;62:1468–1475.

68. Pampallona S, Bollini P. Patient adherence in the treatment of depression. *Br J Psychiatr*. 2002;180:104–109.

69. Samet JH, Libman H, Steger KA, et al. Compliance with zidovudine monotherapy in patients infected with human immunodeficiency virus, type 1: a cross-sectional study in a municipal hospital clinic. *Am J Med*. 1992;92:495–502.

70. Gao X, Nau DP, Rosenbluth A, et al. The relationship of disease severity, health beliefs and medication adherence among HIV patients. *AIDS Care*. 2000;12:387–398.

71. Walsh JC, Horne R, Dalton M, et al. Reasons for non-adherence to antiretroviral therapy: patients' perspectives provide evidence of multiple causes. *AIDS Care*. 2001;13:709–720.

72. Aikens JE, Nease DE, Nau DP, et al. Adherence to maintenance-phase antidepressant medication as a function of patient beliefs about medication. *Ann Fam Med*. 2005;3:23–30.

73. Horne R, Buick D, Fisher M, et al. Doubts about necessity and concerns about adverse effects: identifying the types of beliefs that are associated with non-adherence to HAART. *Int J STD AIDS*. 2004;15:38–44.

74. United States Department of Health and Human Services, Substance Abuse and Mental Health Services Administration. *2003 National Survey on Drug Use and Health*. http://oas.samhsa.gov/nhsda.htm. Accessed August 17, 2009.

75. Gonzales R, Steiner JF, Sande MA. Antibiotic prescribing for adults with colds, upper respiratory tract infections and bronchitis by ambulatory care physicians. *JAMA*. 1997;278:901–904.

76. Watson RL, Dowell SF, Jayaraman M, et al. Antimicrobial use for pediatric upper respiratory infections: reported practice, actual practice, and parent beliefs. *Pediatrics*. 1999;104:1251–1257.

77. Akkerman AE, Kuyvenhoven MM, van der Wouden JC, Verheij TJM. Analysis of under- and overprescribing of antibiotics in acute otitis media in general practice. *J Antimicrob Chemother*. 2005;(July);56:1–6.

78. Jelinski S, Parfrey P, Hutchinson J. Antibiotic utilization in community practices: guideline concurrence and prescription necessity. *Pharmacoepidemiol Drug Saf*. 2005;14:319–326.

79. Avorn J, Solomon DH. Cultural and economic factors that (mis)shape antibiotic use: the nonpharmacologic basis of therapeutics. *Ann Intern Med*. 2000;133:128–135.

80. Flynn EA, Barker KN, Carnahan BJ. National observational study of prescription dispensing accuracy and safety in 50 pharmacies. *J Am Pharm Assoc*. 2003;43:191–200.

81. Barker KN, Flynn EA, Pepper GA, et al. Medication errors observed in 36 health care facilities. *Arch Intern Med*. 2002;162:1897–1903.

82. Davis K, Schoenbaum SC, Collins KS, et al. *Room for Improvement: Patients' Report on the Quality of their Health Care*. New York: The Commonwealth Fund; April 2002.

83. Nau DP, Erickson SR. Medication safety: patients' experiences, beliefs and behaviors. *J Am Pharm Assoc*. 2005;45:452–457.

84. Blendon RJ, DesRoches CM, Brodie M, et al. View of practicing physicians and the public on medical errors. *N Engl J Med*. 2002;347:1933–1940.

CHAPTER 3

The Business Case for Pharmacy Quality

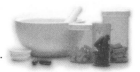

David A. Holdford

INTRODUCTION

Quality of care is a major issue in health care. The Institutes of Medicine stated that quality problems are everywhere resulting in large health care gaps that are better characterized as chasms.[1] It has been strongly argued that for fundamental change to occur, health care providers need to make a compelling "business case" for quality.[2]

However, numerous obstacles have been identified to developing a business case for quality in the U.S. health care system[3,4]:

1. Payment for services within the current system is not linked to quality, while defective care is often rewarded.
2. Consumers are unable to perceive differences between different levels of health care quality.
3. The benefits of quality improvement (QI) are often seen in the distant future and do not accrue to the organizations that finance it.
4. Best practices in health care are often unknown, not accepted, or not feasible to clinicians in practice settings.

5. Changing provider behavior is difficult to do and the methods of behavior change are not well understood.

6. Quality measurement is still a primitive science in that many measures are not available, validated, reliable, or practical.

7. Health care does not have an adequate infrastructure to assess quality and act upon it.

8. There are legal barriers to doing what is necessary.

9. Fiscal concerns make investing in quality problematic.

This chapter explores the business case for quality in pharmacy practice. It will define what a business case is, and it will compare how a business case differs from nonbusiness cases. The chapter will also suggest strategies that pharmacists can use to build a business case for quality in pharmacy practice.

WHAT IS A BUSINESS CASE?

Before starting any discussion, it is important to define what is meant by a "business case." A business case for a health care intervention exists whenever the intervention results in a real or estimated financial return within a reasonable time frame for an investing entity.[3] A key component of this definition is the term financial return.

Financial returns are the profits or losses suffered in an expenditure of money, time, or effort. Profits result when the expenditures are less than the benefits received. Losses occur when the expenditures are greater than the benefits.

Financial returns can be real or estimated. *Real financial returns* are generated when an intervention generates measurable revenue or cost savings. *Estimated financial returns* are only anticipated. They result when an argument can be made that an intervention will probably generate some savings or reduce costs for a business, but that the exact amount can only be anticipated. For example, a chain pharmacy that wants to justify hiring additional technicians to reduce customer wait times for prescriptions might expect to see real financial returns (e.g., additional revenue attributable to the technicians) or estimated financial returns (e.g., anticipated cost reductions associated with employee turnover). The additional real or estimated benefits would need to exceed the costs of those additional technicians to achieve a business case.

IS A BUSINESS CASE NECESSARY?

Is a business case necessary for every health care intervention? The answer to this question depends on the entity judging the intervention's worth. A national, corporately owned retail pharmacy might need different justification for a program than a state-supported pharmacy clinic associated with a university health system or an initiative financially backed by a pharmacy benefit management company.

The funding *organization's mission* is an important determinant in whether a business case is needed – some organizations missions' emphasize benefits, not costs. A case in point might be a charity. Nonprofit charities exist to serve their constituents and may not always worry about the financial bottom line in making decisions. Although

TABLE 3-1. Different Cases Made to Justify Pharmacy Interventions

Case	Definition
Business	When the investing entity realizes a real or estimated financial return within a reasonable time frame
Economic	When discounted financial benefits exceed discounted financial costs whether they accrue to patients, payers, employers, the health care system, or society
Social	When an intervention benefits society regardless of cost

this may impact their viability as a continuing enterprise, viability may not be part of their long-term mission.

Another important determinant in making a business case is the time period (also known as time horizon) over which an intervention is being considered. Some organizations have a longer term view in their decision-making processes than others. Thus, they may forgo short-term profits for long-term returns on their investment. For instance, the federal government is likely to take a longer term view on a diabetes management program than a corporate health insurance program because the government will more likely bear the long-term impact of the disease's negative health consequences. Private health insurance providers are less likely to benefit from a quality investment that pays off in the distant future because enrollees in private health insurance frequently switch plans – often staying only 2 or 3 years before switching to another plan or changing employers. Therefore, any long-term benefits from a quality investment are likely to accrue to someone other than the investing private health plan. As a consequence, a business case may be possible for one provider but not another due to differences in time horizons.

The judging organization may accept other supporting arguments such as an economic or a social case (Table 3-1). The major difference between a business case for quality and these other arguments is perspective, which is driven by the organization's mission. An economic case or social case differs from a business case by who is expected to benefit.[3] An *economic case for quality* can be made if anyone (e.g., patients and society) benefits more than what is spent to achieve those benefits. For example, a pharmacist-managed osteoporosis adherence program could be justified economically if its benefits exceed the costs to a provider, payer, or patient (e.g., reduced hospitalizations and improved patient's quality of life). However, it could also present a poor business case if it ends up costing the pharmacy more money than it receives in revenue and/or nonfinancial benefits. A *social case for quality* differs from the business and economics cases by weighing the benefits of a health care intervention to individuals or society regardless of cost.[3]

The key issue that differentiates business cases from economic and social cases is profit. Businesses seek profits. Therefore, profitability to the investing entity is the goal when developing a business case, whereas economic and social cases do not require such evidence.

BUILDING A BUSINESS CASE FOR PHARMACY

There are some basic foundations underlying the business case for quality.[5] The first is that quality is an investment and therefore must be financially accountable. Quality is not free. It costs something to develop and run a quality intervention. It requires inputs (e.g., pharmacists and medication therapy programs) and processes (e.g., patient counseling and medication therapy management) that result in some outcome(s) (e.g., improved quality of life and revenue). In other words, to achieve quality, we must spend. If we feel that the outcomes resulting from that spending are financially worth it, we have a business case.

Like any other investment, pharmacists should expect a reasonable return on quality (ROQ). This is no different from an investor who chooses to invest money in the stock or real estate markets. When pharmacists put money into QI initiatives, they are investing.

Investments must result in an acceptable financial return. If not, they are a drain on the business's resources and prevent those resources from being spent on something else. It is possible to spend too much on quality – too many people can be hired, too much can be spent on technology, and the like. The goal of developing the business case for quality is to consider QI expenditures the same as any other investment choice.

Many current investments in pharmacy are based on faith, meaning that our belief in the value of pharmacy interventions is based on anecdotes and estimations, not quantifiable results. That faith may not be misplaced if it is based on realistic assessments of the medication-use process and backed up by extensive professional expertise. Nevertheless, investing organizations are increasingly asking for documented evidence of value.

BUSINESS CASE TERMINOLOGY

Table 3-2 describes some common terms and definitions used to describe business cases. These terms are presented for illustrative purposes and not meant to be comprehensive explanations of their foundations and use. For a detailed discussion of calculations behind these terms, see the financial management text by Carroll.[6]

Business case terminology revolves around the financial (e.g., dollars) or nonfinancial (e.g., time and effort) costs and the financial (e.g., dollars) or nonfinancial (e.g., feeling of a job well done) benefits of pharmacy interventions. The terminology becomes slightly more complicated when the costs and/or benefits occur in different years. When this occurs, costs and benefits need to be adjusted to what is called present value (PV). PV is based on the principle that money now is worth more than money in the future, all things else being equal. PV is described by the given equation:

$$\text{Present value} = \frac{\text{Future value}}{(1 + \text{Interest rate})^{\text{No. of time periods}}}$$

TABLE 3-2. Useful Terms and Definitions Used to Describe Business Cases

Terms	Definition
Costs	Total financial (e.g., cost in dollars) or nonfinancial inputs (e.g., aggravation) spent on a quality intervention
Benefits	Total financial (e.g., revenue in dollars) or nonfinancial outputs (e.g., personal satisfaction) received for providing the quality
Present value	Current worth of money (or some other thing of value) received in the future. This future money is discounted to reflect its time value and allow it to be compared to money in the present
Benefits-to-cost ratio	Ratio of benefits to costs from an intervention. An amount equal to 1 "breaks even" and an amount greater than 1 is a positive return on investment
Return-on-investment (ROI)	[(Benefits − Costs)/Costs] × 100 = % ROI

Hence, the PV of a benefit or cost equals the value in the future divided by the compounded quantity of 1 plus an acceptable rate of interest over a number of time periods. This equation illustrates two important conceptual points. One is that as the interest rate demanded on an investment over time increases, the PV of a pharmacy intervention decreases. This might occur if the intervention is perceived to be risky in terms of financial return or if there are other interventions that provide a greater return. A second point is that PV decreases the longer it takes for an investment to pay off. So, a smoking cessation program that costs $10,000 to start up and run in the first year would need to generate returns to cover the $10,000 plus the interest on the $10,000 demanded by an investor over the compounded time period it takes for the benefits to be received. In the case of smoking cessation, benefits such as reduced mortality would accrue at the end of an individual's life many years in the future. If the PV of benefits exceeds the PV of the costs, the smoking cessation program would be deemed to have a positive return on investment (ROI). A positive ROI is the strongest business case for health care,[2] and it is simply the ratio of money gained or lost relative to the amount invested.

The following example illustrates how the PV is worth more than the future value. If a quality investment results in $10,000 savings after 2 years (i.e., future value of $10,000) and the annual compounded interest rate of the investment is expected to be 5%, then the PV of that future $10,000 would be only $9070. Thus, the total personnel, supplies, and other costs invested would need to be less than $9070 to make a business case:

$$\text{Present value} = \frac{\$10,000}{(1+0.05)^2}$$

COMPETING WITH QUALITY

Every pharmacist is competing for consumer dollars. Whenever consumers spend a dollar on one thing, that dollar cannot be spent on something else. Thus, pharmacists are competing with education, national defense, oil companies, and other industries for consumer dollars. Within health care, pharmacists are competing with physicians, nurses, hospitals, nursing homes, and other health care providers for health care dollars.

Pharmacists can compete in two primary ways.[7] The first is by being cheaper than one's competitors in satisfying customer demand. Being cheaper, known as a *cost-based strategy*, attempts to compete by designing workplace environments that simplify work, reduce waste, increase employee productivity, and so on.[8] The problem with an over-reliance on this strategy is that there is always someone cheaper. The second way of competing is by being different. Being different, known as a *differentiation strategy*, occurs when pharmacists compete by offering a mix of products and services that are of higher quality, perform better, or are uniquely desirable.[8] Pharmacies that use differentiation strategies emphasize value over price. To be sure, price is still important because perceptions of value are linked with perceptions that differentiated pharmacies give more for the money. However, quality, not low price, is typically the deciding factor in pharmacy patronage.

An additional argument supporting the use of a quality strategy is that drug therapy is the most cost-effective component of the health care pie. Thus, investments in improving drug therapy can result in greater value than many other interventions. Accordingly, a quality strategy for pharmacists gives them an advantage over other health care providers.

SUPPORT FOR QUALITY'S BUSINESS CASE

Support for the business case for quality depends on how well pharmacists can answer the following question: "How can pharmacists use quality to increase their ROI?" Several quality models from the management literature illustrate how pharmacists can use quality to increase ROI.

Edward Deming is probably the best known proponent of QI. He stated that improving quality can help business compete by starting a chain reaction of events that lowers costs and leads to business success.[9] *Deming's Quality Chain Reaction* (Figure 3-1) starts with some intervention that increases quality. As quality is increased, costs are lowered by reducing the time and expense of fixing mistakes. Consequently, there is less repetition of work that should have been done correctly the first time. There are also fewer delays in service while those mistakes are being fixed and better use of technology, people, and other resources. Although Deming did not state it in his model, fewer mistakes will likely lead to fewer lawsuits.

Because employees spend less time dealing with errors and mistakes, their productivity improves, and they are able to produce a higher quality product at lower cost. This allows the business to offer superior value to customers, attract greater share of the market, and stay in business. It also generates profits that can be used to hire additional

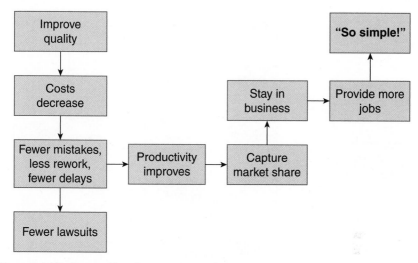

Figure 3-1. The Deming Chain Reaction. *Source:* [9]

employees or pay more to current employees. In sum, the emphasis of this model is on lowering costs. Those savings can be passed on to customers with lower prices or further improved quality, both of which attract more customers.

The *service–profit cycle (SPC)* is an alternative model that makes a business case for quality by presenting a circular process that starts with investments in service and ends with firm profitability (Figure 3-2). The SPC argues that good service starts with attracting and keeping talented employees.[10] This process is called internal marketing.[11] Internal marketing requires employers to provide a good work environment and the opportunity to learn and progress within a job – two benefits of any organization that embraces the practice and philosophy of QI.

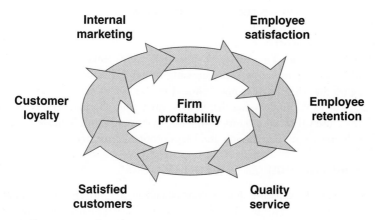

Figure 3-2. The service–profit cycle. *Source:* [16].

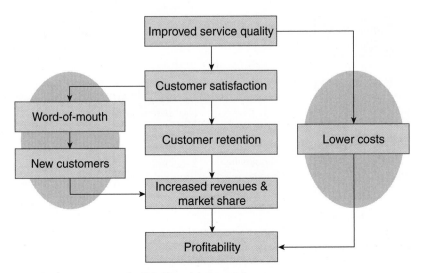

Figure 3-3. The return on quality (ROQ) model. *Source:* [5].

The SPC states further that internal marketing (e.g., improving the work environment and providing better leadership) leads to employee satisfaction and retention. The more desirable the job, the better management is able to select the best employees to serve customers. Employers have fewer issues with job turnover, and when vacancies occur, they are quickly filled due to word-of-mouth recommendations from satisfied employees. Satisfied employees in a well-run organization are more likely to adopt an excellent service attitude and customer-centered behaviors. Those positive attitudes and behaviors are projected to customers who are better served, more satisfied, and loyal. Loyal customers purchase more and require less expenditure for coupons, advertising, and other promotions. This results in greater profit for the firm.

The SPC and Deming models emphasize different ends of the ROI equation. SPC uses QI to generate more revenues through excellent service in contrast to the Deming's model that highlights greater ROI due to cost containment. It has been argued that QI can lower costs *and* generate revenues.

The (ROQ) model (Figure 3-3).[5,12] states that investments in quality can increase profitability by reducing costs and increasing revenue. For pharmacists, the ROQ model argues that the choice is not, "Should we use QI to reduce costs or enhance revenues?" The ROQ model states that in most situations, pharmacists should attempt to do both – use QI to lower costs by increasing efficiency and increase revenues by providing better service that attracts and keeps profitable customers.

LITERATURE FOR PHARMACY'S BUSINESS CASE

Although the business case for quality in pharmacy makes intuitive sense, supporting data are limited. The vast majority of evidence supporting pharmacy services might make social or economic cases, but not necessarily business cases.[13,14] If truth be told, many studies in the literature fail to even make a strong economic case due to methodological limitations such as a weak research design, incomplete collection of clinical and economic impacts, and failure to quantify all input costs (e.g., cost of personnel providing services).[13,14] It may appear obvious to us that increasing the quality of pharmacist services should be profitable given our ability to keep patients out of the hospital, prevent adverse drug events, and influence drug use. However, an intuitive argument may not be sufficient to attract investments in QI. Employers and payers may require actual evidence collected in real life practice settings before they would be willing to invest in QI interventions.

QUESTIONS TO ASK WHEN BUILDING A BUSINESS CASE

Pharmacists need to be able to provide some evidence that their efforts are, in fact, profitable. Thus, the following section discusses key questions to answer associated with building a business case for pharmacy quality.[2] The questions can be grouped under the following interlinking categories: the intervention itself, the benefits received from the intervention, and the stakeholder's motives for funding the quality intervention (Table 3-3).

Does the intervention actually improve quality? An obvious requirement for building a business case for any intervention is that the intervention must actually work. This demands that the intervention be critically appraised for its ability to achieve some desired outcome. Luckily for pharmacists, there is an increasing literature demonstrating that pharmacist interventions do have impact on patient health and economic outcomes, a necessary step toward building a business case.[13,14]

Is the intervention a core component of the business or just an optional feature? A less obvious requirement of most interventions is that an intervention be sustainable and expandable over time. Indeed, pilot QIs cannot sustain the business case for quality. Pilot projects that cannot be expanded profitably throughout an organization are more likely to be cancelled. In a series of case studies of health care interventions, Leatherman

TABLE 3-3. Questions to Ask When Building a Business Case

The quality intervention
• Does the intervention actually improve quality?
• Is the intervention a core component of the business or just an optional feature?
The benefits of the intervention
• Does the intervention make money for anyone?
• What nonfinancial benefits accrue from the intervention?
The stakeholders
• What do stakeholders care about?
• How can arguments be crafted to the interests of stakeholders?

et al.[3] found that interventions that are not seen as a core function of an organization are less likely to succeed in the long term. Optional programs (i.e., nice to have but not essential to the business) are more likely to be canceled because the needed long-term level of commitment is not there.

This can be illustrated with an example from this author's experience. A major pharmacy chain offered a "smoking cessation pilot program" at a single pharmacy. The goal was to build upon the success at this pharmacy and expand the program to other stores. However, smoking cessation services were never seen by the chain's executives or pharmacists to be a key element of the business. Among pharmacists, there was a feeling that this program was not an important aspect of their job and that it took them away from their primary responsibilities: filing prescriptions. Similarly, chain management felt that this "optional" program took resources away from the "core" dispensing business. Consequently, support from pharmacists, managers, and executives dwindled after the program's initial success. Thus, despite the fact that the program was clinically successful (i.e., 25% of the patients enrolled were smoke-free at 1 year) and the program generated some positive public relations for the chain, executives of the firm pulled the plug on the program. The program failed to survive because it was only successful in an economic and social sense.

Does the intervention make money for anyone? An effective health care intervention is likely to result in some financial impact to someone, even though the returns may not be to the one who paid for the intervention. To make a business case, it is important to identify any financial benefits accrued from an intervention.

What nonfinancial benefits accrue from the intervention? It is very difficult to make a business case for most health care interventions on financial benefits alone. The case must often be supported by an intervention's nonfinancial benefits. Hence, a supporting argument might be made for how a pharmacy program helps an organization meet the terms of participation in a contract with health care insurers or to meet performance payment incentives (e.g., generic substitution rates or quality of counseling). A nonfinancial case can also be made if a pharmacy program improves the reputation and image of an organization to help them compete for customers, plan members, and/or patients.

What do stakeholders care about? Many individuals and organizations may have a stake in demonstrating the effectiveness of a pharmacy intervention. These stakeholders may be individuals in the pharmacy organization, insurers, businesses, foundations, professional organizations, governmental bodies, suppliers, and pharmaceutical companies. The key is to identify these stakeholders and craft arguments to appeal to their concerns and desires.

Ultimately, a business case for quality is made if stakeholders perceive sufficient value to support the initiative. One appeal might be to the stakeholder's mission. For instance, a pharmacy QI effort might support a pharmacy organization's claims that its mission is to improve patient health. A case might also be made for a pharmacy program's positive impact on the organization's internal culture. Thus, a pharmacy initiative that emphasizes meaningful efforts to help others can positively impact employee morale and perceptions of professionalism in an organization.

SUMMARY

The business case for quality in pharmacy services needs to be made if pharmacists are going to compete in the health care marketplace. Some pharmacists still question the emphasis of profitability on health care interventions by asking, "Is health care nothing more than a business? Should profit dictate everything?"[15] Is not social responsibility sufficient to justify the pharmacy profession's role in providing pharmaceutical care and other quality interventions?

The answer to this question depends on the viewpoint of one who is paying for pharmacist services. Increasingly, spending on QI efforts will need to be justified financially. Thus, pharmacists will need to be able to persuade payers that their QI ventures provide a bigger bang for the buck than other interventions.

The problem with building a business case is that pharmacy expenditures often do not generate measurable profits. Indeed, many successful pharmacy interventions increase costs (e.g., medication adherence programs), at least in the short term. In addition, many interventions do not have a clearly measurable cause and effect. This means that it can be difficult to unmistakably link what pharmacists do to a specific outcome (e.g., patient adherence) to the exclusion of all other possible influences (e.g., physician, nurse, and family member). Still a case can be made if pharmacists:

- accept that quality must be financially accountable;
- understand that quality can be profitable if it lowers costs, increases revenues, or both;
- identify QI stakeholders and what they care about;
- then, craft arguments to their interests.

Adopting this mindset and process for approaching quality problems will help pharmacists make a strong case for the value of their interventions.

REFERENCES

1. Berwick DM. A user's manual for the IOM's, Quality Chasm' report. *Health Aff (Millwood)*. 2002;21(3):80–90.
2. Bailit M, Dyer MB. *Beyond Bankable Dollars: Establishing a Business Case for Improving Health Care*. Report No. 754. New York, NY: 2004.
3. Leatherman S, Berwick D, Iles D, et al. The business case for quality: case studies and an analysis. *Health Aff*. 2003;22(2):17–30.
4. Blumenthal D, Ferris T. *The Business Case for Quality: Ending Business as Usual in Health Care*. Report No. 715. Boston, MA: Commonwealth Fund; 2004.
5. Rust RT, Zahorik AJ, Keiningham TL. Return on quality (ROQ) – making service quality financially accountable. *J Marketing*. 1995;59(2):58–70.
6. Carroll N. *Financial Management for Pharmacists: A Decision-making Approach*. Philadelphia: Lea & Febiger; 1991.
7. Porter ME. *Competitive Advantage: Creating and Sustaining Superior Performance*. New York: Free Press; 1985.
8. Holdford DA. Marketing strategies. In: *Marketing for Pharmacists*. 2nd ed. Washington, DC: American Pharmacists Association Publications; 2007:177–206.

9. Walton M. *The Deming Management Method*. New York: Perigree Books; 1986.
10. Heskett JL, Jones TO, Loveman GW, Sasser WE, Schlesinger LA. Putting the service–profit chain to work. *Harvard Business Rev*. 1994;72(2):164–174.
11. Sasser ED, Arbeit SP. Selling jobs in the service sector. *Business Horizons*. 1976;19(3): 61–67.
12. Rust RT, Moorman C, Dickson PR. Getting return on quality: revenue expansion, cost reduction, or both? *J Marketing*. 2002;66(4):7–24.
13. Perez A, Doloresco F, Hoffman JM, et al. Economic evaluations of clinical pharmacy services: 2001–2005. *Pharmacotherapy*. 2008;28(11):285e–323e.
14. De Rijdt T, Willems L, Simoens S. Economic effects of clinical pharmacy interventions: a literature review. *Am J Health Syst Pharm*. 2008 15;65(12):1161–1172.
15. Yan J. Health care: a business or responsibility? *Am J Health Syst Pharm*. 2001; 58(May):865.
16. Holdford DA. Managing service performance. In: *Marketing for Pharmacists*. 2nd ed. Washington, DC: American Pharmacists Association Publications; 2007:75.

CHAPTER 4

Health Care Organizations Involved in Quality Improvement

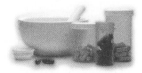

Donna West-Strum

Learning Objectives

At the end of the chapter, the reader will be able to:

1. Describe the various quality functions that different health care organizations are involved in.
2. Describe three government agencies' and three private organizations' involvement in health care quality.
3. Define accreditation and identify three health care accreditation organizations.
4. Describe the structure and activities of public–private partnerships aimed at improving health care quality.

The U.S. health care system spends more per capita on health care than any other country in the world, and yet, the quality is often inferior to other nations and often does not meet expected evidence-based guidelines. There are many reports providing statistics pertaining to care issues in the United States. One study found that 50–60% of patients are nonadherent with medication regimens, especially for chronic, asymptomatic illnesses.[1,2] Moreover, non-adherence is a major cause of hospitalizations, emergency room visits, and repeat physician visits. Other studies show 20–30% of geriatric patients are prescribed potentially inappropriate medications.[3,4] It is these types of reports that cause concern for government agencies, consumers, employers, providers, payers, and others involved in the U.S. health care system. Thus, these various stakeholders are interested in implementing quality improvement programs in the health care system.

Emerging quality improvement and patient safety movements reflect the realization that some patients do not receive important elements of proper care as measured by performance measures. For the past several years, different organizations have been developing and using quality measures to help determine the rates of provision of critical and widely recognized steps in the care of multiple conditions. Other organizations have been focused on quality improvement interventions and how to encourage providers to improve quality of care. Furthermore, the U.S. health care system is moving toward value-based purchasing. Value is the balance of quality and costs, and therefore, private and public payers for health care are starting to demand evidence of quality. As performance measurements continue to evolve, payers and policy makers are becoming increasingly interested in payment models that reward quality and patient safety.

With the health care system so focused on health care quality, it is not surprising that pharmacy is also being targeted. Organizations are developing quality measures that include medications as well as pharmacy service components. Organizations are encouraging retail pharmacies to adopt quality improvement methods. Organizations are including medication issues and pharmacy service quality as part of their accreditation process. Thus, it is imperative that pharmacists are aware of the many organizations involved in health care quality, and specifically quality of medication use and pharmacy services.

In the last 10 years the number of organizations involved in quality measurement and reporting has grown significantly. In the early 1990s, the Joint Commission, the Centers for Medicare and Medicaid Services (CMS), the Institute of Medicine (IOM), and the National Committee for Quality Assurance (NCQA) were focused on health care quality. Then in 1998, the President's Advisory Commission on Consumer Protection and Quality in the Health Care Industry issued their final report titled *Quality First: Better Health Care for All Americans.*[5] The report recommended steps to improve health care quality. With these recommendations came a need for new organizations and for organizations to partner. Now, there are numerous public and private entities interested in quality improvement in health care, and some primarily interested in pharmacy quality.

Because of the many public and private sector groups developing initiatives related to performance measures and reporting data, there was concern that perhaps there would be conflicting initiatives, unnecessary burden for providers, or confusion among consumers with so many measures and reports. Thus, the Quality Alliance Steering Committee (QASC) was formed in 2006 to coordinate the efforts of the existing quality alliances, government, physicians, nurses, pharmacists, hospitals, health insurers, and others working on improving health care quality.[6] This committee is helping to build the initial components of an infrastructure to collect health care quality and cost data nationwide and report it.

The vision of the QASC is to advance high-quality, cost-effective, patient-centered health care through the coordination of various groups that are working to promote public reporting of health care provider information for quality improvement, consumer decision making, and informing policy, including payment policies.[6] The QASC developed a diagram to show the important contributions various organizations are making to improving the quality of health care in this country.[7] We have adapted this diagram, as shown in Figure 4-1, to represent the various tasks and organizations involved in quality and safety, specifically as it pertains to pharmacy.

This chapter provides an overview of some of the major players shown in this diagram. It is beyond the scope of this chapter to highlight all the quality initiatives supported by these organizations; however, a few will be described. Additionally, many providers, hospitals, nursing homes, and pharmacies are implementing quality improvement programs and initiatives. This chapter does not review how all of the providers are implementing

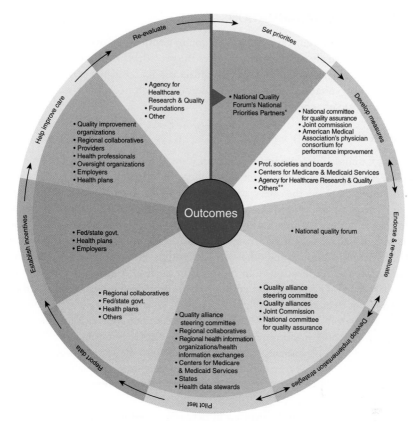

Figure 4-1. Quality Alliance Steering Committee (QASC) Road Map Organizational Wheel.
© 2009, the Engelberg Center for Health Care Reform at the Brookings Institution. Available at
http://www.healthqualityalliance.org/node/189. Reprinted with permission.

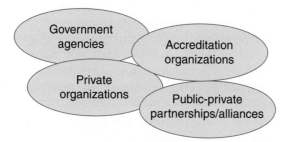

Figure 4-2. Categories of organizations involved in quality.

safety initiatives and quality improvement. The health care organizations discussed in this
chapter have been grouped into four main categories as shown in Figure 4-2. We will
review a few organizations in each of these categories and conclude with a brief discussion
of other entities involved with medication safety and pharmacy quality.

ACCREDITATION ORGANIZATIONS

Accreditation organizations award accreditation to health care providers who meet certain standards. Usually accreditation involves the providers providing documentation and demonstrating at a high level that they meet certain standards as outlined by the accreditation organization.[8] Thus, accreditation is an indicator of high-quality care. It is an external seal of approval.

The Joint Commission

The Joint Commission is a nonprofit organization founded in 1951 by the American Medical Association and the American College of Surgeons. It was established to "continuously improve the safety and quality of health care provided to the public through the provision of health care accreditation and related services that support performance improvement in health care organizations."[9] It accredits hospitals, long-term care, home care, assisted living, critical access hospitals, laboratory services, ambulatory care, networks, and other provider groups. Having the Joint Commission accreditation and certification is an indicator of quality. It means the organization has met certain standards and is committed to providing quality care. Being accredited is not mandatory, although it can affect an organization's reputation and reimbursement status. The Joint Commission accreditation process is moving toward more of an outcome measurement model. Their ORYX initiative is to "integrate outcomes and other performance measurement data into the accreditation process."[10] The ORYX initiative uses core performance measures to measure quality. These quality measures can be used by the providers to facilitate quality improvement processes within the facility.

The Joint Commission is involved in developing performance measures, patient safety initiatives, medical error reporting initiatives, and other resources and tools that health care organizations and providers can use to improve quality of care. A few examples are listed as follows:

- Provide Sentinel Event Alerts to accredited organizations. These alerts identify specific sentinel events, describe their causes, and suggest steps for organizations to take to prevent these types of events.[11]
- Develop medication management standards. Medication management standards are related to the minimum patient information needed to dispense a medication, requirements for preparing and dispensing medications, and storage requirements. Pharmacies within organizations seeking accreditation must adhere to these standards.[12]
- Publish National Patient Safety Goals every year for the public. The 2009 goals include medication goals such as using medicines safely and checking patient medicines.[13]

National Committee for Quality Assurance (NCQA)

The NCQA is a nonprofit organization established in 1990 by a managed care trade association in response to a perceived need to provide standardized quality measurement and reporting.[14] The NCQA reviews and accredits all types of managed health

TABLE 4-1. Examples of HEDIS Measures

Flu shots for adults – measures the percentage of members 50 years of age and older who received an influenza vaccination during the most recent flu season

Follow-up care for children prescribed ADHD medication – measures the percentage of children 6–12 years of age with a prescription for ADHD medication who had one follow-up visit with a practitioner during the 30-day initiation phase

care organizations. The NCQA seal is a widely recognized symbol of quality and is considered a reliable indicator that the organization delivers high-quality care. To earn the seal, organizations have to pass a rigorous, comprehensive review and then annually report on their performance.

To facilitate quality improvement in managed care, NCQA has developed quality standards and measures that are applicable across a broad range of health care organizations. The measures provide an indication of the quality of care provided by an organization. Organizations have to annually report their performance to NCQA using these measures. The provider organization can then use the measures to assess the quality of care delivered and when appropriate develop interventions to improve care.

One of the most recognized set of measures developed by NCQA is the Healthcare Effectiveness Data and Information Set (HEDIS).[15] HEDIS is a set of standardized measures that specifies how organizations collect, audit, and report performance information across various clinical areas, as well as patient experience and satisfaction. It ensures all organizations are measuring the same thing the same way. There are HEDIS measures for various conditions including antidepressant medication management, medication adherence, appropriate medication use in asthma patients, medication reconciliation postdischarge, and appropriate pharmacotherapy for chronic obstructive pulmonary disorder. Table 4-1 provides two other examples of HEDIS measures that are applicable to pharmacy.

URAC

URAC was initially called the Utilization Review Accreditation Commission in 1990 when it was formed; however, in 1996, the formal name became URAC. It is an independent, nonprofit organization that accredits health care organizations.[16] The mission of URAC is to promote continuous improvement in the quality and efficiency of health care management through processes of accreditation and education. To receive accreditation, the organization must have a quality improvement program within the organization and meet other quality standards. Health plans, managed care organizations, pharmacy benefit managers, and other health care organizations seek URAC accreditation in areas related to case management, disease management, call center operations, HIPAA privacy and security, pharmacy benefit management, as well as other specialty services.[16] Some state boards and government agencies refer to URAC accreditation in these various areas.

GOVERNMENT AGENCIES

Although many government agencies at the national and state level are involved with quality care, this chapter focuses on the CMS, the Agency for Healthcare Research and Quality (AHRQ), and the Food and Drug Administration (FDA). These federal health care agencies have been involved with patient safety and quality for many years. However, with the final report from the President's Advisory Commission on Consumer Protection and Quality in the Health Care Industry, there has been increased activity within the government agencies.

Centers for Medicare and Medicaid Services

CMS's vision for quality is the right care for every person every time.[17] As the largest payer of health care, they have taken the position of being a national leader in driving quality improvement in health care and have launched numerous quality initiatives focused on improving the quality of care for Medicare and Medicaid beneficiaries. To guide their efforts, they have developed a Quality Improvement Roadmap, which specifies the destination as a safe, effective, efficient, patient-centered, timely, and equitable health care system.[17] These are the same domains that the IOM uses to define quality. In this Roadmap, they focus on how to work with partners to improve quality of care, how to utilize quality measurements, how to pay in a way to reward quality, how to promote health information technology, and how to bring effective treatments to patients rapidly.[17] Thus, their initiatives encompass various activities including publicly reporting quality measures, collecting physician-reported quality information for benchmarking, encouraging adoption of e-prescribing, and conducting demonstration projects. Since the inception of Medicare Part D, CMS has emphasized the importance of quality care in the medication-use process. They are reporting quality information on prescription drug plans, requiring prescription drug plans to ensure pharmacies are providing quality care, and working with the quality improvement organizations (QIOs) to improve medication use in the elderly.[18]

QIOs contract with CMS to help improve the care Medicare beneficiaries receive.[19] The QIO Program was originally focused on quality assurance and retrospective utilization reviews; however, today it has a quality improvement focus. There is a network of 53 QIOs, responsible for each state, territory, and the District of Columbia. The QIO Program (operated by CMS) thus works with QIOs to (1) ensure payment is made only for medically necessary services, (2) investigate beneficiary complaints about the quality of care received, and (3) develop quality improvement programs.[19] QIOs then work with consumers, physicians, hospitals, home health, nursing homes, pharmacies, and other health care providers to ensure quality care is provided.

To represent the QIOs and help them share information about best practices and other resources, the *American Health Care Quality Association (AHQA)* was formed.[20]

This organization represents the QIOs and professionals working in them to improve quality and patient safety.

Agency for Healthcare Research and Quality

Another large federal agency involved with health care quality is the AHRQ.[21] Initially, AHRQ was the Agency for Health Care Policy and Research formed in 1989. In 1999, the name was changed to AHRQ and it was deemed the lead federal agency for conducting quality research. AHRQ has been involved with quality care since the early 1990s and has begun many patient safety and quality initiatives. Examples of their initiatives include piloting e-prescribing and electronic health records, developing measures to assess inpatient hospital quality, creating informational tools about quality measurement and reporting, educating health care providers about medical errors and patient safety, and educating consumers about health care quality. Although AHRQ is involved in many quality initiatives, this chapter notes just a few programs, listed as follows:

1. *National Quality Measures Clearinghouse*™: AHRQ houses this measures clearinghouse that serves as a public repository for evidence-based quality measures. It provides information about the measures as well as measure development. The purpose of the repository is to promote widespread access to quality measures.[22]

2. *Consumer Assessment of Healthcare Providers and Systems (CAHPS)*: In 1995, AHRQ developed a standardized survey, called CAHPS, that health care plans could use to collect information about the quality of care from the enrollees' perspective.[23] The CAHPS survey allows health care plans to assess the quality of care as reported by the patient and compare patient-reported performance across organizations. A pharmacy CAHPS survey has been developed.

3. *Patient Safety Organizations (PSOs)*: A new function of AHRQ is to oversee the provisions dealing with PSOs.[24] The Patient Safety and Quality Improvement Act of 2005 (i.e., the Patient Safety Act) encouraged the expansion of voluntary, provider-driven initiatives to improve the safety and quality of patient care. Through this Act, PSOs were created to work with providers to identify, analyze, and reduce safety problems associated with patient care. The Patient Safety Act gives PSOs uniform federal privilege and confidentiality protections for patient safety work. Thus, patient-, provider-, and reporter-identifying information that is collected and used for patient safety activities is protected. AHRQ provides information on how organizations can become PSOs and administers the PSO program.[24]

Food and Drug Administration

The FDA has the responsibility for assuring the safety and efficacy of all regulated, marketed medication products.[25] Thus, they are interested in medication safety. The FDA has MedWatch, the FDA Safety Information, and Adverse Event Reporting Program.[26] MedWatch provides a place for health care professionals and consumers to report safety information about specific drug products as well as release important information about the safety of drug products. The FDA encourages pharmacists and other health care

U.S. Department of Health and Human Services

Form Approved: OMB No. 0910-0291, Expires: 12/31/2011
See OMB statement on reverse.

MEDWATCH

The FDA Safety Information and
Adverse Event Reporting Program

For VOLUNTARY reporting of
adverse events, product problems and
product use errors

Page 1 of____

FDA USE ONLY

Triage unit
sequence #

PLEASE TYPE OR USE BLACK INK

A. PATIENT INFORMATION

1. Patient Identifier
2. Age at Time of Event or Date of Birth:
3. Sex
   ☐ Female
   ☐ Male
4. Weight
   _____ lb
   or
   _____ kg

In confidence

B. ADVERSE EVENT, PRODUCT PROBLEM OR ERROR

Check all that apply:

1. ☐ Adverse Event ☐ Product Problem (e.g., defects/malfunctions)
   ☐ Product Use Error ☐ Problem with Different Manufacturer of Same Medicine

2. Outcomes Attributed to Adverse Event
   (Check all that apply)
   ☐ Death: _____ (mm/dd/yyyy)
   ☐ Life-threatening
   ☐ Hospitalization - initial or prolonged
   ☐ Required Intervention to Prevent Permanent Impairment/Damage (Devices)
   ☐ Disability or Permanent Damage
   ☐ Congenital Anomaly/Birth Defect
   ☐ Other Serious (Important Medical Events)

3. Date of Event (mm/dd/yyyy)
4. Date of this Report (mm/dd/yyyy)

5. Describe Event, Problem or Product Use Error

6. Relevant Tests/Laboratory Data, Including Dates

7. Other Relevant History, Including Preexisting Medical Conditions (e.g., allergies, race, pregnancy, smoking and alcohol use, liver/kidney problems, etc.)

C. PRODUCT AVAILABILITY

Product Available for Evaluation? (Do not send product to FDA)

☐ Yes ☐ No ☐ Returned to Manufacturer on: _____ (mm/dd/yyyy)

D. SUSPECT PRODUCT(S)

1. Name, Strength, Manufacturer (from product label)
   #1 Name:
   Strength:
   Manufacturer:
   #2 Name:
   Strength:
   Manufacturer:

2. Dose or Amount | Frequency | Route
   #1
   #2

3. Dates of Use (If unknown, give duration) from/to (or best estimate)
   #1
   #2

4. Diagnosis or Reason for Use (Indication)
   #1
   #2

6. Lot # | 7. Expiration Date
   #1 | #1
   #2 | #2

5. Event Abated After Use Stopped or Dose Reduced?
   #1 ☐ Yes ☐ No ☐ Doesn't Apply
   #2 ☐ Yes ☐ No ☐ Doesn't Apply

8. Event Reappeared After Reintroduction?
   #1 ☐ Yes ☐ No ☐ Doesn't Apply
   #2 ☐ Yes ☐ No ☐ Doesn't Apply

9. NDC # or Unique ID

E. SUSPECT MEDICAL DEVICE

1. Brand Name

2. Common Device Name

3. Manufacturer Name, City and State

4. Model # | Lot # | 5. Operator of Device
   Catalog # | Expiration Date (mm/dd/yyyy) | ☐ Health Professional
   Serial # | Other # | ☐ Lay User/Patient
   | | ☐ Other:

6. If Implanted, Give Date (mm/dd/yyyy) | 7. If Explanted, Give Date (mm/dd/yyyy)

8. Is this a Single-use Device that was Reprocessed and Reused on a Patient?
   ☐ Yes ☐ No

9. If Yes to Item No. 8, Enter Name and Address of Reprocessor

F. OTHER (CONCOMITANT) MEDICAL PRODUCTS

Product names and therapy dates (exclude treatment of event)

G. REPORTER (See confidentiality section on back)

1. Name and Address
   Name:
   Address:
   City: State: ZIP:
   Phone # | E-mail

2. Health Professional? | 3. Occupation | 4. Also Reported to:
   ☐ Yes ☐ No | | ☐ Manufacturer
   | | ☐ User Facility
   5. If you do NOT want your identity disclosed to the manufacturer, place an "X" in this box: ☐ | ☐ Distributor/Importer

FORM FDA 3500 (1/09) Submission of a report does not constitute an admission that medical personnel or the product caused or contributed to the event.

Figure 4-3. MedWatch Form. From Ref.[26]. Available at http://www.fda.gov/medwatch/index.html.

professionals to report medication problems using the MedWatch Form, as shown in Figure 4-3.[27] This form is available on the FDA website. The form asks for information such as outcome attributed to adverse event or error, date of event, description of event, suspect product, strength, dose, patient information, and other relevant information. Also, medical product safety alerts, recalls, withdrawals, and other important labeling changes can be quickly disseminated to the medical community and the general public via this website and the MedWatch E-list. In 2008, FDA launched the Sentinel Initiative.[28] The purpose of this initiative is to provide a mechanism for the FDA to query existing electronic data sources for information about the safety of products on the market. This system would allow for a proactive approach to learning about product safety compared to an approach based mainly on reported data.

PRIVATE ORGANIZATIONS

Private organizations and payers have also developed quality measures, quality reporting systems, and other quality initiatives.

Institute of Medicine

The IOM was chartered in 1970 as a component of the National Academy of Sciences.[29] It is a nonprofit organization that works outside the framework of government. It provides unbiased, evidence-based, and authoritative information and advice concerning health policy to policy makers, professionals, and the public.[29] In 1996, the IOM launched a campaign focused on assessing and improving the nation's quality of care. They define quality as "the degree to which health services for individuals and populations increase the likelihood of desired health outcomes and are consistent with current professional knowledge."[30] The IOM has released many national quality reports including[31]:

- *To Err is Human*: Building a safer health system, that focused on the number of medical errors occurring annually in the U.S. health care system.
- *Crossing the Quality Chasm*: A new health system for the 21st century, that defined six aims for care (i.e., safe, effective, patient-centered, timely, efficient, and equitable) and 10 rules for health care delivery redesign.
- *Preventing Medication Errors*: It highlighted how common medication errors are and provided a comprehensive approach to reducing medication errors.

The IOM continues to put forth reports and recommendations for improving health care quality in this country. They have published reports encouraging information technology use and furthering performance measurement. These additional reports can be found on their website.[31]

United States Pharmacopeia (USP)

The USP is the official public standards-setting authority for all prescriptions and over-the-counter medicines, dietary supplements, and other health care products manufactured and sold in the United States.[32] It is an independent, science-based public health organization. USP has been specifically involved with improving medication safety. In 1995, USP led the formation of the National Coordinating Council for Medication Error Reporting and Prevention (NCC MERP).[33] Between 2001 and 2008, USP analyzed medication error records submitted by facilities participating in its national medication error and adverse drug reactions reporting program, MED-MARX®.[34] The data were compiled, summarized, and presented in an in-depth annual report. Information in the report included types of medication errors, causes, contributing factors, products involved, and actions taken. Now USP has transferred the reporting program to Quantos, a private company.

Institute for Safe Medication Practices (ISMP)

The ISMP is the nation's only nonprofit organization devoted entirely to medication error prevention and safe medication use.[35] It provides education programs and tools for hospital and retail pharmacies to use to prevent medication errors. They provide newsletters, continuing education programs, and other resources to improve medication safety.

The ISMP Medication Errors Reporting Program (MERP) operated by ISMP is a confidential national voluntary reporting program that allows health care professionals to report potential or actual medication errors.[36] ISMP is certified by AHRQ as a PSO, which allows the reported data to be protected. Administrators and practitioners can use the database of errors to study trends and the root causes of medication errors, which then allows for the development of best practices to avoid medication errors.

Institute for Healthcare Improvement (IHI)

The IHI is an independent nonprofit organization that provides many resources pertaining to improving health care quality to health care institutions.[37] The IHI develops programs and tools for health care systems to use to improve patient care. Examples of programs they offer include: IMPACT network where professionals work with IHI to make major changes in their institution to improve quality, IHI Improvement Map that provides guidance to hospital administrators on making improvement changes, and professional development programs that teach people how to lead change in their institution.

PUBLIC/PRIVATE PARTNERSHIPS

The fourth group of organizations discussed in this chapter is the partnerships between both the public and private sectors. Government agencies, businesses, nonprofit organizations, and others are partnering together to improve the quality of health care.

National Quality Forum

NQF was established as a public–private partnership in 1999 in response to the President's Advisory Commission's final report.[38] NQF has broad participation from all parts of the health care system, including national, state, regional, and local groups representing consumers, public and private purchasers, employers, health care professionals, provider organizations, health plans, accrediting bodies, labor unions, supporting industries, and organizations involved in health care research or quality improvement.

NQF is focused on developing a common approach to measuring health care quality and fostering system-wide change to improve health care quality. They have developed a formal consensus process to use when endorsing voluntary performance standards including performance measures, quality indicators, preferred practices, or reporting guidelines. NQF provides the only broad-based consensus-based method by which measures are publicly vetted and broadly endorsed. Thus, CMS depends on NQF's process to determine performance measures to use in their initiatives. Additionally, NQF engages in other activities aimed at promoting the use of such performance standards, linking quality measurement to strategies for quality improvement, providing education and information to stakeholders, and exchanging knowledge and ideas.[38]

Leapfrog Group

After the 1999 IOM report about medical errors was released, the Leapfrog Group was formed by a coalition of Fortune 500 companies and leading health care purchase organizations wanting to improve health care quality and create a market that rewards quality.[39] The Leapfrog Group is focused on reducing preventable medical mistakes, informing consumers and purchasers about quality of care so that they can make informed choices, and rewarding providers for high-quality care. To accomplish these goals, they have developed a Leapfrog Hospital Quality and Safety Survey. This survey specifically addresses computer physician order entry, evidence-based hospital referral, intensive care unit (ICU) staffing, and other best practices.[39]

Hospital Quality Alliance (HQA)

The HQA is a public–private collaboration to improve the quality of care provided by the nation's hospitals by measuring and publicly reporting on that care.[40] The purpose of the alliance is to identify a set of standardized hospital quality measures that would be used by all stakeholders to improve quality of care. Their goal is to identify a set of hospital quality measures that would be recognized by accrediting agencies, payers, and providers. All hospitals would then report these standardized quality measures. They have developed a website called *Hospital Compare* that provides information to the public about hospital quality measures.[41] Currently the hospitals voluntarily report their information on heart attack, heart failure, pneumonia, and surgical care improvement measures.

AQA

In 2004, the American Academy of Family Physicians (AAFP), the American College of Physicians (ACP), America's Health Insurance Plans (AHIP), and the AHRQ joined together to form AQA.[41] AQA is interested in improving performance measurement, data aggregation, and reporting in the ambulatory care setting. The alliance now consists of physicians, consumers, purchasers, health insurance plans, and others.[42] They are working on measuring and reporting performance data at the physician or group level.

Pharmacy Quality Alliance (PQA)

In April 2006, CMS Secretary Mark McClellan announced the formation of the PQA.[43] PQA is a self-sustaining, membership-based quality alliance. It is modeled, for the most part, after other health care alliances. PQA is governed by a Steering Committee of 16 individuals; however, many different organizations (e.g., pharmacy associations, government agencies, pharmaceutical companies, retail pharmacies, employers, health plans, and PBMs) are members of PQA.

To complete the work of PQA, workgroups have been formed listed as follows[43]:

1. a metrics workgroup to develop quality measures for pharmacists and pharmacies;
2. a data aggregation and reporting workgroup to learn how to best aggregate data and develop templates for reporting pharmacy quality data to providers and consumers;
3. a research coordinating council to work with various organizations to pilot test the measures and reporting mechanisms to understand more about quality in pharmacy;
4. an education and communications workgroup to develop educational materials to educate all stakeholders about pharmacy quality.

The PQA has developed performance measures related to medication adherence, patient satisfaction, diabetes care, asthma control, and inappropriate drug use in the elderly.[43] It is likely that pharmacy claims data will be used to calculate many of the performance measures for pharmacists, pharmacies, or health plans. The PQA has also developed templates to report these quality performance measures to providers and to consumers. In 2008–2009, PQA is conducting demonstration projects related to quality improvement in pharmacy.[43]

OTHERS

As one can see from Figure 4-1, there are many other organizations involved with various tasks and functions associated with improving the quality of health care delivered in the United States. Although we do not have time to discuss all of these organizations, it is worth mentioning some other groups focused on quality in pharmacy:

● State boards of pharmacy are interested in patient safety and thus quality. Some states have passed legislation requiring all pharmacies to have a quality improvement plan in place. Some states have passed regulations pertaining to medication errors and reporting. State pharmacy boards may also rely on accreditation processes as part of registering certain providers to provide care in their state.

● National and state pharmacy associations are focused on developing resources and tools to help practitioners improve medication safety and improve quality. For example, the American Society for Health-System Pharmacy has the Resource Center on Patient

Safety. State associations are promoting programs, such as the Pharmacy Quality Commitment, to help pharmacists implement quality improvement programs.

● The National Council for Prescription Drug Programs (NCPDP) is also facilitating quality improvement in the health care system.[44] They promote standards for the transfer of data to and from the pharmacy to the health care industry. They are working toward information technology solutions to improve medication safety.

● Schools of Pharmacy are also involved in the quality improvement initiatives. Pharmacy faculty are involved with many of the organizations listed in this chapter. They are leaders within these initiatives, moving the quality improvement culture forward. They are also conducting research to learn more about medication safety issues and quality issues in pharmacy. They are teaching students how to implement quality improvement programs in pharmacies and how to improve medication safety.

● AHIP is also developing initiatives to improve medication safety and quality of care.[45] AHIP often partners with health care providers and other health care entities to advance quality in the health care system. Examples of their initiatives include using evidence-based decision making, promoting the use of information technology, and empowering patients to make informed choices.

● Insurance companies, PBMs, wholesalers, data companies, and others are positioning themselves to help pharmacists ensure medication safety and improve pharmacy practice. For example, computer software companies may be incorporating quality assurance and quality improvement programs into their pharmacy software. Wholesalers may be developing products and services to help retail pharmacies with quality improvement initiatives. Additionally, many of these organizations are involved in the PQA and other partnerships to improve quality in the health care system.

As one can see, almost everyone involved in health care is becoming focused on improving the quality of care provided. This chapter provides a glimpse of a few key activities by some of the larger organizations. However, the marketplace is constantly changing. Organizations are developing new quality and medication safety initiatives. Quality improvement initiatives are advancing. New organizations are being formed. The reader is encouraged to visit the websites of these various organizations to learn about the new and latest developments in quality improvement. Additionally, for pharmacy activities, it is important to contact state boards of pharmacy and pharmacy associations as they are involved in medication safety and quality improvement initiatives, specific to pharmacy.

REFERENCES

1. Tafreshi JM, Melby MJ, Kaback KR, Nord TC. Medication-related visits to the emergency department: a prospective study. *Ann Pharmacother*. 1999;33:1252–1257.
2. Nichols-English G, Poirier S. Optimizing adherence to pharmaceutical care plans. *J Am Pharm Assoc*. 2000;40:475–485.
3. Pugh MV, Fincke BG, Bierman AS, et al. Potentially inappropriate prescribing in elderly veterans: are we using the wrong drug, wrong dose, or wrong duration? *J Am Geriatr Soc*. 2005;53:1282–1289.

4. Zhan C, Sangl J, Bierman AS, et al. Potentially inappropriate medication use in community-dwelling elderly: findings from the 1996 Medical Expenditure Panel Survey. *JAMA.* 2001;286;2823–2829.

5. *Quality First: Better Health Care for All Americans.* A report by the President's Advisory Commission on Consumer Protection and Quality in the Health Care Industry; July 1998. Available at http://www.hcqualitycommission.gov/.

6. *History.* Quality Alliance Steering Committee website. http://www.healthqualityalliance.org/about-qasc/history. Accessed March 22, 2010.

7. *Quality Alliance Steering Committee Quarterly Meeting;* December 17, 2008. Quality Alliance Steering Committee website. Available at http://www.healthqualityalliance.org/events. Accessed March 22, 2010.

8. *What is accreditation?* URAC website. Washington, DC; 2009. Available at http://www.urac.org/healthcare/accreditation/. Accessed March 22, 2010.

9. *A Journey through the History of the Joint Commission.* The Joint Commission website. Oakbrook Terrace, IL. Available at http://www.jointcommission.org/AboutUs/joint_commission_history. htm.

10. *Facts about ORYX®.* The Joint Commission website. Oakbrook Terrace, IL. Available at http://www.jointcommission.org/AccreditationPrograms/Hospitals/ORYX/facts_oryx.htm. Accessed March 22, 2010.

11. *Sentinel Event.* The Joint Commission website. Oakbrook Terrace, IL. Available at http:// www.jointcommission.org/SentinelEvents/.

12. *Standards.* The Joint Commission website. Oakbrook Terrace, IL. Available at http://www. jointcommission.org/Standards/.

13. *National Patient Safety Goals.* The Joint Commission website. Oakbrook Terrace, IL. Available at http://www.jointcommission.org/PatientSafety/NationalPatientSafetyGoals/.

14. *About NCQA.* National Committee for Quality Assurance website. Washington, DC. Available at http://www.ncqa.org/tabid/675/Default.aspx. Accessed March 22, 2010.

15. *HEDIS and Quality Measurement.* National Committee for Quality Assurance website. Washington, DC; 2009. Available at http://www.ncqa.org/tabid/59/Default.aspx.

16. *About URAC.* URAC website. Washington, DC; 2009. Available at http://www.urac.org/about.

17. *CMS Quality Improvement Roadmap Executive Summary.* Centers for Medicare and Medicaid Services. Baltimore, MD; 2006:1–17. Available at http://www.cms.hhs.gov/CouncilonTechInnov/downloads/qualityroadmap.pdf.

18. *Part D Performance Data.* Centers for Medicare and Medicaid Services website. Baltimore, MD; 2009. Available at http://www.cms.hhs.gov/PrescriptionDrugCovGenIn/06_PerformanceData.asp#TopOfPage.

19. *Quality Improvement Organizations.* Center for Medicare and Medicaid Services website. Baltimore, MD; 2009. Available at http://www.cms.hhs.gov/QualityImprovementOrgs/.

20. *Inside AHQA.* American Health Care Quality Association website. Washington, DC. Available at http://www.ahqa.org. Accessed on March 23, 2010.

21. Agency for Healthcare Research and Quality. U.S. Department of Health and Human Services website. Rockville, MD. Available at http://www.ahrq.gov/. Accessed March 22, 2010.

22. National Quality Measures Clearinghouse. Agency for Healthcare Research and Quality website. Rockville, MD; 2009. Available at http://www.guideline.gov. Accessed March 10, 2010.

23. *Consumer Assessment of Healthcare Providers and Systems.* Agency for Healthcare Research and Quality website. Rockville, MD; 2009. Available at http://www.caphs.ahrq.gov/default.asp.

24. *Patient Safety Organizations.* Agency for Healthcare Research and Quality website. Rockville, MD; 2009. Available at http://www.pso.ahrq.gov.

25. Food and Drug Administration. U.S. Department of Health and Human Services website. Silver Springs, MD; 2009. Available at http://www.fda.gov/.

26. *Medwatch.* Center for Drug Evaluation and Research. Food and Drug Administration website. Silver Springs, MD; 2009. Available at http://www.fda.gov/medwatch/index.html.

27. *Medwatch Form.* Center for Drug Evaluation and Research. Food and Drug Administration website. Silver Springs, MD; 2009. Available at http://www.fda.gov/medwatch/safety/FDA-3500 fillable.pdf.

28. *The Sentinel Initiative: A National Strategy for Monitoring Medical Product Safety.* Food and Drug Administration. U.S. Department of Health and Human Services. Silver Springs, MD; May 2008. Available at http://www.fda.gov/oc/initiatives/advance/reports/report0508.html.

29. *About the IOM.* Institute of Medicine of the National Academies website. Washington, DC; 2009. Available at http://www.iom.edu/.

30. *Crossing the Quality Chasm: The IOM Healthcare Quality Initiative.* Institute of Medicine website. Washington, DC; 2009. Available at http://www.iom.edu/?id=19174.

31. *IOM Healthcare and Quality.* Institute of Medicine website. Washington, DC; 2009. Available at http://www.iom.edu/cms/3718.aspx.

32. The United States Pharmacopeia website. Rockville, MD. Available at http://www.usp.org.

33. National Coordinating Council for Medication Error Reporting and Prevention website. Rockville, MD; 1998–2009. Available at http://www.nccmerp.org/.

34. MEDMARX. Quantros website. Rockville, MD; 2009. Available at http://www.medmarx.com.

35. The Institute of Safe Medication Practices website. Horsham, PA; 2009. Available at https://www.ismp.org/.

36. *Medication Error Reporting Program.* The Institute of Safe Medication Practices website. Horsham, PA; 2009. Available at https://www.ismp.org/orderForms/reporterrortoISMP.asp.

37. Institute for Healthcare Improvement website. Cambridge, MA; 2009. Available at http://www.ihi.org/ihi.

38. National Quality Forum website. Washington, DC; 2008. Available at http://www.qualityforum.org/.

39. The Leapfrog Group website. Washington, DC; 2007. Available at http://www.leapfroggroup.org/.

40. Hospital Quality Alliance website. Available at http://www.hospitalqualityalliance.org.

41. *Hospital Compare.* U.S Department of Health and Human Services website. 2008. Washington, DC. Available at http://www.hospitalcompare.hhs.gov.

42. AQA website. Washington, DC; 2005. Available at http://www.ambulatoryqualityalliance.org/.

43. Pharmacy Quality Alliance website. Washington, DC; 2009. Available at http://www.pqaalliance.org.

44. National Council for Prescription Drug Programs website. Scottsdale, AZ; 2009. Available at http://www.ncpdp.org.

45. American's Health Insurance Plans website. Washington, DC; 2004–2009. Available at http://www.ahip.org/.

Part II
Quality Improvement Concepts

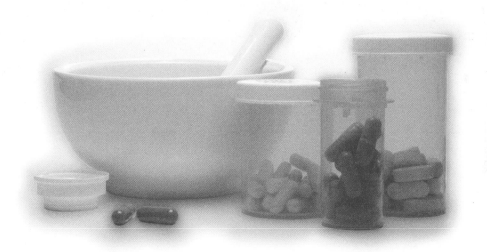

CHAPTER 5

Health Care Quality Improvement

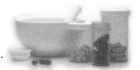

Terri L. Warholak, Ginger G. Scott, and Debra Legner

Learning Objectives

At the end of the chapter, the reader will be able to:

1. Define health care quality.
2. Compare quality by inspection and quality assurance.
3. Compare various quality improvement techniques.
4. Define a framework for improving quality.

INTRODUCTION

In its landmark reported titled *Crossing the Quality Chasm: A New Health System for the 21st Century*, the Institute of Medicine (IOM) stated that "health care has safety and quality problems because it relies on outmoded systems of work. Poor designs set the workforce up to fail, regardless of how hard they try."[1] Let us take a closer look at these outmoded systems of work.

Doctors and pharmacists communicate primarily through a handwritten piece of paper called the prescription. On that prescription, instead of words are abbreviations in the long-dead Latin language. Barriers between doctors and pharmacists make it virtually impossible to immediately clarify those pieces of paper. The prescription does not have the diagnosis, so the pharmacist cannot assess whether the right drug, form, and dosing are appropriate for the patient. Often the names of the drugs look alike and sound alike. Very different drugs may be packaged in very similar containers that are stored right next to each other on pharmacy shelves. A pharmacist shortage created a new person called the pharmacy technician who has been given the responsibilities that a few years ago only a pharmacist could legally complete. In addition, there are no clear standards for educating, training, or credentialing technicians, so the pharmacist never knows whether the technician has baseline knowledge sufficient to assist the pharmacist. Computer systems provide frequent alerts but no clear guidelines on what to do when an alert pops up. Patients expect that the best pharmacies are the fastest and the cheapest. Patient counseling and confidentiality is required, but the pharmacy is not designed to accommodate confidential counseling. Intelligent, conscientious but human people make mistakes because they are stressed, tired, ill, or worried about personal problems that distract them. Finally, administrators, patients, and the public act surprised when pharmacists make mistakes and punish them. (This material is adapted from content developed by *David Brushwood, R.Ph., J.D., professor of Pharmacy Health Care Administration, University of Florida* from Ref.[2]) Punishing the pharmacist does not correct the system.

There should be no surprise that the system just described produces medication errors in any health care system. There is abundant evidence of the negative impact of quality on the U.S. medication-use system. Here are a few examples:

- Research suggests that for every $1.00 spent on a prescription, another $1.33 will be spent on a drug-related illness and complications.[3]
- Medical errors cost $3.5 billion each year. This figure does not include lost wages, compensation, or productivity, and was calculated with 2006 dollars (IOM, 2006).
- Each year 1.5 million Americans experience a medical error (IOM, 2006).
- Medical errors cost Medicare $887 million each year (IOM, 2006).
- Medical errors can cost as much as $15 billion per year, accounting for approximately 7000 deaths and over 770,000 injuries (IOM, 2000).

From looking at this evidence, do you agree that the U.S. medication-use system has quality problems?

HEALTH CARE QUALITY

A definition of health care quality may include the following attributes:

1. increases the probability of positive outcomes;
2. decreases the probability of negative outcomes;
3. corresponds with current medical knowledge;
4. offers the patient what he wants; and
5. provides the patient with what he needs (Warholak, 2008).

The above definition includes several perspectives. It includes the IOM perspective of health care quality as "the degree to which health services . . . increase the probability of desired outcomes and reduce the probability of undesired outcomes."[4,5] A patient perspective "gives patients what they want and need."[6,7]

COMPARE AND CONTRAST QUALITY BY INSPECTION AND QUALITY ASSURANCE

In the 20th century, several terms were used to assure quality. Quality by inspection was used primarily in the manufacturing industry to ensure the quality of manufactured products. Inspectors were hired to inspect the final product prior to leaving the manufacturing plant.[8] If an error were detected, it could be corrected prior to the product reaching the customer. Another method of inspection was to conduct multiple inspections of the same product. The theory behind this method was if an error occurred and was not detected by the first inspection, it would be detected by the second inspection.[8] Thus, fewer errors would occur. An example of this method would be multiple inspections of pharmacy unit dose carts in the mid-1970s. The unit dose cart was filled by the pharmacy technician, checked by the pharmacist prior to leaving the pharmacy, and checked again by the pharmacist and nurse on arrival to the specific nursing unit.

Quality by Inspection

Quality by inspection is often referred to as quality control. Quality control is defined by *Webster's Dictionary* as "an aggregate of activities (as design analysis and inspection for defects) designed to ensure adequate quality, especially in manufactured products."[9]

The limitation of quality by inspection or quality control is that variations or problems within the system will not be detected.[8] For example, the rubber O-rings used on the Challenger failed only under extreme cold conditions. Thus, no amount of inspection prior to takeoff would have detected the problem.[8] In pharmacy, a prescription prepared by the pharmacy technician is verified or inspected by the pharmacist to make sure that the drug to be given to the patient has been accurately filled according to the physician's prescription. If the wrong drug has been filled, the error can be corrected prior to reaching the patient. This action is assuring quality by inspection since the pharmacist is only verifying the right drug and no other patient information such as allergies or duplicate medication, which if present could result in harm to the patient.

Quality by inspection or quality control is a reactive mechanism to detecting variation in a final product but does not assure quality within the system. If the performance level is acceptable, the system is allowed to continue functioning.[10] Deming stated that "inspection with the aim of finding the bad ones and throwing them out is too late, ineffective and costly," and "quality comes not from inspection but from improvement of the process."[11] He emphasized the importance of using data and statistical methods to understand processes to determine where variations occur to bring them under control. Several basic statistical tools used to organize and to display data are flow charts, Pareto charts, run charts, histogram, control charts, scatter to diagram, and cause and effect diagrams.[11-13] Each of these statistical tools will be discussed in detail in Chapter 8.

Quality Assurance

Quality assurance was another term used to assure quality in the 20th century. It is defined as a "program for the systematic monitoring and evaluation of the various aspects of a project, service, or facility to ensure that standards of quality are being met."[9,10] In health care, quality assurance evolved overtime. The American College of Surgeons, formed in 1913, was the first organization to address quality in the American health care system. It developed minimum standards of care for hospitals.[14] This led, in 1918, to the Hospital Standardization Program that eventually became an accreditation process. This program established minimum standards for the medical staff of hospitals including credentials, privileges, and functions, and for adequate equipment and medical records.[14] This accreditation process, in 1951, became known as the Joint Commission on Accreditation of

Hospitals (JCAH). Later, their name was changed to Joint Commission on Accreditation of HealthCare Organizations (JCAHO) and then to The Joint Commission.[14]

In the traditional quality assurance process, health care performance was measured through standards established by regulators.[10,15,16] Deviations and outliers from the standards were identified from performance data and improvement methods were implemented to meet the standards.[16] For example, in pharmacy, the dispensing process should be 100% free of medication errors. If an error occurred, the date of the error, type of error, and name of individual committing an error was documented. This information was reviewed every month to determine deviations in performance by pharmacy personnel from the established standard. Based on the number or extent of the error, individual consequences often punitive in nature resulted.

The quality assurance process is similar to quality control in that it is reactive and defensive.[16] Both quality assurance and quality control require inspection to identify the defect or outlier and improvements focus on the inspection findings. The primary differences in these two terms are quality control relies solely on improvement by inspection and focuses on the defect found, whereas quality assurance is improvement based on performance to meet a specific standard. Improvement is focused on dealing with the outlier[17] in the process rather than improving the process or preventing the variation.[13] Documentation in the literature confirms the shortcomings of using a detection approach to quality.[8,11,18]

COMPARE AND CONTRAST VARIOUS QUALITY IMPROVEMENT TECHNIQUES

Other quality improvement techniques that are more proactive than quality by inspection or quality assurance and not focused on defect detection are continuous quality improvement (CQI), Six Sigma, and International Organization for Standardization (ISO). Each is discussed in detail below.

Continuous Quality Improvement

The CQI approach began in manufacturing. Later, the concept was introduced into health care by Berwick and Leape.[10,19] Shortell et al.[20] defined CQI as "a philosophy of continual improvement of the processes associated with providing a good or service that meets or exceeds customer expectations."[10] CQI is a paradigmatic shift[16] that is proactive and deliberate,[16] continuous or never ending,[21] requires organization-wide participation,[15,16,20] and focuses on preventing and reducing internal sources of variations.[13,16] By promoting a systems perspective, the approach is nonpunitive to an individual member within the organization.[10,15,20,21]

The CQI technique can be applied to individual processes within pharmacy such as monitor medication errors,[22,23] decrease medication errors,[24–27] and implement new technology[28,29] and within different practice settings.[10]

Other terms synonymous with CQI are total quality management (TQM),[4,5,10,18,30] quality control,[4,5,10] and quality improvement process.[4,5,10] A framework for the CQI process is discussed later in the chapter.

Six Sigma

Six Sigma is a quality management methodology[30] and statistical measurement (Chowdury, 2001)[43] created by the president of Motorola in the mid-1980s. The concept of Six Sigma assumes that defects are responsible for the "cost of poor quality"[31] with the overall goal of the program being to decrease defects in all of the organization's processes. If achieved, the results will show better quality, reduced cost, and increased profitability.[12,30,31]

The components of the Six Sigma program include goals, methodology, leadership training, and tools.[12,31] Trusko et al.[30] (p. 36) stated that the program is "divided into four major quadrants: 1) Improvement process, 2) Quality initiatives, 3) Quality measurements 4) Improvement tools." Six Sigma not only refers to the program, but is also the statistical measure used to "compare quality across processes and across organizations."[12] In this program, "sigma" is the same as standard deviation, the distribution of scores from the mean. The goal of the Six Sigma program is "all processes to statistically perform at an error rate no greater than 3.4 errors per million opportunities"[30] (p. 34).

The Six Sigma Leadership program was established to recognize individuals within the organization who excel in promoting the program within the organization. The four levels achievable by individuals based on their knowledge and ability to promote Six Sigma are Champions, Master Black Belt, Black Belts, and Green Belts (Harry, 2000).[12,30,31]

The Six Sigma concept was used primarily in the manufacturing industry until 1988 when Motorola received the Baldrige Award.[30] Afterwards, the methodology spread to other industries including health care. Even though most health care organizations already had implemented CQI or TQM programs, many have begun using the Six Sigma concept within their organizations. Six Sigma only strengthens these programs by focusing on the measurement system.[30] Results from health care facilities who have implemented the program show reduced length of stay, improved customer satisfaction, reduced time to enter the health care unit, reduced inventory, and increased efficiency in the billing system.[12] There are some data that suggest that the Six Sigma statistics in conjunction with control charts can be used in clinical practice to assess baseline performance and amount of improvement with individual patients within an individual practice.[32]

ISO 9000 – Quality Standards

ISO 9000 is recognized worldwide as a family of standards for quality management and quality assurance.[33,34] The standards are maintained by the International Organization for Standardization (ISO). Origination of the standards dates back to 1959 (Mil-Q-9858a), the first quality standard for military procurement in the United States.[35] Later in the 1960s, quality system requirements were developed by the National Aeronautics and Space Administration (NASA) and the North Atlantic Treaty Organization (NATO) accepted the allied quality assurance procedures for the procurement of supplies and equipment.[35] Then in the 1970s, the United Kingdom published standards for quality assurance (BS 9000) and guidelines for quality assurances (BS 5179).[35] Later, the United Kingdom created a series of quality standards for the manufacturing industry known as BS 5750. This series of quality standards (BS 5750) was adopted verbatim by the ISO (1988).[33] The standards were published globally under the name

ISO 9000 in hopes of creating an international definition of quality systems for all organizations within all industries. The standards have been reviewed and revised several times.[33,34] The ISO 9000 series consists of the following standards: quality management systems, fundamentals, and vocabulary (ISO 9000:2005); quality management systems and requirements (ISO 9001:2008); and quality management systems and guidelines for performance improvements (ISO 9004:2000).[33,34] Organizations can voluntarily be certified against the standard for quality management systems.[33,34]

All the quality improvement techniques discussed above have common characteristics. They are continuous, measured, include all personnel in the process being reviewed.

A FRAMEWORK FOR IMPROVING QUALITY

Pharmacists can improve the quality of the medication-use system by employing a systematic CQI process.

> Many CQI models exist. Examples of specific models include the plan, do, check, and act (PDCA) model and the find, organize, clarify, understand, select, plan, do, check, act (FOCUS-PDCA) model, and six sigma.[36,37] Most models include elements that reflect the following core concepts: (1) plan, (2) design, (3) measure, (4) assess, and (5) improve.[38] CQI has been described as a practical application of the scientific method.[21] Planning in both processes is similar. In this manner, one can think of the steps in the CQI cycle as parallel to the sections of a scientific article: background, methods, results, conclusions, and recommendations. Considering CQI in this manner diminishes the need to memorize additional terminology.[10]

It is important to note before we get into details that small changes can have big impact. Also, the CQI cycle should be short and relatively contained to ensure rapid progress and sustained motivation (Figure 5-1).

Now, let us add additional details about the QI process. See Figure 5-2 for an example of a preliminary timeline and Figure 5-3 for a copy of these questions in worksheet format.

Background

When doing background work, it is important to investigate the issue to ensure you know and are able to define the following:

● *What is the problem?* Problem definition is essential. You need to be sure you are working on the *right* problem. Problem definition can be accomplished through root cause analysis or other in-depth investigation into the cause of the problem as discussed in Chapter 7. Be sure to identify the *cause*(s) of the problem and not a symptom. This is where you will need to gather background data to prove to yourself and others that the problem exists.

● *Why is the problem a problem?* This sounds like metacognition but in fact it is really straight forward. You need to be able to state *why* an issue is important to focus on. Why is the problem worthy of your attention?

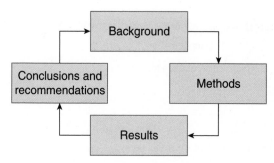

Figure 5-1. A framework for improving quality. No matter the CQI model, the steps in the CQI cycle parallel the sections of a scientific article: background, methods, results, conclusions, and recommendations.

● *What solutions have been tried?* This is important and can be derived from the literature. If someone else has tried a solution and it has worked, it may be able to be adapted for your practice setting. This could be a *huge* time saver. Alternatively, you could use a novel approach. Take a look at the research worksheet for a partial list of some data collection techniques.

● *State the global goal of the project.* The global goal should relate to the project stated in #3 above. Some options may include: (1) discovery; (2) frequency estimation; (3) measure of a change; or (4) a combination.

Timeline												
	Week											
Step	1	2	3	4	5	6	7	8	9	10	11	12
1	×											
2	×	×										
3			×									
4				×								
5				×								
6					×	×						
7						×						
8							×					
9								×				
10			×						×			
11										×	×	
12											×	×
13											×	×

Figure 5-2. Example time line for a quality improvement project.

Quality Improvement Planning Worksheet #1

Date of meeting: _____

Name and contact information of each team member
1. _____ 2. _____
3. _____ 4. _____
5. _____ 6. _____

Introduction

1. Brainstorm possible areas of study (list here) _____
_____

2. Rank and select an area of focus from the list above
3. Provide a detailed description of the area chosen for study
   Area or project: _____
   Setting: _____
   Portion of the medication use process involved: _____
   Baseline data (if available): _____
4. State why the proposed project is important
_____

5. Relate the proposed project to the literature
_____

6. State the global goal of the project *(Hint – Some options may include: 1. Discovery; 2. Frequency estimation; 3. Measure of a change; or a combination)* Note: Goal should relate to project stated in #3 above.
_____

7. State the specific goal(s) of the project
_____
_____
_____

Methods

8. List possible interventions (some options may include: reduce reliance on memory, simplify, standardize, use constraints or forcing functions, use protocols of checklists, improve access to information, decrease reliance on vigilance, reduce handoffs, differentiate or automate)
_____

9. Select best intervention to accomplish goals (listed in #7 above)
_____

10. List process and/or outcome measures necessary to determine if goal(s) were met
_____

11. Determine what data are all ready being collected and what measures exist.
_____

12. Plan data collection methods *(Hint – May choose from: 1. Inspection points; 2. Focus groups; 3. Monitoring for markers; 4. Chart review; 5. Observation; and 6. Spontaneous report)*
_____

13. Plan statistical analysis – make sure you will collect all information needed.
_____

14. Break the project into steps and detail practical considerations

Figure 5-3. Quality Improvement planning worksheet.

Step	Who	What	Where	When	How

15. Sketch preliminary timeline for project.

Timeline										
	Week									
Step	1	2	3	4	5	6	7	8	9	10

16. List challenges to be addressed before the next meeting

  1. _____

  2. _____

  3. _____

17. Assign a responsible party to address each challenge listed above.

Challenge	Person responsible	Due date
1.		
2.		
3.		

18. Set date for next team meeting _____

Figure 5-3. *Continued*

Methods

When thinking about the methods you might use to solve – or begin to solve – your QI problem, consider the methods that you discovered when thinking about solutions in the background work.

Think about the methods that others have used in the past to solve similar QI problems and adapt them for your needs and practice situation. For example, you might list possible interventions, such as: reduce reliance on memory, simplify, standardize, use constraints or forcing functions, use protocols of checklists, improve access to information, decrease reliance on vigilance, reduce handoffs, and differentiate or automate.

Select the best intervention to accomplish the global goals listed in the background work.

List process and/or outcome measures necessary to determine if global goal(s) were met.

Determine what data are already being collected and what measures exist.

Plan data collection methods. You may choose among (a) inspection points; (b) focus groups; (c) monitoring for markers; (d) chart review; (e) observation; and (f) spontaneous report.

Plan the statistical analysis, making sure you will collect all information needed.

Break the project down into steps and detail practical considerations of what steps are needed, and determine the who, what, where, when, and how each will be accomplished.

Sketch the preliminary timeline for project.

List any challenges to be addressed before the next meeting, and assign a responsible party to address each challenge listed above.

Results

For this portion, you need to put the plan developed in the section "Methods" into action:

1. Measure your chosen measures.
2. Enter data and analyze them. Usually, MS Excel can handle the calculations you will need for most QI projects [descriptive statistics such as measures of central tendency (mean, median, and mode), frequency, and percents, as well as measures of dispersion (range, standard deviation, etc.)]. These statistics can be *very* useful and are often times all you need. If more sophisticated analysis is needed, it may be helpful to get someone from your local college of pharmacy involved to assist you.

Conclusions and Recommendations

At this point you need to take some time to think about your results and what they mean. What is the bottom line? What worked? What could be done better? What recommendations for further improving the process can you make now? This reflection will help you plan your next QI cycle as well as rate the success of this one.

Let us look at an example of the process and how it can be used in a grocery store pharmacy practice setting to improve quality. Please note that the example is fictitious.

EXAMPLE

Background

- *What is the problem?* Many prescriptions are being dispensed to patients without proper counseling, and this poses a potential risk for medication error reaching the patient.
- *Why is the problem a problem?* Medication errors can harm patients. Research has shown that a common dispensing error is choosing the wrong medication.[39]
- *What solutions have been tried?* There is evidence to suggest that up to 83% of dispensing errors may be identified before they leave the pharmacy by having the pharmacist counsel the patient using the Indian Health Service (IHS) "show and tell" patient counseling technique. This counseling technique involves asking the patient three open-ended questions, opening the medication bottle to show the patient the medication, and making sure that the patient repeats everything back to the pharmacist.
- *State the global goal of the project*: Frequency estimation.
- *State the specific goal of the project*: The specific aim of this study was to measure the impact of "show and tell" counseling on error identification.

Methods

List possible interventions.

Possible interventions include: reducing reliance on memory by posting the counseling steps in the counseling window, standardizing the counseling procedure (and training pharmacists how to use it), or developing a protocol for counseling every new prescription.

Select the best intervention to accomplish the global goal:

1. Standardize the counseling procedure (and train pharmacists how to use it).
2. Develop a protocol for counseling every new prescription.

List process and/or outcome measures necessary to determine if global goal(s) were met.

Determine the number of errors identified during counseling before and after implementing the interventions listed in the previous question.

Determine what data are already being collected and what measures exist.

No measures currently exist.

Plan data collection methods.

This will be an observational pre/post-study. The researchers will observe the pharmacists' counseling during all store hours for 7 days. They will then educate the

TABLE 5-1. Example of quality improvement project steps

Step	Who	What	Where	When	How
1	Whole group	Meet with pharmacy manager to discuss plan and achieve buy-in	At the pharmacy	One month before data collection	Researcher A will call the pharmacy manager to find available times for this meeting and will work with the remainder of the team to schedule a time that is acceptable for all
2	Whole group	Create and test data collection forms and delineate data collection procedures	At researcher #2's house	Etc.	Subsequent boxes for the remaining steps would be completed in a similar fashion to the line above. To save space this table has been abbreviated. Only the tasks appear for the steps below
3	Collect predata				
4	Obtain IHS counseling training materials				
5	Create and test new counseling policy				
6	Get approval of manager on all materials (training, counseling policy, and data collection procedures)				
7	Practice (a) teaching pharmacists to counsel and (b) explaining the new counseling policy				
8	Teach all pharmacists to counsel using the IHS technique and explain the new counseling policy to all pharmacy staff members				
9	Collect postdata				
10	Enter data into spread sheet, check for accuracy, analyze, and interpret				
11	Write report				
12	Disseminate results to pharmacy staff, stakeholders, and other interested parties				
13	Plan next quality improvement study				

pharmacists on how to perform IHS counseling and will inform all pharmacy staff of the new counseling policy; every patient picking up a new prescription will receive medication counseling by a pharmacist. The researchers will then observe the counseling process for a second week.

Plan the statistical analysis.

The number of errors identified during counseling will be compared before and after the intervention. A Chi-square test will be used and the alpha will be set a priori at 0.05.

Break the project down into steps (Table 5-1).

Sketch the preliminary timeline for project (Figure 5-2).

List any challenges to be addressed before the next meeting, and assign a responsible party to address each challenge listed above.

Getting buy-in from the manager and the pharmacists is important but may be challenging. We will need to discuss strategies for successfully accomplishing these tasks.

Results

During the pre-phase, counseling was not completed in a standardized manner; not all pharmacists counseled patients on new prescriptions and the counseling techniques of those who did counsel patients varied widely (some used open-ended questions and some used close-ended questions). Three errors were identified via counseling. During the post-phase all pharmacists complied with the new counseling procedure. A total of 854 new prescriptions were dispensed and all patients were counseled. Twelve errors were identified via counseling in the post-phase. Chi-square 5.4, df = 1, $p = 0.02$.

Conclusions and Recommendations

This study concluded that by counseling patients on their prescriptions, the potential for medication errors significantly decreased. The pharmacy should continue this policy.

REFERENCES

1. Kohn LT, Corrigan JM, Donaldson MS, eds. *Crossing the Quality Chasm: A New Health System for the 21st Century. Institute of Medicine Committee on Quality of Health Care in America.* Washington, DC: National Academy Press/Sage Publications; 2001 [Executive Summary, pp. 1–23].

2. Ukens C. How to create the worst possible pharmacy.. *Drug Top.* 2004;7(June):148. *Source*: David Brushwood, R.Ph., J.D., professor of Pharmacy Health Care Administration, University of Florida.

3. Johnson JA, Bootman JL. Drug-related morbidity and mortality: a cost-of-illness model. *Arch Intern Med.* 1995;155:1949–1956.

4. Lohr K. Health, health care, and quality of care. In: Lohr K, ed. *Medicare: A Strategy for Quality Assurance.* Washington, DC: National Academy Press; 1990.

5. Lohr KE. Concepts of assessing, assuring and improving quality. In: *Medicare: A Strategy for Quality Assurance.* Washington, DC: National Academy Press; 1990:45.

6. Lohr KN. Outcome measurement: concepts and questions. *Inquiry.* 1988;25(Spring): 37–50.

7. Ovretveit J. *Health Service Quality.* Oxford, England: Blackwell Scientific; 1992.

8. Aguayo R. Foreword by W. Edwards Deming. In: *Dr. Deming: The American who taught the Japanese about Quality.* New York: A Fireside Book by Simon and Schuster; 1991.

9. Merriam-Webster's Collegiate Dictionary. *Merriam-Webster Dictionary*. 11th ed. Springfield, MA: Merriam-Webster; 2003.

10. Warholak T. Ensuring quality in pharmacy operations. In: Desselle S, Zgarrick D, eds. *Pharmacy Management*. 2nd ed. New York: McGraw Hill; 2008:125–149.

11. Walton M. Foreword by W. Edwards Deming. In: *The Deming Management Method*. New York: Berkley Publishing Group; 1986;96.

12. Carey RG. *Improving Healthcare with Control Charts Basic and Advanced SPC Methods and Case Studies*. Milwaukee, WI: ASQ Quality Press; 2003:151–158.

13. Johnson SP, McLaughlin CP. Measurement and statistical analysis in CQI. In: McLaughlin CP, Kaluzny AD, eds. *Continuous Quality Improvement in Health Care Theory, Implementation and Applications*. 2nd ed. Gaithersburg, MD: An Aspen Publication; 1999:93–138.

14. DesHarnais SI, McLaughlin CP. The outcome model of quality. In: McLaughlin CP, Kaluzny AD, eds. *Continuous Quality Improvement in Health Care Theory, Implementation and Applications*. 2nd ed. Gaithersburg, MD: An Aspen Publication; 1999:59–61.

15. Godwin HN, Sanborn MD. Total quality management in hospital pharmacy. *Am Pharm*. 1995;NS35:51.

16. Leebov W, Ersoz CJ. *The Health Care Manager's Guide to Continuous Quality Improvement*. Chicago, IL: American Hospital Publishing, Inc., an American Hospital Association Company; 1991;11–13.

17. Teboul J. *Managing Quality Dynamics*. Englewood Cliffs, NJ: Prentice-Hall; 1991.

18. Henshall E. The application of quality techniques achieving a balance. *Total Qual Manage*. 1990;1(3):355–363.

19. Berwick DM, Leape LL. Reducing errors in medicine. *Br Med J*. 1999;319:137.

20. Shortell SM, Bennett CL, Byck GR. Assessing the impact of continuous quality improvement on clinical practice: what it will take to accelerate progress. *Milbank Q*. 1998;76:593.

21. Blumenthal D, Kilo CM. A report card on continuous quality improvement. *Milbank Q*. 1998;76(4):625–648, 511.

22. Braithwaite RS, DeVita MA, Mahidhara R, et al. Use of medical emergency team (MET) responses to detect medical errors. *Qual Saf Health Care*. 2004;13:255–259.

23. Newland S, Golembiewski JA, Green CR, et al. Continuous quality improvement approach to reducing hydromorphone PCA programming errors. *Am J Health Syst Pharm*. 2001;36:7–10.

24. Briggs FE, Mark LK, Faris RJ, et al. Innovative solutions to a missing dose problem. In: *American Society of Health System Pharmacy Summer Meeting*; 2002; Baltimore, MD.

25. Farber MS, Palwlicki KS, Tims PM, et al. Proactive root cause analysis in a multi-hospital system. In: *ASHP Summer Meeting*; 2002; Baltimore, MD.

26. Hritz RW, Everly JL, Care SA. Medication error identification is a key to prevention: a performance improvement approach. *J Healthcare Qual*. 2002;24:10.

27. Rozich JD, Haraden CR, Resar RK. Adverse drug event trigger tool: a practical methodology for measuring medication related harm. *Qual Saf Health Care*. 2003;12:194.

28. Gambone JC, Broder MS. Embedding quality improvement and patient safety: the UCLA value analysis experience. *Best Pract Res Clin Obstet Gynaecol*. 2007;21:581–592.

29. Karow HS. Creating a culture of medication administration safety: laying the foundation for computerized provider order entry. *Jt Comm J Qual Improv*. 2002;28:396.

30. Trusko BE, Pexton C, Harrington HJ, Gupta P. *Improving Healthcare Quality and Cost with Six Sigma*. Upper Saddle River, NJ: Financial Times Press; 2007:21, 31–57, 241–260.

31. Harry M, Schroeder R. *Six Sigma*. New York: Currency; 2000:20–21.

32. Staker LV. The use of run and control charts in the improvement of clinical practice. In: Carey RG, ed. *Improving Healthcare with Control Charts Basic and Advanced SPC Methods and Case Studies*. Milwaukee, WI: ASQ Quality Press; 2003;159–163.

33. International Standardization Organization. *Management Standards*. http://www.iso.org/iso/management_standards.htm. Accessed September 8, 2009.

34. International Standardization Organization. *Selection and Use of the ISO 9000 Family of Standards*. 11 pp. http://www.iso.org/iso/iso_9000_selection_and_use-2009.pdf. Accessed September 8, 2009.

35. Emerson P. *History of ISO 9000*. http://ezinearticles.com/?ISO-9000-History&id=352837. Accessed July 30, 2009.

36. Lazarus IR, Butler K. The promise of Six Sigma: part 1. *Manag Healthcare Executive*. 2001;10:22–26.

37. Lazarus IR, Stamps B. The promise of Six Sigma: part 2. *Manag Healthcare Executive*. 2002;1(January):27–30.

38. Coe CP. An overview of the Joint Commission's improving organizational performance standards. In: *Preparing the Pharmacy for a Joint Commission Survey*. Bethesda, MD: ASHP; 1998:189.

39. Leape LL, Bates DW, Cullen DJ, et al. Systems analysis of adverse drug events. *JAMA*. 1995;274(1):35–43.

40. Asher JM. A structured approach to continuous improvement. *Total Qual Manage*. 1990;1(3):403–408.

41. Aspden P, Wolcott J, Bootman J, Cronenwett L. *Preventing Medication Errors: Prepublication Copy; Uncorrect Proofs*. Washington, DC: National Academies Press; 2006.

42. Bisgaard S. Continuous improvement of quality improvement tools: building on Taguchi's ideas and going beyond. *Total Qual Manage*. 1993;4(2).

43. Chowdhury S. *The Power of Six Sigma*. Chicago: Dearborn Trade; 2001.

44. Kohn L, Corrigan J, Donaldson M. *To err is human: building a safer health system*. Washington, DC: National Academy Press; 2000.

45. Snee RD. Why should statisticians pay attention to Six Sigma? *ASO Qual Prog*. 1999;9:100.

CHAPTER 6

Recognizing and Defining Quality Problems

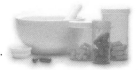

David A. Holdford

Learning Objectives

At the end of the chapter, the reader will be able to:

1. Contrast linear thinking with systems thinking.
2. Identify three ways that quality problems are typically recognized in pharmacy practice and their implications for solving them.
3. Discuss why improperly framing a quality problem will result in a poor solution.
4. Delineate the elements of a good problem statement for a quality problem.

INTRODUCTION

This chapter discusses how pharmacists identify problems with "quality" in pharmacy practice settings and how they go about approaching these problems. Specifically, it deals with recognizing and defining quality problems and addresses how pharmacists can improve the process of effective problem recognition and definition.

Quality improvement (QI) in pharmacy practice encompasses a sequence of actions taken by pharmacists to solve complex problems. The effectiveness of QI depends a great deal on the process employed. The process of QI begins with the way a problem is approached.

HOW DO PHARMACISTS APPROACH QUALITY PROBLEMS IN PRACTICE?

There are three broad approaches to dealing with quality problems: not dealing with them, tackling them using a linear approach to problem solving, and addressing them using a systems approach. These three approaches will be described in the following sections.

Not Addressing Quality Problems

The first broad approach is to not address a problem at all by avoiding the problem, denying the problem exists, judging the problem to be unimportant, rejecting responsibility for the problem, or putting the problem off through procrastination. In many cases, not dealing with a problem is the right thing to do, such as when problems are likely to resolve themselves or when they are not worth the effort of addressing. However, there are many problems that should be addressed, such as problems that have the potential to result in patient harm. This section focuses on quality problems in pharmacy practice that should be dealt with but are not for various reasons.

Avoidance.

Pharmacists might avoid quality problems in pharmacy practice because problems appear to be so overwhelming and unsolvable that it is not clear where to start. Indeed, many quality issues are entrenched within the system, making efforts to solve them appear futile. Nevertheless, that does not make it acceptable for pharmacists to reject their professional obligation to take action. Pharmacists may also avoid quality problems because they do not have confidence in solving the problems, especially if they have not had training in QI techniques.

Denial.

Some problems are not attended to because pharmacists deny that they exist (e.g., "We don't have a drug interaction problem because we have a computerized notification system in place"). In other instances, the severity of a problem is minimized (e.g., "We do miss some drug interactions but only those that are not clinically significant"). These are poor excuses unless they can be backed up by credible evidence. Indeed, if the statements can be backed up by evidence (e.g., no errors were found by secret shoppers bringing in prescriptions for drugs that interact), there really is no problem. However, without supporting evidence, any denials lack credibility, especially when anecdotal reports to the contrary are available.

Unimportant.

Some quality problems are dismissed because of the belief that they are not important enough. It costs money, time, and effort for pharmacists to intervene to improve quality. If the return on those efforts is not deemed to be worth it, the pharmacist's focus will be redirected to some other productive use of time and money. Because resources are limited, some quality problems may be seen as an inevitable cost of doing business.

Denying responsibility for the problem.

Pharmacist responsibilities are not entirely clear in many practice situations. Leaders in the profession state that pharmacists are supposed to be responsible for drug use control throughout the entire health care system.[1] However, physicians often disagree with this characterization of the pharmacist's role,[2] as do many employers, legal experts, legislators, patients, and even pharmacists. Thus, pharmacists often deny that some quality problems are their concern declaring, "I am only responsible for the dispensing process. I can't be expected to worry about problems that occur because some physician did not choose the right drug for the patient or some patient can't adhere to his medication therapy. I have enough problems dealing with what goes on in this pharmacy to worry about what occurs outside of it!"

Procrastinating.

Many quality problems are not dealt with because of procrastination. Pharmacists plan to address the problem, "When I get time." The problem is that there is never enough time in daily practice and there is always something more urgent. The consequences of procrastinating are illustrated by the following example.

A patient drops off a prescription for clonidine 0.1 mg twice daily for high blood pressure. When the technician enters the prescription into the computer using the letters "CLO," he or she mistakenly selects the antiseizure medicine clonazepam 1 mg from the choices on the computer screen. Consequently, the technician fills the prescription for clonazepam 1 mg every morning and evening with refills. Although the pharmacist catches the error in the process of reviewing the prescription, the problem within the computer system remains. And even though the pharmacist recognizes and plans to address the problem when he or she gets time, it gets put off until the error occurs again resulting in serious patient harm.

Linear Thinking

The second broad approach to problem solving in pharmacy practice uses the process of linear thinking. Linear thinking is a simplistic approach to problem solving that, in its simplest form, assumes that (1) each problem has a single cause, (2) the solution will only affect the problem and nothing else, and (3) once implemented, a solution will remain "solved."[3] A pharmacist manager who uses linear thinking to resolve the problem of lost revenue due to decreasing dispensing fees for pharmacists might conclude that the solution is to "fill more prescriptions." The manager might say, "If we can double the number of prescriptions we fill at this pharmacy, my problem would be solved."

However, linear thinking such as this often results in ineffective solutions. Several difficulties are associated with the solution "fill more prescriptions." Implementing the solution might require the hiring of more technicians or utilizing ATM-type dispensing machines. Other strategies include moving more prescriptions to mail order or isolating pharmacists from patients to reduce interruptions of dispensing process.

The difficulty with "fill more prescriptions" is that doing so may lead to other unexpected problems for the manager. Hiring more technicians could complicate personnel management for the manager. Moving to mail order, using ATM-type dispensing machines, or isolating the pharmacist would change the way patients are served and potentially affect the patient–pharmacist relationship. Pharmacists might have fewer opportunities to impact patient care, employee satisfaction could be affected, and the professional image of pharmacists may well be hurt. Even when linear solutions resolve problems in the short run, they can cause greater, more persistent problems in the future.

Problems with linear thinking.

A difficulty with linear thinking is that problems usually have multiple causes. The problem of shrinking dispensing fees originates from numerous sources. One stems from the delivery and finance structure of the health care system. Another comes from strategic choices made by pharmacy providers to focus on dispensing drugs rather than pursuing a service- or patient-focus to pharmacy practice. Other causes include previous acceptance of small dispensing reimbursements, the refusal of many pharmacists to accept responsibility for patient outcomes, contradictory messages to payers from pharmacy leaders, and more third-party involvement in paying for drugs. The solution "fill more prescriptions" does little to address these causes.

Another trouble with linear thinking is that it focuses on *intended* consequences of a solution, rather than those that are *unintended*. One well-known example of an unintended consequence associated with a managed care solution comes from a state Medicaid program that tried to reduce drug costs by implementing a three-drug limit per enrolled patient.[4] A study of the program found that drug costs decreased as intended. However, the program savings were more than offset by the additional unintended increase in non-drug costs due to nursing home admissions associated with drug-related problems. Numerous other examples of unintended consequences can be found in the pharmacy and medical literature.[5,6]

Lastly, linear thinking often makes the false assumption that once solutions are implemented, problems are "solved" and therefore require no further action or follow-up. The trouble with this assumption is that things change. An effective solution at one time may become ineffective in the future as circumstances and the world change.

Why do people engage in linear thinking? There are several reasons for the prevalence of linear thinking.[7] One reason is mental laziness. Some people just do not want to expend the effort on deep contemplation. It is easier to jump to quick conclusions than to put serious effort into analysis and thought. Another reason is that people often want quick and easy answers to problems. It is much more comforting to have a problem with a single unambiguous answer. That way, people can solve the problem and move on (although the problem may not really be "solved"). It is also human nature for us to try and simplify complex issues in our minds. If we did not, life would be too complicated and overwhelm our capacity to cope with it. Finally, people often do not recognize or suffer the consequences of their poor decisions. For instance, a pharmacist may never realize that his or her failure to effectively resolve a quality problem (e.g., insufficient screening for drug interactions) has resulted in a serious harm to a patient. Consequently, he or she will not learn from his or her mistake and change the behaviors that resulted in patient harm.

Linear thinking is common in pharmacy practice. If there is any doubt in one's mind, watch how frequently the same quality problems occur over and over again in pharmacy. Then observe how these problems are addressed by pharmacists. You will see linear problem solving processes in place.

Systems Thinking

The third broad approach to problem solving, systems thinking, is the one that is preferred for dealing with complex quality issues in health care. Systems thinking differs from linear thinking by assuming that causes of problems are complex and solutions can have both intended and unintended consequences.[3] Thus, any solution from this approach is evaluated for how well it solves the problem (i.e., intended results) with minimal negative unintended results. A systems approach considers the way that different systems are linked together instead of assuming that they exist as separate silos with no influence on each other. It further assumes that neither problems nor solutions remain constant – situations change, problems change, and new solutions are constantly necessary.

A systems thinker approaches problems by considering the interrelationships among different systems before implementing a solution. Pharmacists who practice systems thinking always ask before attempting to solve any quality problem, "Who will be potentially affected by this problem and any possible solution, and how will they be affected?" "How will they react to potential solutions to the problem, and what can be done to increase acceptance and success of these solutions?" "How might things work out in an unexpected way, and how would this influence my decision?" Answers to these questions can help mitigate any negative consequences and enhance any positive ones.

For example, Jeanne, the pharmacist in charge at a community pharmacy, recognizes a problem with drug interaction screening in her pharmacy. To use a systems approach, Jeanne should consider all the people who might be affected or need to be involved in any solution she proposes. This includes the other pharmacists, technicians, software experts, her boss, and her boss's boss. If any of these people are ignored, they may resist her efforts and even effectively block her, no matter how good her ideas may be. She will also miss out on their expertise and counseling. At the minimum, Jeanne will need to identify any potential resistance to her ideas and develop strategies to neutralize opposition to her plans. Even better, she can recruit allies to assist with her plans.

INITIAL STEPS IN SOLVING ANY QUALITY PROBLEM

Like all complex decisions, QI follows a process with specific steps (e.g., plan, do, check, and act). Although the specific steps may vary depending on the QI framework chosen (e.g., Juran, Deming, and Six Sigma), two key steps are necessary. First, recognize that there is a problem and second, clearly define what that problem is. If these two steps are done well, a more effective solution is likely, because they help minimize the biases and bad habits that blind our thought processes.

Recognize the Existence of a Problem

To solve a problem, one must first be aware that it exists. This may appear obvious and unnecessary of further consideration, but many quality problems exist of which we are unaware. Recognizing problems can be difficult because many are the result of gradual change. Gradual change is more difficult to detect, because human beings are programmed through evolutionary processes to react to sudden dangers – such as an attack from a grizzly bear or mountain lion – threats rarely faced by modern man.

Today, the primary threats to our jobs and safety come not from sudden events but from slow, gradual processes.[8] Indeed, many more people are killed from gradual processes such as poor health habits each year than auto accidents, murders, or other risks. Yet, we rarely react to these threats until our health and safety are at acute risk.

Few people consciously think about the risks of poor eating behaviors or lack of exercise until something bad occurs. On the other hand, we respond emotionally to relatively rare but sensational tragedies in the news.

Many quality problems in pharmacy practice could be prevented if pharmacists were able and willing to recognize quality problems and correct them. But human nature often prevents us from recognizing these gradual changes. Thus, if 100 people are killed by a tornado, it is big news. On the other hand, when thousands of people die every month due to drug errors, the deaths are virtually ignored. There are several ways to recognize existing problems.

Deviation from the past.

Problems are often identified when people recognize that things are not the way they used to be. A pharmacist may declare that, "Dispensing errors are greater than usual" or "Patient complaints seem to be increasing." Individuals often rely on personal memory to detect deviations from the past, but memories can fade or distort reality.

Deviation from the plan.

Problems are also identified when things differ from the way they were planned (e.g., "We didn't expect so many people to show up for our cholesterol screenings"). Faulty memories are also relied upon often to detect deviations from the plan.

Outside criticism.

Criticism by others is the worst way to learn about problems. When a problem, such as medication errors, is so bad that outsiders recognize and criticize it, pharmacists are forced to not only deal with the problem, but also respond to the criticism and its impact on their reputations. The last thing any pharmacist wants is for a reporter from "USA Today" or the television program "60 Minutes" to show up on his or her doorstep asking for an interview about medication quality at his or her pharmacy.

Many problems are never recognized because of an overreliance on memory to detect deviations from the past or plan. Indeed, our memories often let us down, so we fail to act until outside critics identify our problems for us. The solution to this predicament is to employ statistical process control in problem identification.

Statistical process control (discussed in Chapter 8) analyzes collected data using statistical techniques to detect desirable and undesirable changes in systems. Statistical process control requires that key quality measures be collected and followed over time. Any negative trends in these measures identified through statistical analysis may indicate a problem. If statistical process control systems are in place in pharmacies to identify and deal with quality problems, it is much less likely that outsiders will recognize a problem and criticize it. Statistical process control is essential in overcoming the problems of faulty memory and inability to detect gradual changes.

Clearly Defining the Problem at Hand

The second step to solving a quality problem is to define it correctly. There is a lot of truth to the aphorism, "a problem well-defined is half-solved," because the way a problem is defined helps determine how it will be approached and therefore answered.

If defined imprecisely or incorrectly, the proposed solution may solve the wrong problem. Thus, special care must be taken in how one frames the problem.

Framing the problem.

Framing refers to how a question is set up to be answered. It considers issues such as the perspective taken, elements of the problem to be considered, and criteria used to choose one solution over another. Framing helps simplify the problem by including some information and excluding others. For example, when purchasing a car, one frames the problem of which car to choose by listing a limited number of key characteristics that are desired (e.g., color, safety, and gas mileage) and other characteristics are ignored (e.g., type of spare tire and cleanliness of undercarriage).

Consider how the following ways of framing a car-buying decision affect the final choice:

- "What American car should I choose?" versus "What car should I choose?" "Which car will result in the most affordable monthly payment?" versus "Which car can be purchased for the lowest price?"
- "Which is the best car for me?" versus "Which car will my family want for me?"

Framing biases.

Poor solutions to problems result when pharmacists and other decision makers let themselves become influenced by common framing biases. Framing biases are ways of looking at problems in a way that negatively prejudices the final solution. They can result in poorly defined problems, because they inappropriately hinder the assumptions involved in the decision. A pharmacist may frame a drug cost question as, "How can we cut drug costs?" Or it may be framed as, "How can we provide more cost-effective drug therapy?" These two contrasting frames to the question may result in completely different solutions. Table 6-1 lists some common framing biases: defining problems with solutions, anchoring, confusing symptoms with problems, seeing the world from a pharmacist's viewpoint, and knowing the "truth."

Framing biases hurt good problem solving by closing one's mind to important aspects of an issue and preventing him or her from getting at the real problem. For instance, identifying problems with solutions occurs when an individual already has a solution in mind when defining a problem. When a solution is part of the problem statement, pharmacists no longer explore for better alternative solutions. Anchoring biases decision making by limiting solution options due to events that occurred previously. This occurs when a frame is restricted by a statement similar to, "We can't do X because we already spent too much time and effort on Y."

One reason pharmacists have framing biases is that we have a pharmacist-centric view of the world. Our professional identity makes us see everything from a pharmacist's interests and concern. There is a common saying, "When the only tool you have is a hammer, every problem begins to resemble a nail." This can be reinterpreted here to mean, "When your primary focus is drug use, the solutions tend to revolve around the role of pharmacists and pharmaceuticals." Therefore, we are more likely to advocate for pharmacy-centered solutions to problems of health, medicine, and

TABLE 6-1. Common Framing Biases

Framing Bias	Description	Examples
Defining problems with solutions	When a pharmacist already has a solution in mind when defining a problem blinding him or her to other potential solutions	"The problem with medication errors is that we do not have sufficient staff" "The problem with pharmacist turnover is that we need to increase pharmacist salaries"
Anchoring	When initial data or impressions anchor subsequent thoughts and decisions	A pharmacist with a difficult-to-read prescription says, "This looks like a prescription for Valium. What do you think?" Framing the question this way biases the individual asked toward seeing Valium. A less biased frame would be, "What does this prescription say?"
Confusing symptoms with problems	Symptoms such as employee stress or feelings of being overworked often indicate the presence of a greater underlying problem within the system. Treating the symptoms may do little to resolve the cause	"The problem at work is that our employees are too stressed" "The problem with medication errors is that pharmacists are overworked"
Seeing the world from a pharmacist's viewpoint	When a pharmacist's professional identity blinds him or her to relevant information or limits his or her viewpoint to the boundaries of a pharmacist's position	A pharmacist might frame a problem as "the patient is not compliant with his medication," while the patient frames it as "I am having trouble balancing the need to take my medication with my family and work responsibilities"
Knowing the "truth"	Truths are deeply ingrained assumptions and generalizations about the world that can blind pharmacists if left unchallenged. These truths influence how we understand the world and how we take action. The problem is that they are often partially or totally wrong	"Pharmacists are too busy to check for drug interactions" "Patients only care about low drug prices and fast service" "People are motivated by pay"

policy. The way to overcome this bias is to redefine problems from alternative perspectives, physician, nurse, patient, payer, and others. If the definitions differ, they need to be reconciled.

We are also biased because our experience and education in pharmacy often leads to deeply ingrained assumptions and generalizations about the world. In some cases, these assumptions are faulty, only partially true, or just wrong. Consequently, any decision-making processes based on these assumptions and generalizations blind us and affect our decisions. For example, a common refrain from pharmacists is, "Pharmacists are too busy to _____." In many cases, it is true. However, in other cases, it is just an excuse for not addressing a problem. Surely, pharmacists are busy for a substantial portion of the day. However, it is also likely that with better time management, many problems could be worked out within a pharmacist's work day. Good problem solving requires pharmacists to challenge their deeply ingrained assumptions about practice in order to avoid framing bias.

DEVELOPING GOOD PROBLEM STATEMENTS

When defining a problem, it is important to write a good statement of the problem. Good problem statements are concise and hit the heart of an issue. Avoiding framing biases is also important.

It can be recommended that a good problem statement define the broad problem in a single short sentence. This helps provide focus and clarity and avoid distracting side issues such as symptoms. One way of determining if the problem statement as defined is getting at the real problem is to ask, "What would happen if the problem, as I defined it, was fixed?" For example, to assess the problem statement "Pharmacists are missing potentially dangerous drug interactions because they are too busy," ask if the problem will be fixed if pharmacists had more available time. If the problem is likely to continue even if more time were made available for pharmacists to check for drug interactions, the problem statement may need to be redefined.

Another way to get at the real problem is to repeatedly ask, "Why?" If a problem is defined as "the employees are complaining," ask "Why?" The answer might be "Because they are unhappy at work." "Why?" "Because they don't feel they are being paid enough." "Why?" "Because their friends at other pharmacies claim that they are being paid more." "Ahah!" The real problem at hand might be that employees are unhappy because they perceive that their peers are being paid more for the same work. To resolve this problem, the manager can identify how the pay and work differs at other pharmacies. Only then can the manager identify if salaries should be increased to remain competitive, or if he or she needs to have a frank discussion with employees about their perceptions of their job and the job market.

A single problem statement about a broad, complex problem often requires a series of statements of subproblems that relate to the broad problem. The purpose of identifying these subproblems is to break the overall problem into more manageable pieces. To attack a major problem such as "How do we improve employee morale?" can be overwhelming. However, attacking subproblems (e.g., "How much are our competitors paying?") can be easier to handle if they are dealt with one by one.

It can also be useful to explicitly state the perspective of the decision maker in any problem statement. The solution of a problem may differ depending on whether it is defined from one's personal perspective or that of one's boss, coworkers, or patients. Ideally, any problem statement should be acceptable to all perspectives, but this is not always possible for people with competing interests.

CONCLUSIONS

QI is most effective when it follows a proven process. Proven techniques for identifying and defining QI problems are discussed in this chapter. To identify problems well, it is important to have a method for collecting key variables that signal quality and analyzing them statistically to identify undesirable trends. Using judgment and an analysis of the data, a systems approach should be used to explore the problem in depth. That systems approach should guide how the problem is framed and eventually resolved. Understanding various framing biases can help pharmacists to develop strategies to avoid prejudicing the problem-solving process. If pharmacists adopt the recommendations in this chapter, good solutions are more likely to result.

REFERENCES

1. Hepler CD, Strand LM. Opportunities and responsibilities in pharmaceutical care. *Am J Hosp Pharm.* 1990;47(3):533–543.
2. American College of Physicians, American Society of Internal Medicine. Pharmacist scope of practice. *Ann Intern Med.* 2002;136(1):79–85.
3. Montana P, Charnov B. Management decision making: types and styles. In: *Management.* New York: Barrons Educational Series, Inc; 2008:70.
4. Soumerai SB, McLaughlin TJ, Ross-Degnan D, et al. Effects of limiting Medicaid drug-reimbursement benefits on the use of psychotropic agents and acute mental health services by patients with schizophrenia. *N Eng J Med.* 1994;331:650–655.
5. Hsu J, Price M, Huang J et al. Unintended consequences of caps on Medicare drug benefits. *N Engl J Med.* 2006 1;354(22):2349–2359.
6. Ash JS, Sittig DF, Dykstra RH, Guappone K, Carpenter JD, Seshadri V. Categorizing the unintended sociotechnical consequences of computerized provider order entry. *Int J Med Inform.* 2007;76(suppl 1):S21–S27.
7. J. Edward Russo, Paul J.H. Schoemaker. *Decision Traps. The Ten Barriers to Brilliant Decision-making and How to Overcome Them.* 1st ed. New York: Simon & Schuster; 1989.
8. Senge PM. *The Fifth Discipline. The Art and Practice of the Learning Organization.* 1st ed. New York, NY: Currency Doubleday, 1990.

CHAPTER 7

Identifying Causes of Quality Problems

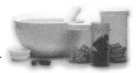

Terri L. Warholak and Ana Hincapie

Learning Objectives

At the end of the chapter, the reader will be able to:

1. Recognize problems associated with identifying quality issues and solutions.
2. Select an appropriate topic for analysis.
3. Support the use of root cause analysis.
4. Support the use of Healthcare Failure Modes and Effects Analysis (HFMEA^SM).

Key Definitions

- *Detectable hazard*: A very evident potential risk that will be promptly discovered before it hampers the completion of an activity (e.g., an IV bag that is leaking).
- *Effective control measure*: A barrier that eliminates or substantially reduces the likelihood of a hazardous event occurring (e.g., the pharmaceutical form of some medications prevents its use via the wrong administration route such as I tubing that only connects for IV catheter, not nasal cannula).
- *Failure mode*: Different ways that a process or subprocess can fail to provide the anticipated result.
- *Failure mode cause*: Different reasons as to why a process or subprocess would fail to provide the anticipated result.
- *Hazard analysis*: Identification and evaluation of potential hazards that are likely to produce harm in a specific process if not controlled.
- *Healthcare Failure Modes and Effects Analysis (HFMEA^SM)*: A systematic approach to identify and prevent product and process problems before they occur.
- *Single point weakness*: A step in the process so critical that its failure would result in system failure or an adverse event (e.g., the prescriber order is processed for the wrong patient; this would result in the preparation, delivery, and administration of the wrong medications).

In this chapter, we will talk about how to identify the causes of quality problems.

IDENTIFYING PROBLEMS ASSOCIATED WITH IDENTIFYING QUALITY ISSUES AND SOLUTIONS

There are many problems associated with identifying quality issues and solutions; many of these are called heuristics and judgmental biases. In many cases, decision makers rely on a limited number of heuristic principles (or simple decision rules) to reduce cognitively complex decision-making tasks to simpler judgmental operations.[1,2] Although many heuristics exist, only those more commonly mentioned in the literature will be described. Some common heuristics are included in Table 7-1.

Often, humans prefer to use heuristics rather than utilizing more complex cognitive processes such as decision making.[2] Heuristics can be useful or can lead to error, depending on the situation (Tversky and Khaneman, 1982b).[1,2,7] It is important to recognize these common heuristics as potential sources of error so that decision-making techniques can be implemented to reduce the impact of these cognitive biases.[3]

For example, when using the availability heuristic, the decision maker confuses the ease of remembering an incident with the probability that an incident will occur. This and other definitions appear in Table 7-2.

To illustrate this, let's look at a case of confirmation bias. A physician ordered a heparin flush bag for a 6-year-old child. The pharmacist approved the order and gave it to a technician for sterile compounding. The technician selected a stock vial from the shelf and prepared the bag. The technician pulled the syringe plunger back to the amount of the medication that had been added to the IV bag and placed the stock bottle and IV patient label with the bag for pharmacist final check as per pharmacy protocol. The pharmacist looked at the final preparation, checked the label, confirmed that the correct amount of medication had been added to the bag, and approved the medication for dispensing to the pediatric ward. The bag was delivered to the ward and the nurse set the drip rate for the patient as prescribed. In approximately 2 hours the

TABLE 7-1. Problems Associated with Assigning Causes and Choosing Solutions

Biases
• Availability
• Representative
• Ego
• Hindsight
• Confirmation bias
• Ignoring negative evidence
• Framing

Data from Refs.[3–8], Tversky and Khaneman 1982b.

TABLE 7-2. Selected Heuristic Definitions

Heuristic	Definition
Availability	Confuses the ease of remembering an incident with the probability that an incident will occur
Representativeness	The decision maker assesses the likelihood that an object or a person belongs to a given class
Ego bias	The decision maker warps probability estimates in a self-serving way
Hindsight bias	The decision maker can easily predict an event after it has occurred
Regret	The decision maker would regret a decision, and thus may overestimate the probability of its occurrence
Confirmatory bias	The decision maker acknowledges only evidence that will confirm his or her hypotheses
Ignoring negative evidence	The decision maker can more easily consider the presence of evidence than the absence of evidence
Framing	The context in which the information is considered

Data from Refs.[3-8], Tversky and Khaneman (1982b).

patient began to be shaky and irritable. This prompted the nurse to check the blood sugar and it was noted that his blood sugar levels were low. On investigation, it was discovered that an error had occurred. On root cause analysis, it was discovered that the technician had mistakenly put insulin in the IV bag, not heparin. Because insulin and heparin are both frequently used in sterile compounding, they were on the same shelf and the technician selected the wrong drug. The pharmacist confirmed that the correct volume was drawn up but failed to check to ensure that the correct medication was used.

SELECTION OF A TOPIC FOR ANALYSIS

There are several different ways to identify quality problems suitable for analysis. For example, one could examine a significant error that has occurred in your practice setting or one might look at a particular process that has not yet produced an error to determine how to prevent an error from happening. Errors that are caught before they leave the pharmacy or before they reach the patient are also important because they are good indicators of what types of errors the system is creating. These could also be selected for analysis.

Another alternative is to use statistical process control charts to identify topics or areas that may benefit most from quality improvement interventions. These charts can be created by examining internal error reporting programs. The words statistical process control sound intimidating but, as you will learn in Chapter 8, they are simple charts and graphs that can help you determine where your quality improvement activities might have the most impact.

It is important to keep in mind the biases mentioned in the above-mentioned section. Once topics are narrowed down or selected, take a fresh look at them; are they biased in an important way? Might you have a better effect with your project if you selected another topic? The topic selected should be important, timely, and actionable.

Let's examine the process you might take if you decided to thoroughly examine a significant error in order to put processes in place to prevent this error from happening again. A significant error if it involved "death or serious physical or psychological injury, or the risk thereof" is called a sentinel event by the Joint Commission on Accreditation of Healthcare Organizations (JCAHO but now they are referred to simply as the Joint Commission). The Joint Commission is an accrediting body for health systems whose mission is to continuously improve the safety and quality of care provided to the public through the provision of health care accreditation and related services that support performance improvement in health care organizations (http://www.jointcommission.org/AboutUs/).

In order to make health care safer, we need to learn from the mistakes of others and identify potential problems in the system. That is, leaders must ensure that an ongoing, proactive program for identifying risks to patient safety and reducing medical/health care errors is defined and implemented (JCAHO Standard LD.5.2). This reduces the risk of sentinel events.

The following is an example of a sentinel event: if a baby is given an insulin overdose and dies. As you can see from this example, sentinel events should be avoided.

If a sentinel ever happened at your facility – or if a sentinel event is reported in several facilities – then this may be a good topic to select for analysis. In fact, the Joint Commission requires hospitals to *respond* to all sentinel events.

ROOT CAUSE ANALYSIS

Root cause analysis is a mandatory component of the response to a sentinel event because it is intended to prevent reoccurrence. However, institutions can learn from sentinel event from other institutions or they can select a topic for analysis that specifically addresses an internal issue that has the potential to cause harm. This is why it is essential that near misses (errors that are identified before they reach the patient) or errors are logged and analyzed; this information lets the pharmacy or other portion of the institution know where they need to focus QI activities.

Once you select a topic for analysis, what techniques can be used to determine the *true cause*(s) of the error? There are two major categories: (1) root cause analysis and (2) health care failure modes and effects analysis. Both of them help the user to identify *what* is or *could* go wrong in the system that may contribute to an error. However, they are used in different situations. That is, root cause analysis is done *after* a sentinel event to determine *why* the error happened while failure mode and effects analysis is done *before* a sentinel event to assess what *could* go wrong with a process.

Root cause analysis is done *after* a *sentinel event* to determine *why* the error happened. The goal is to identify the cause – or *all* of the factors that contributed to the error (identifying the *underlying* reason for an event) – so that actions can be taken to prevent recurrence. The root cause analysis process is lengthy but in general it is a systematic process of examining *all* factors that could have contributed to the problem and determine if they did – why they did – and determine what can be done to prevent recurrence. In root cause analysis, we ask "Why, Why, Why?"

The steps include:

- identify the *underlying* reason for an event;
- identify causes and analyze related processes/systems;
- identify ways to improve processes/systems to reduce chance of reoccurrence;
- create action plan for implementing process/system improvements;
- implement improvements;
- evaluate effectiveness of improvements.

There are two commonly used formats for root cause analysis:

1. The Joint Commission has a three-page form that can help guide a user through the process (http://www.jointcommission.org/SentinelEvents/Forms/).
2. The Veteran's Administration National Center for Patient Safety (NCPS) offers a concise, complete set of flip cards to assist the user (http://www.va.gov/ncps/CogAids/ Triage/index.html or http://www.va.gov/ncps/CogAids/RCA/index.html).

Let's use the NCPS triage questions with an example. A pharmacist working in a community pharmacy finds out that he or she has been involved in a significant medication error; he or she did the final check on the medication. The error entailed a wrong drug error. That is, the physician ordered zidovudine for a patient who has human immunodeficiency virus (HIV) but the prescription was filled with azathioprine instead (the abbreviation AZT has been used for both of these medications). The medication was new for the patient and she took it for a month. At the end of that month, she was admitted to a local hospital because she was feeling "run down." On examination of the situation, the physician discovered that a wrong drug error had occurred. The pharmacist who made the error is very upset by this and begins to engage in root cause analysis to determine what factors contributed to the error. Once these are determined, he or she intends to put procedures in place to prevent similar errors from happening again.

Note that in the interest of brevity and clarity, only the specific questions deemed applicable to this example will be reviewed below. For a more in-depth look at all root cause questions and the full procedure, please see the VA NCPS website (http:// www.va.gov/ncps/CogAids/Triage/index.html). All materials are readily available for public use through this site and the reader is encouraged to view for additional information.

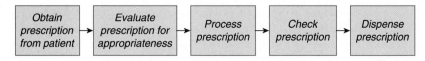

Figure 7-1. Cognitive steps in the medication dispensing process.

First, was this a criminal act? If so, the root cause process might not need to be undertaken. Once it is assured that the act was not intentional, the root cause procedure should be begun.

Step 1. Familiarize yourself with the triage questions.

Step 2. Create a flowchart that depicts the activities surrounding the event (Figure 7-1).

Step 3. Evaluate your situation with the triage questions. Your answers on the triage questions will lead you to more in-depth questions as appropriate. The following triage questions are verbatim from NPCS:

a. "Were issues related to patient assessment a factor in this situation?"
b. "Were issues related to staff training or staff competency a factor in this event?"
c. "Was equipment involved in this event in any way?"
d. "Was a lack of information or misinterpretation a factor in this event?"
e. "Was communication a factor in this event?"
f. "Were appropriate rules/policies/procedures – or the lack thereof – a factor in this event?"
g. "Was the failure of a barrier designed to protect the patient, staff, equipment, or environment a factor in this event?"
h. "Were personnel or personnel issues a factor in this event?"

In the case of our example, all triage questions except for "c" (referring to equipment) would be answered with a "Yes" and would therefore justify further in-depth evaluation.

Step 4. Use the triage questions to identify additional specific questions that will help you delve into the root cause(s) of the event. Let's look at each root cause triage question for which the answer was "Yes," discuss it in detail, and examine the subsequent questions for further evaluation.

a. "Were issues related to patient assessment a factor in this situation?"

Because we responded "Yes" to this question, the root cause process leads us to evaluate the human factors/communication questions with this item. When looking at these questions, which, again, in the interest of brevity and clarity are not reprinted here (see VA NCPS), it seems that there are a few issues in this category that could have caused the error. Specifically, these are: "Was information from various patient assessments shared and used by various members of the treatment team on a timely basis?" "Was the correct technical information adequately communicated 24 hours a day to the people who needed it?" "Did management establish adequate methods to provide information to employees, who needed it, in a manner that was easy to access/use and timely?" These apply to our example, at least in part, because if the pharmacist had known the patient's diagnosis was AIDS, this information might have helped him or her select between the two medications for which AZT has been used as an abbreviation. There was no policy, law, or rule to require the physician to indicate the diagnosis on the prescription and this information was not communicated to the pharmacist in any other manner. In addition, the AZT abbreviation should not have been used because there is the possibility of two different interpretations.

b. "Were issues related to staff training or staff competency a factor in this event?"

We responded "Yes" to this item because the pharmacist should have recognized that there were two medications that have been referred to as AZT and he or she should have recognized the need to clarify the medication and/or diagnosis with the provider and/or the patient.

c. "Was equipment involved in this event in any way?"

Our answer to this question was "No," so it can be skipped.

d. "Was a lack of information or misinterpretation a factor in this event?"

For our example, the answer to this question is "Yes" because of the fact that the AZT abbreviation can refer to two different medications and is easily misinterpreted. This triage question refers the root cause analyst to the same human factors/communication questions that were answered for the first triage question in reference to patient assessment. Therefore, these questions have been addressed and do not need to be reconsidered here.

e. "Was communication a factor in this event?"

The answer to this question is also "Yes" for reasons similar to those stated for the above-mentioned question. This triage question also refers the root cause analyst to the same human factors/communication questions that were answered for the first triage question in reference to patient assessment.

f. "Were appropriate rules/policies/procedures – or the lack thereof – a factor in this event?"

I would also answer this question in the affirmative when thinking about our example. In this case, the root cause analysis procedure as delineated by NCPS guides the analyst to the rules/policies/procedure questions. After considering these questions, it is apparent that in this situation the error would not have been identified by an audit or review because the pharmacist did not have access to the patient diagnosis. In addition, there should have been a policy to require that the pharmacist contact the prescriber to confirm the medication in a situation in which a medication abbreviation may refer to more than one medication. Alternatively, a policy might be implemented to indicate that pharmacists clarify all medication abbreviations in the future. Either way, all personnel should be adequately trained on these policies.

g. "Was the failure of a barrier designed to protect the patient, staff, equipment, or environment a factor in this event?"

Let's assume that a policy for checking an unclear abbreviation on prescriptions did exist to provide a barrier to misinterpretation errors at the pharmacy where the error occurred. In this event, the policy was not followed, so it could be said that a barrier to errors failed.

h. "Were personnel or personnel issues a factor in this event?"

Because personnel were involved, the answer to this triage question is also "Yes." Therefore, we need to assess the human factors fatigue/scheduling questions. While answering these questions, and subsequent interviewing with the pharmacist involved in the error, we find out that there were several distractions to the pharmacist during critical decision-making points when processing this prescription. For example, the pharmacist tells us that he or she was interrupted during his or her final check of the prescription as well as during counseling. Both of these might have contributed to the pharmacist's ability to identify the error before it left the pharmacy.

Step 5. If necessary, gather additional information from interviews, documents, or references. We went a bit out of order and interviewed the pharmacist for triage question but this can be done concurrently with step 4 or sequentially as step 5.

Step 6. Make a list of the root cause(s) of the event. As discussed before, root cause analysis should help the user determine why an error occurred and suggest what can be done to prevent a recurrence in the future, so at this point the root cause analyst should look at the issues identified in the above-mentioned steps and use these to create the list. In the case of our AZT error example, the root causes we identified include:

- insufficient patient diagnosis information (the pharmacist did not have this information and did not use it to determine appropriateness);
- use of an abbreviation that could be misinterpreted;
- failure to recognize that AZT is used as an abbreviation for two different medications;
- failure to clarify medication;
- absence of a policy requiring the pharmacist to clarify an unclear medication order;
- multiple interruptions during the decision-making process.

Make sure these statements show the cause and effect relationship for *each* error. The statements should be phrased in a positive manner. It is important to note that violations of procedure are not considered a root cause and failure to act is considered a root cause only when there was a duty to act. So, let's modify our statements:

- The patient information available to the pharmacist increased the probability that if the wrong medication was selected to fill the AZT prescription, it would not be identified. This contributed to a wrong drug error.

- The pharmacist's assessment of medication appropriateness was performed with available information that increased the chances that wrong drug errors would not be identified. This contributed to a wrong drug error.
- An abbreviation that could be misinterpreted was used, thus increasing the probability of a wrong drug error. This contributed to a wrong drug error.
- The pharmacist's level of training concerning medication abbreviation errors increased the likelihood that he or she failed to recognize that AZT is used as an abbreviation for two different medications. This contributed to a wrong drug error.
- Due to lack of encouragement and high workload expectations, an informal norm has been created such that few prescriptions are clarified with the prescriber.
- The pharmacist was interrupted multiple times during crucial points in the prescription processing system, increasing the possibility a problem or error could be overlooked. This contributed to a wrong drug error.

Step 7. Delineate actions to be taken and outcome measures to assess the impact of the actions. Actions are taken to prevent or minimize reoccurrence. Outcome measures are collected to determine if interventions worked. Based on our above-mentioned list above, what actions should we take? How about the following:

- Provide the pharmacist additional patient information. Options for this include: (a) having the provider put the diagnosis or reason for use on each prescription (written or electronic – if e-prescriptions are used, ensure that the diagnosis is displayed to the pharmacist); and (b) implementing a policy for the pharmacy technician to gather additional patient information when taking the prescription from the patient (diagnosis or reason for use).
- Ensure the pharmacists use the additional information (diagnosis) to assess medication appropriateness. Create protocol and train all personnel.
- Educate providers that medication abbreviations increase the chances of wrong drug errors and ask that they write out the full name of the medication (or use e-prescribing).
- Educate all pharmacists about abbreviations that may be interpreted in several different ways. Create a policy to require all pharmacists to verify the medication needed in these instances, and educate all staff about policy.
- Create a policy that pharmacists should not be interrupted when performing important cognitive tasks in the medication dispensing process (prospective drug utilization review, final check, counseling, etc.).
- Provide managerial support for pharmacists to take the extra time required to clarify prescriptions when necessary. These new expectations must also be communicated to the patient so that they will understand the need for an occasional delay in the processing of their prescriptions.

Step 8. Take action to prevent reoccurrences of the error(s). Implement the changes suggested above.

Step 9. Monitor and reassess the process periodically. A few ideas for the above-mentioned problems include: gathering data concerning policy adherence, percent of prescriptions for which diagnosis was obtained, percentage of abbreviations used over a period of time, and which prescribers most frequently use abbreviations.

In the previous section, we examined an analysis that focuses on errors after the fact (ex post facto); however, it is very important to prevent potential errors and identify what could go wrong with a process (i.e., a proactive assessment before events occur). The Healthcare Failure Modes and Effects Analysis (HFMEA^SM) is a prospective risk analysis system that can be used for such a purpose.

HEALTHCARE FAILURE MODES AND EFFECTS ANALYSIS

This analysis is derived from Failure Mode and Effect Analysis (FMEA™) used in the engineering sector to assess risks in manufacturing processes. HFMEA^SM was adapted by the Veterans Affairs NCPS.[9]

HFMEA^SM is defined as "A systematic method of identifying and preventing product problems BEFORE they occur." Therefore, HFMEA evaluates health care processes and anticipates harmful events.

There are, in general, five steps required to conduct a HFMEA^SM analysis:

Step 1. *Define the topic*: In order to develop a thorough analysis, its process and scope have to be clearly defined. Consider in this step topics categorized as high risk in your organization.

Example: This HFMEA^SM is focused on preparing and delivering total parenteral nutrition (TPN) for the neonatal intensive care unit (NICU) for preterm infants. In my experience as pharmacist, I found this patient population very vulnerable. I consider that any mistake in the process of producing TPN could become a hazard that might seriously affect preterm newborns (Figure 7-2).

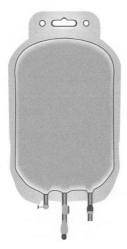

Figure 7-2. Total parenteral nutrition for neonatal intensive care unit.

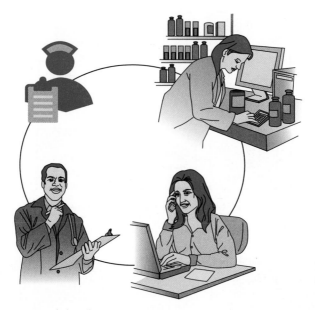

Figure 7-3. HFMEA^SM multidisciplinary team.

Step 2. *Assemble the team*: The team should be multidisciplinary and include subject matter expert. Expertise cooperation may present better feedback of potential undesired events and provide a more comprehensive analysis. Outside observes (e.g., medical assistant) may provide critical review and identify potential flaws that experts might fail to see. Ideally the team should not include more than 12 participants to facilitate focusing in the analysis. A leader should be assigned. The leader is meant to keep the team motivated, encouraging participation, and if possible he or she should be able to obtain resources necessary for the team (e.g., computer and data). Additionally, a designated facilitator within the team keeps it focused on its objectives and helps the leader. It is important to delegate a member of the team who documents and registers all the activities of the *HFMEA^SM*.

For our example, we might want to include practitioners from the clinical nutrition department, a pediatrician, pediatric nurse, pharmacists, ..., a pharmacy technician (Figure 7-3).

Step 3. *Graphically describe the process*: This step involves three subprocesses. This approach will help to narrow the analysis to avoid an overwhelming project that will be difficult to finalize in a reasonable time frame.

a. First gather information to develop a flowchart that depicts the steps in the process (Figure 7-4).

b. Successively, number each process step identified in the process flow diagram (Figure 7-5).

c. Identify all subprocesses under each block of the flow diagram in Figure 7-6 and letter them.

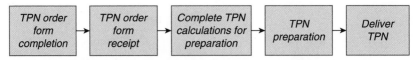

Figure 7-4. HFMEA^SM step 3a, process depiction.

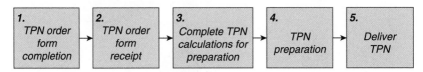

Figure 7-5. HFMEA^SM step 3b: Numbering each step in the process.

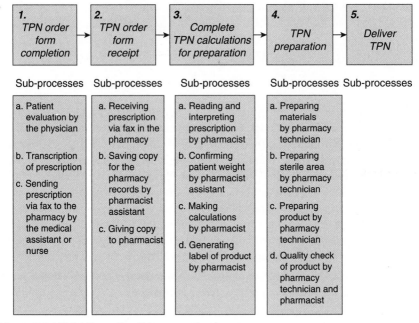

Figure 7-6. HFMEA^SM step 3c: Subprocess identification.

Determine if the process you selected is too large to manage at once. If so, determine what steps you will focus on first (Figure 7-7).

Step 4. *Conduct a hazard analysis*: For the specific part of the process the team decided to analyze, list all potential failures for each subprocess (e.g., 3A1, 3A2, …, 3E1)

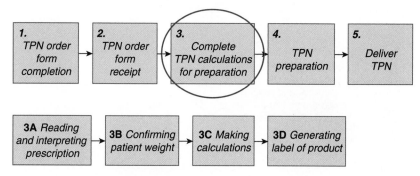

Figure 7-7. Determining the step on which you will focus for the HFMEA^SM.

(in this step, use all the expertise of the members of the team; their particular past experiences contribute to the brainstorming activity):

(3A)   prescription not legible or misinterpretation;
(3B1) weight cannot be obtained;
(3B2) obtaining weight from a different patient or using incorrect weight;
(3B3) using birth weight versus actual weight;
(3C1) using wrong equations;
(3C2) putting wrong numbers on the spreadsheet;
(3C3) computer does not work;
(3C4) using laboratory results from a wrong patient;
(3D1) generating label for wrong patient or incorrect label.

Once you finish with the potential failures identification, establish the severity and probability of each one of them. For doing this, use:

1. the Hazard Scoring Matrix HFMEA^SM (Table 7-3);[10]
2. HFMEA^SM Decision Tree (Figure 7-8).[10]

TABLE 7-3. The Hazard Scoring Matrix HFMEA^SM

	Severity			
Probability	Catastrophic	Major	Moderate	Minor
Frequent	16	12	8	4
Occasional	12	9	6	3
Uncommon	8	6	4	2
Remote	4	3	2	1

Scores of 8 or higher mean sufficient likelihood of occurrence and severity of the hazard. Thus, actions to prevent the hazard need to be taken.
Reproduced with permission from Veterans Administration National Center for Patient Safety; http://www.patientsafety.gov

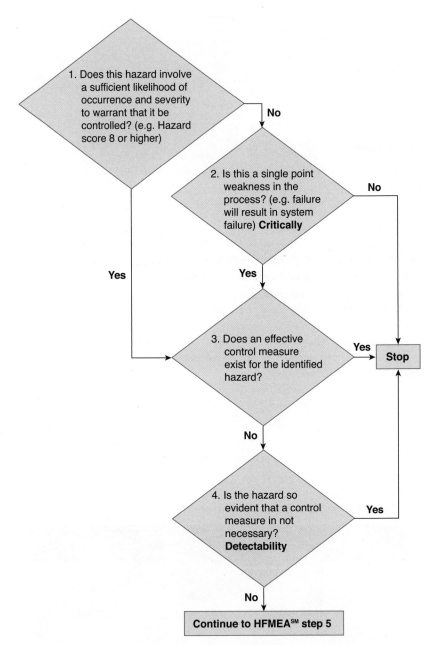

Figure 7-8. HFMEA^SM Decision Tree. (Redrawn with permission from Veterans Administration National Center for Patient Safety; http://www.patientsafety.gov.).

Severity refers to the potential effect of failure on patients. As can be seen in Table 7-3, severity varies from minor, moderate, and major to catastrophic.

Probability is defined as the number of events expected to occur during a certain period of time: frequent (several times in 1 year), occasional (several times in 2 years), uncommon (sometimes in 2–5 years), and remote (5–30 years).

To follow our example, let's assign the hazard score of the previously identified potential failure 3A: prescription not legible or misinterpretation. If this process fails, the results can be disastrous because overdose or subdose of any of the ingredients (i.e., amino acids, lipids, proteins, and electrolytes) could result in malnutrition, toxicity, or TPN chemical instability. The team decided that the probability of occurrence is "occasional" because the institution uses a fax system to send the prescription to the pharmacy and therefore legibility could be inappropriate. However, if the failure occurs, the severity would be "catastrophic." The resulting hazard score is 12.

After giving the score, now we should proceed to conduct a decision analysis using the HFMEA^SM Decision Tree.

The HFMEA^SM Decision Tree helps us to determine the actions that have to be taken for each potential failure previously identified. It narrows the course of actions; therefore, it optimizes team effort when evaluating a process. This Decision Tree ascertains the need of further action based on three characteristics:

1. *Criticality*: A potential failure is classified as critical when the complete process is hindered if this potential failure occurs. This is also known as single point weakness in the process.

2. *Controlled*: It ascertains whether there is an effective control measure that eliminates or reduces the probability that the failure occurs.

3. *Detectability*: If a potential failure is readily evident, it is most likely to be discovered before it affects the entire process.

If the result of the decision tree analysis indicates to advance with the failure mode assessment, you should proceed with the next step where specific actions are carried out to eliminate, accept, or control the potential failure mode. Using the worksheet presented Figure 7-9 will help to complete the mentioned steps.

Following our example, the potential failure 3A obtained a hazard score of 12. There is no effective control measure for this step. This potential failure is not easily detected; therefore, actions need to be taken.

Step 5. In this step, for each failure mode you proceed to describe the actions needed to eliminate the hazard. To do this, develop an action plan. The plan should be specific, designate the person responsible for completing each action, and identify the outcome measure to demonstrate accomplishment. This would help to keep track of the hazard.

This institution might consider changing the current fax system to a Computerized Physician Order Entry system (CPOE) or implement a control measure where the prescription is always confirmed by phone before beginning the process of TPN preparation.

HFMEA step 4 - Hazard analysis													
Failure mode: First evaluate failure mode before determining potential causes	Potential causes	Severity	Probability	Haz score	Single point weakness?	Existing control measure?	Detectability	Proceed?	Action type (control, accept, eliminate)	Actions or rationale for stopping	Outcome measure	Person responsible	Management concurrence
		Scoring			Decision tree analysis								
3. Errors in the TPN calculations for preparation	→	Catastrophic	Occasional	12	Y	N	N	Y					
	3A Prescription not legible, misinterpretation												
	3B1 Weight cannot be obtained												
	3B2 Obtaining weight from a different patient or using incorrect weight												
	3B3 Using birth weight versus actual weight												

Figure 7-9. Health care Failure Mode and Effect Analysis worksheet.[10] (Reproduced with permission from Veterans Administration National Center for Patient Safety; http://www.patientsafety.gov.).

REFERENCES

1. Cook RI, Woods DD. Operating at the sharp end: complexity of human error. In: Bogner MS, ed. *Human Error in Medicine.* Hillsdale, NJ: Lawrence Earlbaum Associates, Inc; 1994:255–309.

2. Reason J. A framework for classifying errors. In: Rasmussen J, Duncan K, Leplat J, eds. *New Technology and Human Error.* New York: John Wiley & Sons; 1987:5–14.

3. Dawson NV, Arkes HR. Systematic errors in medical decision making: judgment limitations. *J Gen Intern Med.* 1987;2:183–187.

4. Perow C. *Normal Accidents: Living with High-risk Technologies.* New York: Basic Books, Inc; 1984.

5. Reason J. *Human Error.* New York: Press Syndicate of the University of Cambridge; 1990:40, 44.

6. Taylor SE. The availability bias in social perception and interaction. In: Kahneman DK, Slovic P, Tversky A, eds. *Judgment under Uncertainty: Heuristics and Biases.* Cambridge: Cambridge University Press; 1982:190–200.

7. Tversky A, Khaneman D. Judgment of and by representativeness. In: Kahneman DK, Slovic P, Tversky A, eds. *Judgment under Uncertainty: Heuristics and Biases.* Cambridge: Cambridge University Press; 1982:85–98.

8. Wolf FM, Gruppen LD, Billi JE. Differential diagnosis and the competing-hypothesis heuristic. *JAMA.* 1985; 253:2858–2862.

9. DeRosier J, Stalhandske E, Bagian JP, Nudell T. Using health care failure mode and effect analysis: the VA National Center for Patient Safety's prospective risk analysis system. *Jt Comm J Qual Improvement.* 2002;28(5):248–267.

10. Veterans Administration National Center for Patient Safety. Available at www.patientsafety.gov/. Accessed January 2009.

CHAPTER 8

Statistical Process Control

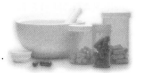

Leticia R. Moczygemba and
David A. Holdford

Learning Objectives

At the end of the chapter, the reader will be able to:

1. Explain the rationale for statistical process control.
2. Describe and learn how to utilize the following tools for statistical process control:
   - histograms;
   - Pareto charts;
   - scatter diagrams;
   - run charts;
   - control charts;
   - sampling;
   - benchmarking.
3. Discuss how statistical process control tools can be incorporated into the steps of quality improvement.

INTRODUCTION

Pharmacy is comprised of complex systems. It is important that these systems are reliable in order to deliver quality pharmacy services. Statistical process control (SPC), the use of statistical techniques to measure change in systems, is one method of monitoring quality in pharmacy practice. SPC is particularly useful because a key determinant of quality in products and services is consistency. Statistical analysis can be utilized to improve quality by identifying inconsistency in systems, and SPC tools, such as histograms, Pareto charts, scatter diagrams, and run and control charts, can help distinguish between acceptable and unacceptable inconsistencies in pharmacist services. This chapter will describe the rationale for SPC, commonly used SPC tools, and how to incorporate SPC into the steps of quality improvement.

THE RATIONALE FOR SPC

Repeated measurements of the same process within a system will have variable outcomes over time.[1-4] The inherent variability within all systems is the foundation for SPC. Two types of variation exist, common-cause variation and special-cause variation.

Common-cause variation is always present within a system and consists of modest changes that occur randomly. Common-cause variation in a pharmacy can be a result of things such as differences in individual pharmacists and technicians, patient populations, situations, and chance. Despite the myriad of factors that can influence variations in pharmacy practice, over time, a predictable pattern of variation emerges. Think about 100 random measurements repeated over a 3-month period of the time it takes to fill a prescription at a pharmacy. If it takes somewhere between 5 and 25 minutes to fill 95 out of the 100 sampled prescriptions, the variation in fill times due to common cause would be 20 minutes assuming that no major changes to the system have occurred over the 3 months. As long as the system stays the same (e.g., personnel and workflow processes), common-cause variation stays the same. A system is considered to be in a state of statistical control when only common-cause variation is present.[1-4] Nevertheless, a state of statistical control is not sufficient if the variation in output does not align with the system goals.[1,2,5] Consider a pharmacy that has an average prescription wait time of 1 hour with times ranging from 55 to 65 minutes. Although the wait times may be predictable to within 10 minutes, the pharmacist-in-charge (PIC) may not consider the wait time to be acceptable given that the average wait time is 1 hour. It is also likely that patients would not be satisfied with the 1-hour wait.

In contrast, special-cause variation occurs when there is an interruption to the regular process. This may be due to a deliberate event, such as implementation of a new policy, or an unexpected occurrence, such as a pharmacy technician calling in sick. In addition, special-cause variation could be desirable or undesirable. For example, if the PIC in the scenario described above receives patient complaints regarding prescription wait time, he or she may take action to reduce waits. If he or she hires a new technician to help decrease prescription wait times to shorter, more predictable periods, reductions in special-cause variation would be desirable and deliberate. On the other hand, if a pharmacy technician calls in sick for his or her shift, it is likely that a transient undesirable increase in prescription wait times due to the call-in will occur. Special-cause variation is not predictable, and it fluctuates over time. When special-cause variation is present, the system is considered to be out of the state of statistical control.[1-4]

SPC can be used to interpret the type of variability within a system to determine what changes need to occur to facilitate system improvement.[1,2] Often times eliminating special-cause variation will bring a system back to statistical control to produce the desired outcome. If a system is already in statistical control, management may need to make a change to make the system better,[1,2,5] such as hiring new staff as described above. A variety of common SPC tools are available to help pharmacists monitor and interpret the type of variability within their practice settings. They are described in the following section.

SPC TOOLS

The process of SPC should not be intimidating because many of the statistical tools necessary are descriptive (e.g., mean, standard deviation, median, and percent) and already known to most pharmacists. Most are readily available in spreadsheet programs such as Microsoft Excel. If one has a basic understanding of how to use spreadsheets, most tools in SPC should be easy to use. The following discussion will be spent showing the tools and how to interpret them. For specific directions on how to build SPC charts and other analysis tools, consult the Microsoft Excel website or other reference.

Histogram

A histogram is a graph that displays frequency distributions for unique categories of measure.[1] Histograms are useful for determining the overall shape of the data, data distribution, and variation in data. For example, the histogram in Figure 8-1 shows the range and frequency of times that it takes for new prescriptions to be ready for waiting patients at a community pharmacy. It appears that the majority of prescriptions were ready between 16 and 30 minutes after receiving the prescription. This information can be used to determine if the range is acceptable for prescriptions to be ready. It may also prompt an investigation to figure out why some prescriptions took so long to get ready (i.e., >50 minutes).

Pareto Chart

A Pareto chart, a type of histogram, categorizes data according to the most frequent issues on the left to the least frequent issues on the right.[1] The Pareto principle, which

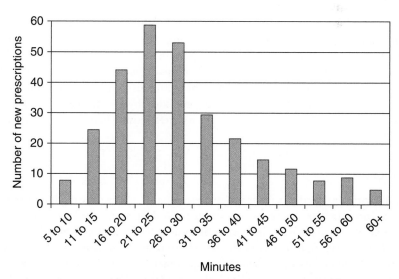

Figure 8-1. Histogram: time in minutes for new prescriptions to be filled in a community pharmacy.

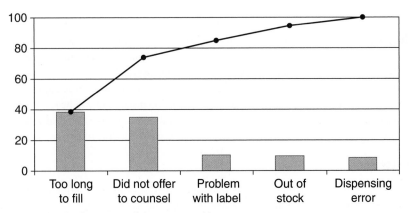

Figure 8-2. Pareto chart: types of dispensing problems.

states that 80% of your quality output comes from 20% of what you do, is the foundation for the chart. Pareto charts can assist in deciding which issues should be emphasized for problem-solving, thereby having a larger impact on quality improvement. The Pareto chart in Figure 8-2 reveals that 75% of dispensing problems can be attributed to two categories, too long to fill prescription and did not offer to counsel. Focusing on improvement in these two areas is likely to have a large impact on quality improvement in the dispensing process.

Scatter Diagram

Scatter diagrams show patterns in data and relationships between two variables for a unit of analysis (e.g., a patient). A statistical program can be used to plot the matching variables on a chart and conduct a regression analysis of the data on the chart. Analysis of the data allows a regression line to be drawn that shows the relationship between variables in the scatter diagram. The scatter diagram in Figure 8-3 illustrates how overall patient satisfaction relates to patient loyalty for each patient responding to a survey. In this instance, there is a positive relationship between satisfaction and loyalty.

Run Chart

A run chart can identify performance patterns and trends by showing how a variable changes over time. In Figure 8-4, you can tell that the percentage of patients receiving counseling prior to discharge from a hospital was stable for the first 5 months and then began to increase. Run charts can also be used to make comparisons among trends by using multiple variables. For example, the percentage of patients experiencing an adverse drug event can be compared with the percentage of patients receiving discharge counseling to see if they are related.

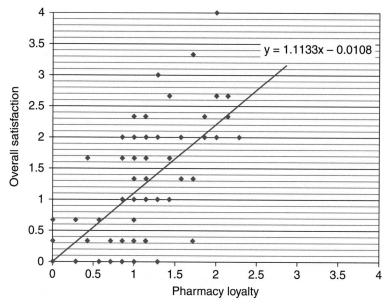

Figure 8-3. Scatter diagram: the relationship between pharmacy loyalty and overall patient satisfaction.

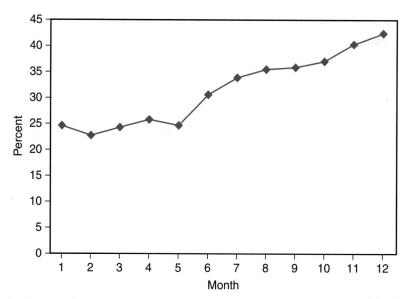

Figure 8-4. Run chart: percentage of patients receiving medication counseling prior to discharge from a hospital.

Control Chart

A control chart is a type of run chart. It is a key tool in SPC and serves as a visual aid to distinguish between common- and special-cause variations. A control chart is comprised of a series of measurements over time and three horizontal lines, which represent the upper control limit (UCL), mean, and lower control limit (LCL).[1,2] Variation that occurs between the UCL and LCL is considered to be acceptable and will not trigger a review of the system. Therefore, potential causes for the variation will not be investigated. Only the events outside the acceptable control limits are pursued. The control limits are typically set at 3 SD around the mean, which says that 99.97% of measures will fall within the control limits.[2] This approach allows only meaningful changes in the process to be captured and greater confidence that a measure observed outside of the control limits is really due to special-cause variation.

Figures 8-5 and 8–6 are examples of control charts of prescription fill times for two pharmacies in the same chain. Figure 8-5 depicts the average time it takes for a prescription to be filled at ABC Pharmacy. During the 12-month period shown, the times appear to be under control because they fluctuate around the mean between the UCL and LCL. On the other hand, Figure 8-6 depicts the average time it takes for a prescription to be filled at XYZ Pharmacy. The chart indicates that delivery times for the 8th and 11th months of the year are out of control, meaning that they fall way outside of what is expected by normal forms of variability. This may signify a problem with the prescription fill process and trigger an investigation to determine the cause of the variation.

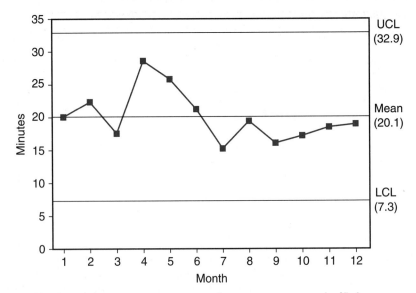

Figure 8-5. Control chart: average time in minutes for a new prescription to be filled at ABC Pharmacy.

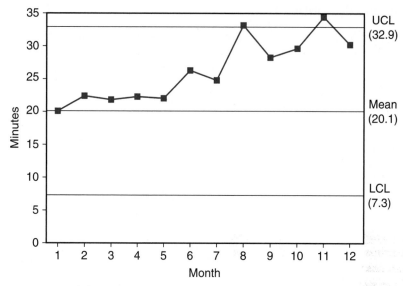

Figure 8-6. Control chart: average time in minutes for a new prescription to be filled at XYZ Pharmacy.

Sampling

Sampling is a technique that can be employed to measure a portion of the output of a system in order to judge its quality. Rather than testing the entire system, which can be time-intensive and expensive, a sample can be a quick way to assess system performance. Additionally, statistics can be used to extrapolate the results from a sample to predict the impact on the entire system with some level of confidence (e.g., ±2.5%).

Benchmarking

Benchmarking is used to make comparisons of an organization's processes and outcomes with the best practices of others. It is useful for an organization to know how it measures up against comparable entities to ensure that it is meeting or exceeding accepted best practices. Benchmarking also promotes learning by exposing an organization to new ideas and methods. The key is to benchmark oneself to an organization that can highlight one's performance, strengths, and deficiencies. Comparisons might be with departments within an organization (e.g., pharmacy and medicine departments), with competitors or peers (e.g., CVS and Walgreens), or across industries (e.g., Wal-Mart and Bank of America). Comparisons attempt to answer the following key questions: "How do the results of our benchmarks compare to us, and why?" "What can we learn from how they achieve their results?"

PERFORMANCE INDICATORS

The type of SPC tool that is utilized to detect variation within a system is often determined by the measures used to evaluate performance in an organization. These measures are called performance indicators and include sentinel event and aggregate data indicators. A sentinel event is defined by the Joint Commission on the Accreditation of Healthcare Organizations as "an unexpected occurrence involving death or serious physical or psychological injury, or the risk thereof." Sentinel events are generally rare within a system, but serious. Immediate action is required. Therefore, a sentinel event indicator would need to alert administrators that an event has occurred so that action can be taken. Aggregate data indicators, which can be rate-based or continuous, summarize the frequency of an outcome for a specific process. A rate-based indicator measures the rate of occurrence of an outcome, such as the number of dispensing errors per number of prescriptions dispensed, and can be presented in ratios or percentages. Continuous indicators are comprised of normally distributed data that typically provide an average score of a particular outcome. An example of a continuous indicator is average overall patient satisfaction scores. Performance indicators vary among pharmacy systems; however, good performance indicators have the following five characteristics:

1. accurate;
2. quantitative;
3. reliable;
4. sensitive;
5. simple.

A performance indicator must provide an accurate assessment of the quality process in order to be useful in detecting problems or areas for improvement. The indicator should also be able to be counted to provide a quantitative measure for statistical analysis. A performance indicator should only change when a condition changes, so reliability is also important. Sensitivity, which means significant differences can be detected over time or conditions, is another key quality of a performance indicator. Finally, the indicator must be simple for most people to collect, use, and understand.

INCORPORATING SPC INTO THE STEPS OF QUALITY IMPROVEMENT (PLAN, DO, CHECK/STUDY, ACT)

The Shewhart Cycle is a four-step approach [i.e., Plan, Do, Check/Study, Act (PDCA)] to improving quality in an organization.[1] SPC can be used at each step in the cycle. Below is a description of each step and an example of how to apply the PDCA approach with SPC tools to solve a quality problem. Figure 8-7 depicts a diagram of the cycle.

Plan

First, a plan is developed to study a system to find out how it can be improved. Once an area for improvement is identified, multidisciplinary teams of individuals are gathered to determine what type of change is necessary. The following are some questions to consider: What changes might be beneficial? What data are currently available? Are additional data necessary? If additional information is needed, a change or test can be

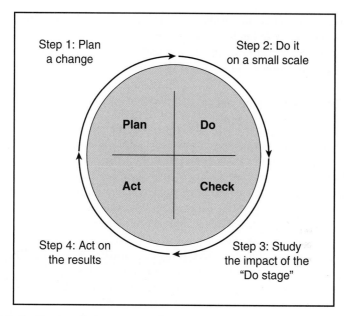

Step 1: Plan
a change

Step 2: Do it
on a small scale

Plan   **Do**

Act   **Check**

Step 4: Act on
the results

Step 3: Study
the impact of the
"Do stage"

Figure 8-7. The Shewhart Cycle: steps in quality improvement.

planned.[1] A histogram or Pareto analysis can be utilized in this step to pinpoint the problems that have the greatest impact on quality.

Do

If a change or test is necessary, it should be tested on a small scale.[1] This approach minimizes disruptions to the rest of the current system and allows the effectiveness to be evaluated before system-wide implementation of a new idea. Sampling can be used to test the new idea on a small scale, and a scatter diagram can be used to evaluate the relationship between new inputs into the system and the outcomes.

Check/Study

Next, the small-scale change or test should be checked to see if it works.[1] The new method should be compared with the old one to see if it makes the desired impact. Control charts are useful in this step to evaluate the consistency of data. The data can be compared visually using graphical analysis, and statistical analyses, such as T-tests, ANOVA, and group comparisons, may also be conducted.

Act

Finally, act on the findings of the small-scale study. If successful, the small-scale study should be implemented on a larger scale based on lessons learned in the "Do" and "Check" steps of the Shewhart Cycle. Sometimes, it might be necessary to collect additional information before deciding to implement a new idea on a larger scale. In these situations, the cycle can be repeated to perform more tests or continue to fine-tune a new process. Benchmarking can be a useful tool to compare the new process with other processes within and outside of the system.

A Case Example of Using SPC

The Director of Pharmacy at a hospital in the southeastern United States had received numerous complaints from physicians and nurses in the intensive care unit (ICU) regarding an increase in IV delivery times from the pharmacy. The Director was concerned about the complaints and decided to investigate the extent of the problem. Since the hospital staff just completed training in quality improvement, he or she decided to create a control chart from existing data to determine whether or not IV delivery times were unacceptable. Figure 8-8 shows a control chart with average IV delivery times by month to the ICU. Looking at the control chart, it can be seen that the delivery times were stable for the first 8 months and then they started to deteriorate. The delivery times increased in months 9 and 10, but they were still within acceptable limits of variability. However, the average delivery time in months 11 and 12 exceeded the UCL, indicating that IV delivery times had become unacceptable.

Next, the Director decided to create a committee to pinpoint the reason for the increase in delivery times. The committee consisted of the Director, a staff pharmacist, a pharmacy technician, and nurse. At the first meeting, the committee decided to use the PDCA approach to determine how to improve IV delivery times. They brainstormed to figure out reasons for the increase in delivery times. At the end of the brainstorming session, it was concluded that several reasons could be causing the increase: lack of a

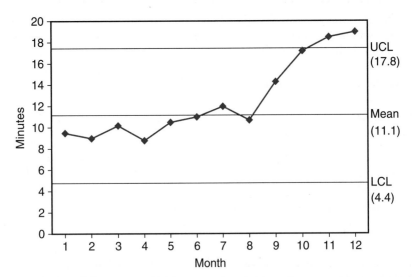

Figure 8-8. Control chart: average IV delivery times by month from pharmacy to intensive care unit.

standardized workflow, interruptions due to phone calls, a delay in pharmacist review of ICU orders since implementation of new computer system, or inadequate training. Since the committee was uncertain about how to prioritize the potential causes for the increase in delivery times, they decided to observe the process. The staff pharmacist on the team observed five ICU orders per day from the time it was received until the time of delivery for 2 weeks. The pharmacist reported that 58 out of 70 orders exceeded the UCL of 17.8 minutes and documented the reason (i.e., one of the four reasons described above) for the increased delivery time. The pharmacist created a Pareto chart to identify the most common causes of the increased delivery times for the orders that exceeded 17.8 minutes. The Pareto chart revealed that 54% of the increase in delivery times was due to a delay in pharmacist review, 30% was due to lack of a standardized workflow, 10% was due to phone interruptions, and 6% was due to inadequate training. The team further investigated the cause for the delay in pharmacist review. The old computer system had prioritized ICU orders by placing them first in the pharmacists' queue; however, the new system prioritized orders by time of entry. Therefore, nonurgent orders were being reviewed before the ICU orders, causing a substantial increase in delivery times. The committee met again to discuss the *plan* for improving the time of pharmacist review, and a member of the information technology (IT) team was asked to join the team.

During the meeting, it was decided that the new computer system should prioritize ICU orders by placing them first in the pharmacist's queue. This would require the IT team to create an update to the new program. In order to avoid interruptions to the entire system, the IT representative decided to test (*do*) the update with the staff pharmacist on the team. The team *checked* the update by a creating a run chart (Figure 8-9)

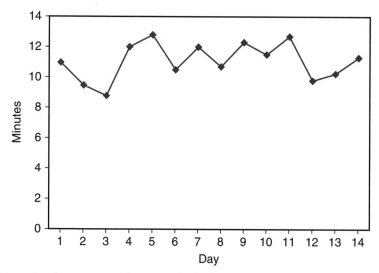

Figure 8-9. Run chart: average delivery times by day from pharmacy to intensive care unit after installation of update.

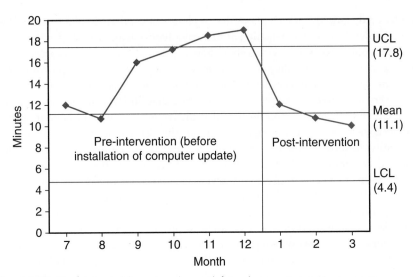

Figure 8-10. Control chart: delivery times by month from pharmacy to intensive care unit pre-intervention and post-intervention.

of the delivery times for the staff pharmacist's ICU orders over a 2-week period. The new computer program that prioritized ICU orders was successful in reducing IV delivery times; therefore, the update was installed on all pharmacists' computers (*act*). After just 1 month, the delivery times decreased to acceptable times once again and this was sustained for 2 more months (Figure 8-10). It was agreed that a control chart would be evaluated on a monthly basis to provide monitoring of ICU delivery times. The team decided to meet again and utilize the PDCA process to determine how to improve the workflow of the system, with the goal of decreasing the mean delivery time.

Incorporating SPC tools in the PDCA cycle was useful for identifying unacceptable variability in IV delivery times, identifying reasons for the increase in delivery times, and determining which problems were most responsible for increased delivery times. This allowed the team to focus their efforts on problems that were likely to have a meaningful impact on decreasing delivery times.

CONCLUSION

Monitoring variation in pharmacy systems can help identify areas for quality improvement. SPC is one method that can be used to interpret variation in pharmacy systems. SPC tools, such as histograms, Pareto charts, scatter diagrams, and run and control charts, can be incorporated into various steps in the quality improvement process to help monitor current systems to ensure quality performance and test new ideas for improvement.

REFERENCES

1. Walton M. *The Deming Management Method*. New York: Pedigree Books; 1986.
2. Benneyan JC, Lloyd RC, Plsek PE. Statistical process control as a tool for research and healthcare improvement. *Qual Saf Health Care*. 2003;12:458–464.
3. Thor J, Lundberg J, Ask J, et al. Application of statistical process control in healthcare improvement: systematic review. *Qual Saf Health Care*. 2007;16:387–399.
4. Kahn MG, Bailey TC, Steib SA. Statistical process control methods for expert system performance monitoring. *J Am Med Inform Assoc*. 1996;3:258–269.
5. Matthes N, Ogunbo S, Pennington G et al. Statistical process control for hospitals: methodology, user education, and challenges. *Qual Manage Health Care*. 2007;16(3):205–214.

Part III
Quality Measurement

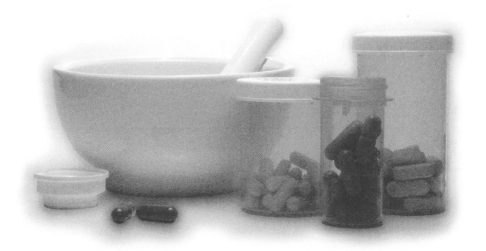

CHAPTER 9

Measuring Medication Safety and Quality

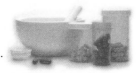

Susan J. Skledar and Robert J. Weber

Learning Objectives

At the end of the chapter, the reader will be able to:

1. Describe the importance of measurement of quality in health care and pharmacy.
2. Provide three examples of measures that can be used to assess pharmacy quality measures in pharmacy.
3. Propose a quality measure for pharmacy.

INTRODUCTION

During the 1990s, significant emphasis was placed on defining and evaluating medication errors and adverse drug events (ADEs). Researchers were published on the definition, incidence, and severity of these events.[1] The incidence and severity of medication errors discovered by these researchers prompted a federal review of errors as published in the first Institute of Medicine (IOM) report.[2] This report clearly showed the causes of medication errors and adverse events to be the result of faulty systems; it was also a call to action to implement systems to improve quality by reducing medication errors. Inherent to implementing systems to improve patient safety was to also develop a system for measuring the effectiveness of these system process and outcome measures.

At the beginning of the new millennium, the Agency for Healthcare Research and Quality (AHRQ) began funding research that measured the impact of patient safety interventions on the occurrence of medication errors and adverse events.[3] These research studies focused on equipment such as computerized physician order entry (CPOE). In addition, the Joint Commission on Accreditation and Health Care Organizations [now, The Joint Commission® (TJC)] placed a greater emphasis on organizations developing and implementing interventions to improve quality and safety, with the advent of national core quality measures and National Patient Safety Goals. Further, the second IOM report published in 2006 described ways to prevent medication errors, and stressed the importance of developing surveillance and reporting systems to track the effectiveness of patient safety interventions.[4] As the second IOM report gained more publicity, measuring quality and safety in health care became more important.

Organizations such as TJC required a specific quality organization improvement plan that measures the quality and safety of their patient care processes. As a result, most hospitals and health care organizations implemented quality improvement programs and applied them to medication-use processes. Many hospitals and health systems dedicated significant resources to quality improvement departments, and appointed Chief Quality Officers and/or Patient Safety Officers to assume responsibility and oversight for process improvements. Within the last 5 years, health care payors and the federal government are offering pay-for-performance programs for quality, with significant financial incentives attached to measuring and demonstrating improvement in patient care processes. In 2004, the national core quality measures of TJC and the Centers for Medicare and Medicaid Service became the same, helping to further focus hospital quality improvement efforts. Finally, continuous quality improvement (CQI) has been incorporated into most of TJC standards, particularly those related to medication management. Most of the current TJC standards for clinical departments require a comprehensive quality improvement plan.

CQI is defined as a systematic, organizational approach for continually improving all processes that deliver quality services and products.[5] CQI efforts must provide information and answer questions in the following areas: (1) primary aim of the improvement; (2) key stakeholders in affecting change; (3) measures showing that improvement has occurred; and (4) taking actions to ensure and sustain improvement. Developing an effective working team, creating and applying sound CQI methodology, promoting data integrity, and developing effective analysis tools are integral to the structure and process of quality improvement.

During their accreditation surveys, TJC examines a health care organization's program on quality improvement, and makes recommendations for new and innovative ways to improve it. Many recommendations of TJC are in the design of the quality improvement program; often the hospital or organization cannot show credible or sustainable results from process improvement projects since their design process was fundamentally flawed. For example, an organization may have initiated a quality improvement effort to improve the reporting of medication errors without analyzing the current state of reporting errors (describing the current problem). As a result, they are surprised when their efforts are minimal in sustaining a system for promptly catching medication errors. More surprisingly, TJC surveyors noted that many hospitals did not understand fully the individual components of a quality improvement program. The TJC also focuses on results of CQI efforts, and how those have been disseminated and learned from. They frequently ask clinicians to give examples of successful CQI efforts and ask leadership to explain how CQI data are maintained and disseminated.

It is critical to have a quality or performance improvement methodology that guides all CQI efforts within a health care organization. To make this matter more challenging, the economic downturn in the country has focused resources to patient-centered activities and has integrated, consolidated, and even eliminated resources for functions such as quality improvement. As a result, organizations must use their resources wisely and correctly and efficiently apply the techniques of quality improvement. As concerns for patient safety grow and as health care financial resources become more scarce, stakeholders (e.g., physicians, payors, hospital trustees, patients, etc.) expect that new systems (e.g., computers, pharmacy automation, and intravenous infusion pump technology) will maintain safety and quality.

A key part of the CQI process is *measurement*. A team cannot be successful in improving a process unless they can effectively measure the improvement; conversely, no CQI process is credible without a successful method of measurement. This chapter will describe several ways to measure improvement in medication safety that can be successfully incorporated into the CQI process.

This chapter focuses on methods and examples for measuring the quality and safety of the medication process. The aims of this chapter are to (1) review methods of measuring the quality of the medication process; (2) explain how failure modes and effects analysis (FMEA) is used to identify problems in health care; (3) describe the two most common CQI models, Lean/Toyota Production System and FOCUS-PDCA; and (4) provide two case examples of applying the FOCUS-PDCA process. This chapter will hopefully provide the reader with the tools to appropriately conduct and measure a quality improvement process in their organization.

MEASUREMENT METHODS IN MEDICATION SAFETY

The methods of measuring improvements in medication use are varied and should be tailored to the scope of the improvement project and its devoted resource and expertise. Importantly, however, results of measurement must be interpreted in the context of standard and accepted methods of defining medication errors and ADEs. There are essentially three methods of measurement that can be used in assessing both the baseline practice patterns and the impact of a new patient safety intervention: direct observation, surveillance, and voluntary reporting systems. The advantages and disadvantages of each method must be considered in measuring quality and safety. This section describes various ways to define medication errors, describes methods of measuring the incidence of errors, and discusses the management of data as a component of proper measurement.

Defining Medication Errors and Adverse Drug Events

Much time and effort has been spent on defining medication errors and ADEs. To many, this definition was a critical piece in proving real improvement in medication safety as well as a way to gain acceptance of medication safety efforts in a litigious environment. In reality, too much time has been spent on defining these terms. Dr Lucian Leape, a renowned expert in medication safety, has long believed that health care needs to get beyond defining and proving the incidence of medication errors, ADEs, and ADRs; the real work is in preventing medication errors and ADEs by fixing our broken medication systems.[6] Measuring the incidence of ADEs is a way to prove that our medication systems have been fixed.

Medication errors and ADEs must be clearly defined before any system of measurement can be effectively employed. These terms have been defined more completely and the reader is referred to several key references.[7,8] A medication error can be defined very broadly as any discrepancy in the ordering, preparation, dispensing, administration, and monitoring the effects of medications. An ADE is defined as any harmful event occurring as a result of a drug, and more specifically due to a medication error.[9] Not all medication errors lead to its most serious consequence such as an ADE; however, preventing medication errors at any point in the medication process has the potential to reduce ADEs.

An example illustrates the differences between medication errors and ADEs. Consider the case of two patients (Patient A and Patient B) who both receive a dose of digoxin that is too high for the compromised renal function of the patient. A medication error in prescribing occurred in Patient A and Patient B since the incorrect dose was prescribed for each patient. However, harm from this prescribing error (digoxin toxicity) occurs only in patient A. The events in these two patients would be documented as a medication error and ADE in patient A and a medication error in Patient B. An additional way to explain the differences between medication errors and ADEs is to say that medication errors describe process errors and ADEs describe clinical outcomes consequences.

Medication errors in the drug procurement (ordering of inventory) process consist of failing to order adequate stock of a medication to meet patient needs; ordering expired or adulterated medication; confusion with substitutions during product shortages and recalls; and ordering the incorrect product, strength, or dilution. Medication errors in drug preparation include preparing the incorrect drug, dose, or dilution of a product. Medication dispensing errors are defined as any discrepancy between the medication dispensed and the original prescriber's order. Likewise, a medication administration error is defined as any discrepancy between how the medication is given to the patient and the administration directions from the physician or hospital guidelines. Medication errors involved in monitoring and evaluating the effects of medication are defined as not assuring for proper follow-up of the therapeutic effect of a medication, or failing to recognize a medication side effect. Most importantly, medication errors in prescribing occur when the drug selected, the dose, frequency, or duration is not appropriate for the patient's disease or physiologic condition. A clear example of this is prescribing penicillin for a patient with a known allergy.

Direct Observation

Direct observation is one of the oldest methods used in demonstrating improvement in the medication process.[10,11] Observation has been shown to be the best method for detecting a variety of medication errors and their potential unique causes. In the early 1960s, Dr Kenneth Barker and associates used direct observation to determine the incidence of medication errors. Observation involves a person trained in *both* observation methods and the medication-use process to witness steps (medication preparation, dispensing, or administering) and document objectively how the process is carried out. For example, a person trained in observation and conducting a study of the effect of bar-code medication administration on errors would observe and document the following activity of the health care practitioner (nurse or other professional):

(1) review of the medication record; (2) selection of medication; (3) electronic scanning of the medication; and (4) administration of the medication.

An important point to consider when conducting observations to determine medication errors is that the observer must be completely blinded to any information related to the medication process, including if a medication error is occurring during the observation. In addition, the sample observed must be randomly selected. For example, a study was conducted to determine medication errors in a mail-order pharmacy.[12] The researchers reviewed the process of medication dispensing (refills, new orders, and stock medication) and objectively documented the activities of the dispensing pharmacy staff. They were totally blinded to the original prescription order as written by the physician and did not review the observed filled orders for medications until 1 week after the medication was dispensed. As a result, their observation would capture the true process occurring in medication dispensing.

The observation technique for medication error detection/measurement is offered by several proprietary vendors as well as colleges and universities in pharmacy and industrial sciences. While a powerful technique to measure the incidence of medication errors, it does not detect ADEs, or medication errors related to prescribing, or monitoring and evaluation of medication side effects. Medication errors related to medication administration, however, can be a useful quality indicator for many hospitals and health care organizations. Medication administration observations conducted across a relatively large sample of patients (e.g., 50–100 patients) produce a very reliable measure of medication administration accuracy.

Surveillance

Surveillance of the medication process is a passive approach to detecting medication errors. The most common surveillance method includes reviewing signals, triggers, or tracers for the incidence of medication errors and ADEs. Based on these signals or triggers, data can be reviewed manually, or electronically, to determine the error or ADE rate. Examples of electronic surveillance include: (1) electronic review of medication orders filled for "antidote" medications that may indicate a medication error or ADE (e.g., flumazenil for benzodiazepine overdose, naloxone for opioid overdoses, protamine for unfractionated heparin overdosing, and vitamin K_1 for warfarin dosing errors) or (2) electronic review of common laboratory side effects of medications (e.g., elevated creatinine, low glucose, or low platelets).

In general, surveillance methods identify situations with the potential for a medication error or an ADE; review of the situation and analysis must be completed to definitely determine whether an ADE or medication error occurred.

Voluntary Reporting Systems

Using voluntary reporting systems is the most common method for reporting medication errors. By definition, if a medication error or ADE is discovered, the person discovering the error reports the incident in a voluntary manner. The medication errors and ADEs are reported anonymously to a local, regional, or national depot of information.

Examples of this include an MS Excel™ spreadsheet for reporting at the local (hospital) level, database reporting of errors at the state-wide level (e.g., Pennsylvania Patient Safety Authority, www.psa.state.pa.us/), or the national FDA MedWatch™ reporting program (www.fda.gov/Safety/MedWatch/default.htm). These systems depend on health care workers to report medication errors and ADEs committed by themselves or others. As a result, very few medication errors and ADEs are reported through this process. Despite the fact that all voluntary reporting systems are anonymous, health care workers may be fearful to report medication errors and adverse events due to disciplinary concerns at their job or legal concerns from affected patients.

To track quality indicator progress over time, hospitals can create graphs, databases, or dashboards to represent data. In these formats, the baseline data are included, as well as the ongoing progress marked by data per day, week, or month, and the threshold (goal) for improvement. The threshold could be an internal benchmark based on prior performance, or could be a national target set by a safety or regulatory agency or published in the literature. Displaying the impact graphically is important to trend progress over time, and visual cues can be used within the data management plan to show performance above target (usually displayed in green), performance near target (displayed yellow), and performance below target (displayed red). These dashboards can be used daily to provide immediate feedback on performance and can also be used weekly, monthly, or quarterly to trend progress over time. Often, hospitals will use combined methods for displaying data.

PROBLEM IDENTIFICATION IN HEALTH CARE

Failure Modes and Effects Analysis

A key component of solving problems using a quality improvement model is to identify the correct problem, and choosing a problem that, if solved, will significantly improve the quality of a process. A method for identifying problems is called FMEA. This process is also called Healthcare Failure Mode and Effects Analysis (HFMEA), although the terms FMEA and HFMEA are used on an interchanging basis. FMEA analyzes processes to identity potential modes of failure along with the consequences of those failures. Simply stated, it identifies what could happen when something goes wrong.

The formal definition of FMEA is a method that "looks at a given process, identifies possible errors, and gauges what their effects could be, even before they take place."[13] Historically several key industries whose operations have critical consequences for failure – airlines, aerospace, transportation, water, gas, oil, and nuclear power – use FMEA. These industries realize that although systems can be made as fail-safe as possible, honest accidents and mishaps happen.[14] The FMEA process recognizes that errors may occur, but seeks to prevent the error from becoming an accident, through the use of a safety system, or "error trap."[15] The error trap is a series of actions that can improve the detection of the error, eliminate alternative processes that are dangerous, provide barriers for unsafe practices, and mitigate the adverse outcome of an error.[15]

As is the case with all successful collaborations to improve quality, FMEA is most effective when conducted through a multidisciplinary team of health care providers and administrators who are the major stakeholders for a given process. It is important to enlist "front-line" staff participation, as they can "map" the true workflow involved in the process being studied versus what ideally *should* be happening.

The steps in conducting an FMEA are summarized as follows. An individual or an organization identifies a process to be examined. In the realm of CQI, this process could be one with quality problems or the potential to have a significant impact on the quality of processes. The FMEA team of experts is then assigned to design an outline (or diagram) of the specific process flow, including as much relevant detail as possible. From this diagram or outline, the team decides which processes are key "functions"; functions are activities that contribute to a part or whole of a process. The team of experts then analyzes these functions to determine any and all modes of failure – and from this failure determine the potential outcome, or adverse consequences. Next the factors that contribute to the failure mode are identified along with controls or measures that manage a contributory factor to cause a failure. The impact of that contributory factor in causing the failure along with the ability to manage (or solve) the contributory factor is assessed. The contributory factors and their risk are prioritized using techniques such as a Pareto chart to determine the problem (contributory factor) that needs to be addressed in an improvement cycle along with the degree of risk (failure and adverse consequence) associated with the problem. The CQI team then uses this problem as the springboard to an applied CQI technique (lean production and FOCUS-PDCA).

The following brief case demonstrates the practical use of FMEA: an organization is implementing a system of patient-controlled analgesia (PCA) and is evaluating a series of infusion devices. The team is composed of experts from various areas of medication use, pain management, and biomedical engineering. The group knows of the reported issues associated with PCA and wants to avoid them. The group outlines the PCA clinical process and identifies three functions that may be error-prone and result in devastating consequences: loading of opioid PCA cartridge into the device, programming the correct drug dosing and concentration, and appropriately educating patients and families on using the device. The expert team decides that if the incorrect drug or concentration of the opioid were incorrectly loaded into the PCA device, errors would occur without recognition by the nurse; as a result, this function is placed as the highest potential for serious error. The factors associated with this error include the nurse not checking the medication to the physician order. The control identified to remedy this error is to have the capability of bar-code recognition of the medication cartridge by the PCA device. As a result of the problem identification along with the potential solution (bar-coding) through the HFMEA process, the organization specifically requests a required functionality of any PCA device purchased by their organization in bar-code reading of medication by the PCA device.

HISTORY OF CONTINUOUS QUALITY IMPROVEMENT

Measuring quality in health care dates back to the 19th century, with original work on gathering data, and then progression to managing quality pioneered by Ernest A. Codman. Quality improvement began as a science in the post-World War II era, with the industry work of a statistician, Walter Shewart. He focused on the incidence of process variation, determination of the cause of the variation, and elimination of that or those causes. He is most well known for creation of the of the Plan–Do–Check–Act (PDCA) cycle, which is a framework still used today that directs process change planning, implementation, check (or study) of that change, and action to sustain, spread, and/or adapt the change.[16] He also realized the importance of trending change impact over time, creating the statistical process control chart, which displays data over multiple measurement time points and incorporates upper and lower control limits to the data, capturing 95% of the variation in any given process. This chart can help to identify usual process variation, or "common noise" in a process, from special process variation, so CQI teams can focus on the special causes within their action plans. In any process, normal small variation should occur.

A colleague of Shewart was W. Edwards Deming. Deming was responsible for using the PDCA framework of Shewart and introducing this after World War II to the Japanese automobile industry.[17] Deming's fundamental philosophy is built on the principle that identification of problems is not a negative, but should be viewed as an improvement opportunity. The team should focus their efforts on the causes of the problem(s), specifically those causes that are in their control to affect change. Acknowledging that some causes are not within the scope of the teams' responsibility or purview is a reality. Once the causes are identified for action, then changes can be implemented as a pilot, or test, to hopefully eliminate, or at least reduce, the cause of the problem. Continual monitoring of process outcomes continues to be the backbone of CQI programs today, to enhance efficiency, improve quality, and maximize resources and output.

A physician, and scholar, named Donabedian, more than three decades ago, created what is still the fundamental method for measuring quality in health care: the structure–process–outcome (SPO) model.[18,19] He is known for challenging the health care industry to ask: "How can you tell if you have good quality health care?" He theorized that processes depend on structure within the health care environment, which can be resources, systems, and even philosophy. The process is the activity, method, or procedure used to deliver care. These processes can be often based on best practice in the literature or established national standards. The outcome then depends on the care provided. Measurement of these outcomes can include consequences of care such as readmissions, length of stay – morbidity and mortality measures – or humanistic outcomes such as patient satisfaction.[20] Simply stated, solid structure plus defined processes equals improved outcomes. Donabedian also is credited with expanding quality improvement beyond data management and process change to include the human element of impacting and managing change. Quality improvement transitioned into quality management, including people, access to care, and continuity of care.[21] He created what is known today as the "seven pillars of quality," which are characteristics of quality health care and how it should be provided: efficacy, effectiveness, efficiency, acceptability, optimality, equity, and legitimacy.[22] It is interesting that these principles coined years ago are similar to those from the 2001 IOM report of what health care should be: "safe, effective, patient-centered, timely, efficient, and equitable." These quality pioneers set the groundwork for what is still used in health care quality improvement strategies today.

CONTINUOUS QUALITY IMPROVEMENT MODELS

Lean/Toyota Production System

Since the era of World War II in the 1960s, the Japanese have founded what are still many basic elements of quality improvement today. The concepts include use of statistics to identify product or process defects, participation in quality efforts across all levels in an organization or group, the importance of communication and training, interdisciplinary teams, and real-time process changes. These principles are similar with CQI models, but industrial models of improvement, such as the lean production principle, also differ. Donabedian noted that the industrial model of health care QI is beneficial because of its focus on consumer (or customer) requirements and expectations, attention to system and process design to deliver and improve care, involvement of practitioners in addition to physicians in monitoring processes, increased role of management, and in-depth use of statistics.[23] He also noted several limitations of this model, including, but not limited to, the following:

- it may ignore how complex the clinical–patient relationship can be;
- more focus is on support or process activities than clinical ones;
- there is decreased emphasis on practitioner education and training.

Industry-like processes are suited best for workflow where the output is identical, and desired to be identical, every time, such as manufacturing of parts or assembly of motor vehicles. In pharmacy practice, examples of such processes are checking medications for cart fill or completing inventory orders. Repetitive steps, repeating cycles, and minimum worker discretion are evident. Laboratory workflow and operations are somewhat like an assembly line, in great contrast to diagnosis of patients' conditions, which requires professional clinical judgment. The assembly line should be defect-free and with minimal variability. The clinician and patient, however, will together do whatever is needed for promoting wellness and health.[5] Their workflow and processes have variable input (the patient condition), need for flexibility with standardized treatment plans (for unique and/or complex patient scenarios), and very high worker discretion and decision making.

Lean production models are centered on cost, time, and quality, at the same time. This model is derived from the Toyota Production System.[24] Originally called "Just in Time," to reflect having supplies available only on demand, the terms have changed to the Toyota Production System in the 1980s. The system realizes the key importance of the front-line worker to the daily processes, and the need to change processes to reflect a changing industry (at that time, automobiles). Factory workers could help with problem solving. The need to adapt to changing markets and allow for product variation was important. The model focuses on "reducing setups," with respect to decreased time to make a product and breaking it into small, simple, repetitive steps, and making "small batches" of product versus large quantities. This helps to reduce variation and also allows for rapid changes to product that may be needed due to changing times or technology. In the 1980s, American industry groups began to learn and embrace this process, and in the 1990s, the "principles of lean manufacturing" were coined. Lean manufacturing rests on five key principles[25]:

◖ *Cellular manufacturing*: Self-contained work units responsible for similar product lines.
◖ *Pull scheduling*: Replacing orders or inventory based on daily movement of product.
◖ *Total quality management*: Management of total process planning and assurance.
◖ *Rapid setup*: Creating small, predictable, rapid tasks versus large, infrequent processes.
◖ *Team development*: Knowledgeable and efficient team of problem solvers.

The overarching concepts of lean manufacturing are to minimize process steps, reduce or eliminate waste, harmonize people and technology, and zero-defect work. In contrast to CQI, the lean production model is relatively new to health care, and is only within the last 5–10 years being applied to health care quality improvement. Although much of health care is patient-specific, identification of processes that require identical output and have standardized procedures will lead to more opportunity to integrate lean production methodology into the health care administrator and medication safety officer's CQI thought process.

FOCUS-PDCA

The cycle of FOCUS-PDCA is a commonly used CQI method in health care delivery systems today. By using an integrated effort of work teams, data-driven analysis, careful planning and implementation, and measurement, this method successfully shows improvements in quality. FOCUS-PDCA is an acronym for F – find the problem, O – organize a team, C – clarify the current problem, U – understand the causes of process variation, S – select an opportunity for change, P – plan the change, D – do the change, C – check for improvement, and A – act to hold the gains.

Finding the problem involves using systems in your organization to detect unsafe, inefficient, or ineffective processes. To identify the problem in a hospital, several approaches can be taken. A review of voluntarily reported MEs and ADEs can be done. A baseline, or "snapshot," audit of practices related to medication prescribing, for example, can identify real-time opportunities for improvement. Data from clinical information systems or charge records can also be used to identify and focus the problem. Reports from the literature and safety organizations, such as the Institute for Safe Medication Practices (www.ISMP.org), can also be used to identify problems that may not have occurred in your organization. Continuing with the FOCUS-PDCA steps, organizing a team helps to further clarify the problem while also taking part in subsequent steps such as determining quality indicator measures, gathering and analyzing baseline compliance data, reviewing the literature for best practices, benchmarking other facility approaches to the problem, and determining the implementation plan. Having the team comprised of the major stakeholders in the process, and the content experts, as well as front-line staff who do the work each day, is critical to ensure that all possibilities for improvement are discussed.

Clarifying the problem and, in particular, simplifying the issue at hand is necessary to make the work of the team efficient and effective. This requires making a process flow diagram that clearly outlines steps in the process. Importantly, having content experts and staff workers involved will also depict most accurately the nature of the problem. It is important to understand the current practice as it exists, not as practitioners think it ideally happening. Understanding the variation in the current process to determine the frequency of the problem further directs the solution for change as well as resources necessary to make the change.

Selecting which change to make to improve quality must center on a change of such a magnitude as to practically see a tangible improvement in the process. The team often can be aided by tools used to prioritize problems, such as a Pareto chart or frequency chart. This chart will help to rank the specific causes in highest to lowest frequency of occurrence, to graphically target what causes have the most impact. Returning to this diagram after process improvement actions are implemented is also helpful, as next steps for action can be determined around the next most frequent causes identified.

Improvements in processes often failing are the crux of planning the change; the change can be in the form of a wide-scale or pilot change. The pilot change must be defined in terms of length of time, so as to properly quantify the effects of the pilot and to identify successes and barriers. The pilot change should not be continued unnecessarily when it could be expanded. Stopping points in the pilot should be identified at the outset also, in case the impact of the change is not what was intended. Attempting wide-scale, complex changes will fail, and most likely cause larger and more difficult problems to solve. Wide-scale changes in a process to improve quality are most successful if they include a very concrete change that can be easily implemented in a variety of areas throughout an organization.

Doing the change, or implementation, can be challenging, but it is at the heart of a successful improvement project. This step involves taking the actions in the planning phase and carrying them out. Time must be allowed for implementation, as this includes training, process and system change, and updation or creation of materials for education. Implementation can depend on the right composition of the team, selecting appropriate communication strategies, and appropriate time delineation for learning and testing. Optimal methods for implementation have been studied in the literature, and have been reported, for example, to include computerized reminders and focused education in small groups as generally effective strategies, retrospective feedback as variably effective, and passive education programs (didactic lectures without case application) as least effective.[26]

Checking the results of the change in the post-implementation period involves measuring processes in a manner consistent before the change was completed. For example, any quality indicator data that were collected before the change should be again measured against the baseline performance. Additional quality measures can be added to the data collection process, especially as the data begin to be generated and problems are identified. Holding the gains, or *a*cting to sustain the improvement (A in FOCUS-PDCA), is also challenging, but tests the rigor of the conducted quality improvement process. All too often, an improvement effort works very well at the outset, but then processes and behaviors change over time to what was happening prior to the change. Continued diligence with monitoring, education, and feedback are important to sustaining, or holding, the gained benefit. To achieve this result, accountability to team members for ongoing data collection should be assigned. If the improvements are ongoing, and nearly all of them will be, as situations change, the next cycles of improvement can be planned. Even after the improvement in quality is achieved and sustained, the team often will stay as a functioning unit, but may meet less regularly or even electronically to review the compliance data.

CASE EXAMPLES IN QUALITY IMPROVEMENT MEASUREMENT

CASE EXAMPLE 1: IMPLEMENTING DECENTRALIZED PHARMACY SERVICES

Find the problem.
At your facility, there have been numerous concerns expressed from nurses, physicians, and even patients related to timeliness of medication delivery and appropriateness of dosing. There is a perception that it takes greater than 6 hours on the average for a newly ordered medication to arrive on the unit for patient administration. The medication administration records that the nurses are using to pass medications to patients are also often incorrect or outdated with current therapies. The pharmacy services are currently centralized, with central operations on the first floor of the hospital, geographically distant from the inpatient care units. You are charged with designing a decentralized pharmacy services plan that would provide a solution to both problems.

Organize the team.
The team should include the Pharmacy Director and Nursing Administrator as advisors, or the "Guidance Team" and also may include a physician as well. The project team should include pharmacists, nurses, pharmacy technicians, a Pharmacy Manager, and at least one Nursing Director. It may also be necessary to include a pharmacy information systems person, as decentralization of workflow will require enhanced technological capabilities. Customers and their expectations also should be defined, as this helps to ensure you have the right membership on the team. Figure 9-1 and Table 9-1 describe the geographic issues and considerations for customers and their expectations.

Clarify the current problem
A flowchart, or process map, should be prepared to walk through the current medication ordering and delivery process. This will shed light on the current workflow and stimulate brainstorming as to where the process can be improved and/or re-evaluated. Figure 9-2 is an example flowchart of this process. To further define the problem, the team must determine quality indicator measures

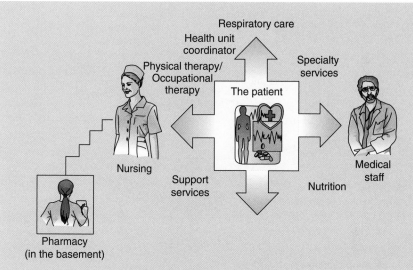

Figure 9-1. Pharmacy's challenge regarding geographics.

that will appropriately track the impact of process improvements. Key quality indicators (or measures) are determined to be:

◯ nursing satisfaction with pharmacy services;

◯ medication delivery turnaround time;

TABLE 9-1. Customers and Expectations

Customers	Expectations
Patients	Right medication at the right time Medication safety
Pharmacists	Safe and non-distracting work environment Job satisfaction and challenge
Pharmacy technicians	Improved workflow Job satisfaction
Nurses and physicians	Safe medication practices Timely responsiveness to patient care needs
Pharmacy administration	Improved recruiting for new staff Improved retention of experienced staff
Risk management Patient relations	Decreased medication errors and adverse events Decreased complaints

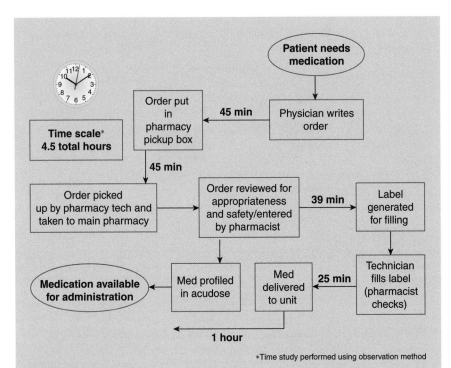

Figure 9-2. Process flow.

● missing dose calls to pharmacy;
● documentation of pharmacist interventions.

Data sources for these indicators are a satisfaction survey (designed and administered pre-improvement, and then again post-improvement), observations, missing dose tracking log kept by pharmacy, and the pharmacy's intervention database, respectively. Measurement will be done pre- and post-implementation via audit (snapshot) method, as well as monthly data collection. Pharmacy will have the responsibility for data collection and monthly reporting. Baseline data reveal that nursing satisfaction is poor, and that delivery time is greater than 4 hours. Eighty percent of calls to pharmacy are for missing doses, and pharmacists are only documenting approximately 10% of their potential interventions. Initial targets for each indicator were set with the team, and these can be modified as the data post-implementation are generated. Benchmarking pharmacy services across hospitals with similar bedside and patient populations also can yield helpful information, so the team decides to do a survey on the pharmacy listserv to gather that information. Questions asked include: bed size, automation support, satellite pharmacy support, information systems detail, and wireless technology

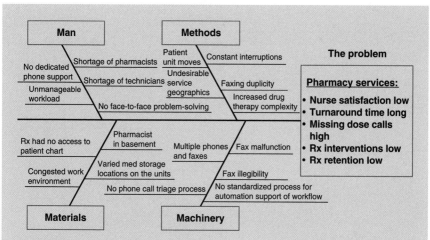

Figure 9-3. Understand practice variation.

extent. The final part of the "C" step is to evaluate the current literature on decentralized pharmacy service models and solutions to improving pharmacy services. Studies noting impact of pharmacists on reducing adverse events and improving patient care delivery also should be reviewed, and service models in those articles discussed. Key journals for these types of articles are the *American Journal of Health-system Pharmacy, Pharmacotherapy, Hospital Pharmacy,* and the *Journal of the American Medical Association.*

Understand causes of process variation.
The multidisciplinary team brainstorms causes of the problems with pharmacy services, and puts the ideas into a cause-and-effect diagram, to group the causes into like categories (Figure 9-3). Causes include multiple distractions in the pharmacy for pharmacists with competing demands, extended delivery times, pharmacy's location in relation to patient units, and different storage locations for medications on the units. These brainstormed causes were grouped into three major categories: workload burden in the central pharmacy, geographics, and medication distribution process flow issues.

Select opportunity for change.
The team decided that the focus of the improvement should be to plan for decentralizing the pharmacists onto the patient units, in service-based care teams, with a pharmacist and pharmacy technician partnership for the nurses and physicians (Figure 9-4).

Plan the change.
The team begins regular weekly meeting, with attendees in-person (versus teleconferences) to work out the building blocks for decentralized service options.

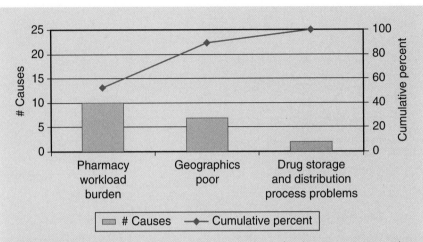

Figure 9-4. Select opportunity for change. The major reasons for pharmacy services needing improvement are workload burden and the physical removal of daily activities from the direct care of patients.

The team gathers additional data on which units are the most medication-intensive, and where service complaints have been placed. Clarification of roles of the pharmacists and pharmacy technicians is established. In-depth discussions occur regarding consolidation of medication drop-off areas on the units, automated medication station stock, and mechanisms to contact pharmacists if drug information is needed. Use of technology is evaluated, including the logistics of remote order entry from the patient unit to the central pharmacy, which is as many as eight floors away. The use of pagers versus phones is discussed, and the team decides they would like the use of pagers, to allow the pharmacists to rotate through their service units freely during their shift. The pharmacy technician also will have a pager, so they can be the main point of contact for missing doses and drug storage/location questions. The pharmacist will be paged for clinical and patient medication therapy information. With the extent of these changes, the team decides the best approach is to initiate decentralized services via a pilot, or test. One surgical intensive care unit and one surgical ward are chosen for the pilot, which will last 3 months.

Do the change.
The team designs promotional materials and team contact signs for the project, and attends pharmacy and nursing leadership and staff meetings to promote the initial pilot service plans. A timeline grid is created to keep the tasks needing to be done on track, and this grid is reviewed and sets the agenda for the continued weekly meeting. The informatics team estimated that it will take them a month to set up pagers, phones, and computer access on the

units to the information system, and during that time, order entry stations were identified for the pharmacist. Medication rooms were reorganized and consolidated also for ease of medication access on the pilot units. Pharmacists also asked for educational modules to review therapeutics concepts and basic clinical knowledge. A staff education program was created by a working group of the larger team, focusing on medication safety, review of analgesia and antibiotic management, and hospital formulary decisions, since the pilot would be in surgical care areas. Planning for the pilot took 6 months. Once the pilot completed, it was estimated that new teams could be decentralized monthly until the key hospital service areas were covered. Administration was supportive of obtaining new pharmacist positions to sustain this service model, and filling current vacancies as well. The analysis of full-time equivalents needed for the service is facility-dependent, and is beyond the scope of this chapter. It is key though that this topic be addressed early on in planning, as it may have impact on decisions of how quickly the decentralization plan can be implemented. The data generated from the pilot can also help to facilitate staffing decisions.

Check the change.

Once the pilot was implemented, data are generated to show the impact of service enhancements. A repeat satisfaction survey was administered to nurses on the pilot units at the end of the third month, and observations of turn-around time were again collected. The calls to pharmacy for missing doses were reduced, and the pharmacists were able to document many more interventions due to their workload being more focused and balanced on the units. Sample graphics shown in Figures 9-5 to 9-7 demonstrate results and examples of how to display the data to show the success of the decentralized model. The team also uses these data to discuss barriers that have arisen, for example, data showing that turnaround time is improved during decentralized service hours, but continues to need improvement during off-shifts. Also, nurses expressed concern with having to remember multiple pager numbers, so a plan to have one pharmacy contact number (the technician) to triage calls was implemented, to further allow the pharmacist to focus their clinical work. Tracking the calls to the decentralized pharmacy team showed that the majority of calls were better handled by the technician related to missing doses and automation questions, so the nurses were comfortable with the technician being the first point of contact.

Act to hold the gains.

In this case, the data generated in the pilot showed that turnaround time improved, as well as nursing satisfaction. The pilot was determined to be a success, and decentralization continued across the hospital over the next year. It was important that pharmacist and pharmacy technician satisfaction with this

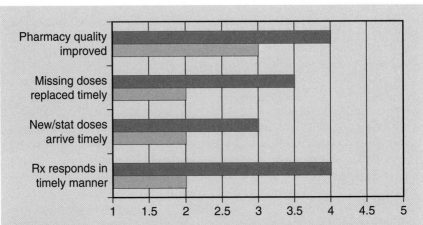

Figure 9-5. Survey of nursing satisfaction in the intensive care unit. Lightly shaded bars represent pre-model and darkly shaded bars represent post-model. Scale (median): 1, strongly disagree; 5, strongly agree.

enhanced clinical role was measured, so new quality measures were designed to track this as well as tracking of pharmacist turnover and vacancy rates. Once the decentralization efforts were completed, impact of pharmacist activity on medication errors and adverse events was also analyzed as the outcome indicator measures. The team continues to meet monthly to discuss successes, failures, and lessons learned.

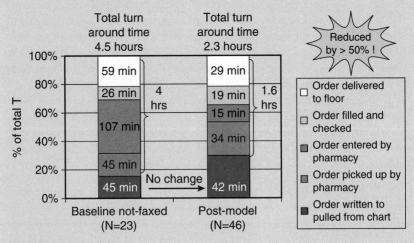

Figure 9-6. Turnaround time.

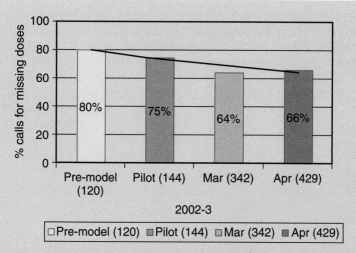

Figure 9-7. Missing dose calls. Each number in parentheses represents the total number of calls recorded.

CASE EXAMPLE 2: REMOVING MEPERIDINE FROM THE HOSPITAL FORMULARY

Find the problem.
The Pain Nurse Specialist for the surgical services at your facility approaches you about ADEs she has witnessed as well as anecdotal concerns that patients are having seizures related to overuse of meperidine (MEP) for postoperative analgesia. She asks if you are willing to work with the Pain Service on a proposal to remove meperidine from the hospital formulary. With other effective and safer opioid analgesics available, you are charged to help with this important safety initiative.

Organize the team.
The team should include a pharmacist content expert, a Pain Service nurse and physician, a surgeon, an Emergency Department physician, and a pharmacist or nurse who would know or have access to adverse event data for your hospital. Anesthesiology physicians or nurse anesthetists also may want to be involved since much of their focus is pain management. Customers and expectations can include patients (expect pain relief), nurses (expect analgesics to be readily available and appropriate for individual patients), physicians (expect protocols and safe practice enforcement), pharmacists (expect evidence-based practice and adequate analgesia), and risk/patient safety (expect reduced ADEs and harm).

Clarify the current problem.
To describe the current process, a flow diagram is created to explain how an order for meperidine is generated. The team discusses the therapeutics of analgesia and

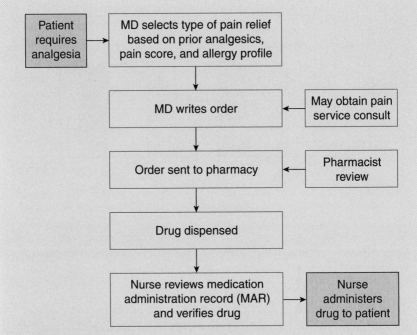

Figure 9-8. Flowchart for selection of analgesic drug.

how a prescriber would decide that meperidine may be a viable option for the patient (see Figure 9-8). The team must ensure that if meperidine is removed from the formulary, or categorized as a restricted medication, alternative analgesic choices are available with dosing strategies provided for clinicians. Quality indicator measures chosen relate to process and outcome: percent use of meperidine by route of administration (process), percent versus total opioid (process), and meperidine adverse events by severity (outcome). Initial data show 12 ADEs reported in the last year, including idiosyncratic allergies, and neurotoxic effects of seizures and hallucinations, which validates the anecdotal reports of the nurses. In a snapshot audit of meperidine usage, or a drug use evaluation, only 20% of the use of meperidine is clinically appropriate. Other opioids could be used in the majority of cases. If the proposal is accepted to completely remove from formulary and designate meperidine as a "no buy" opioid, then meperidine use should decrease to zero doses as the target. See Table 9-2 for a list of indicators. Literature support for the dangers of using meperidine is compiled; key references are provided in Table 9-3.

Understand causes of process variation.
The causes of the problems of meperidine adverse events and overuse were brainstormed by the team (Figure 9-9). Causes included lack of knowledge of the

TABLE 9-2. Meperidine Quality Measures

Example measures
Meperidine adverse drug events (per total meperidine doses dispensed)
Severity III meperidine adverse drug events
Compliance with meperidine guidelines (avoiding meperidine use)
Meperidine use by route of administration (avoiding IM, patient-controlled analgesia, and PO meperidine)
Meperidine use versus total opioid use

safety profile of meperidine, and its availability as a choice on the hospital formulary, although there was no specific hospital protocol available currently. An analysis of the adverse events showed that neurotoxic adverse events occurred most frequently, other than allergic reactions. The team determined that the

TABLE 9-3. Evidence in the Literature

Source	Role of Meperidine
American Pain Society (6th ed. Glenview, IL: 2008)	Do not prescribe for chronic pain; do not use for >48 hours for acute pain; do not exceed 600 mg/24 hours
"Beers" list (Fick DM, Cooper JW, Wade WE et al. *Arch Intern Med.* 2003;163:2716–2724)	Inappropriate medication for elderly patients; not an effective oral analgesic; may cause confusion
ASHP/SCCM Guidelines (*Am J Health Syst Pharm.* 2002;59: 150–178)	Do not use repeated doses in the critically ill adult; use hydromorphone, morphine, or fentanyl
Meperidine: A Critical Review (Latta KS, Ginsberg B, Barkin RL. et al. *Am J Ther.* 2002;9:53–68)	Narrow therapeutic niche (<24th), if at all, for procedural use; gold standard analgesic is morphine or hydromorphone; PCA option is fentanyl
Acute Pancreatitis Guidelines (Toouli J, Brooke-Smith M, Bassi C et al. *J Gastroenterol Hepatol.* 2002;17(suppl):S15–S39; Banks PA. *Am J Gastroenterol.* 1997;92:377–386)	Does not state meperidine preference over other analgesics for control of acute pancreatic pain

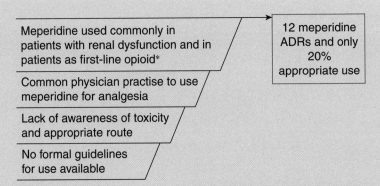

Figure 9-9. Analysis of root causes. (*) Inappropriate indications according to the literature review.

focus of the work would be to eliminate meperidine as a formulary choice, and also ensure that appropriate allergy checks were in place for patients with opioid allergies. The team gathered existing informal protocols and physician inservice materials and began to determine the extent of the revisions that would be needed.

Select opportunity for change.
The adverse event data, literature, and anecdotal concerns support the concept of removing meperidine from formulary, or at least placing tight restrictions on its use. A review of other institution practices also found several sites that restrict meperidine use to Pain Service and Anesthesiology content experts, in the case that a patient has a combined hydromorphone/morphine allergy and fentanyl cannot be used on a non-monitored unit, as is the case in many hospitals. Several sites have had success at removal of select dosage forms of meperidine from the formulary, specifically PCA, since it is high doses at repeat intervals that can lead to meperidine and its neurotoxic metabolite, normeperidine, accumulation and neurotoxicity. As the work begins to plan the safety improvement, the team is reminded that medication-use protocols must be endorsed by the physicians in the involved service areas (in this case anesthesiology, surgery, emergency medicine, trauma, and gastroenterology), but that the Pharmacy and Therapeutics Committee will have the final approval on a restriction protocol or designation as a "no buy" non-formulary medication.

Plan the change.
Planning involved the pharmacist creating the evidence-based document that compiles the data and literature on the dangers of meperidine, along with viable therapeutic opioid alternatives. Time is needed to create the document, as well as gather content expert input on additional published practices guidelines and

safety literature to include. Although no formal, approved hospital protocols exist that include meperidine, six different printed and typed order sets were found that included meperidine as an option. These needed to be changed. The hospital also was beginning its work on CPOE, so the electronic protocols and formulary had to be matched to the decision that was about to be made. Additionally, training materials for physicians (both leaders and trainees), nurses, and pharmacists had to be created to explain the reason for the formulary change, since meperidine was thought of as a relatively safe agent. Case examples of adverse events were de-identified and used as this information was presented to hospital committees and physician groups. A timeline was created with action steps for the group to follow. This served as the agenda for the biweekly meetings that were in place. It took the team 3 months to compile the data and finalize the written document and its accompanying educational pieces.

Do the change.

The evidence-based review was supported by the physicians at every level of the organization. One physician group had concerns that in the setting of pancreatitis, meperidine provided an advantage of causing less sphincter of Oddi pressure than other opioids. It was discussed that the latest practice guidelines (see references in Table 9-3) denote that morphine and hydromorphone can be used in this setting with equivalent analgesic efficacy and lesser safety concerns. One-time use of meperidine for postoperative shivering and drug-induced rigors was permitted, and other meperidine uses were deemed non-formulary. Meperidine PCA, for the reasons noted above (and see also Figure 9-10), was removed from formulary and designated as a "no buy" agent. Educational inservices were completed once the proposal was accepted, and computer support was revised and aligned. Pharmacists would have the responsibility to contact prescribers if they ordered meperidine outside of these guidelines. Table 9-4 lists the complete list of the multifaceted implementation strategy used. Figure 9-11 displays the post-implementation process flow changes that occurred.

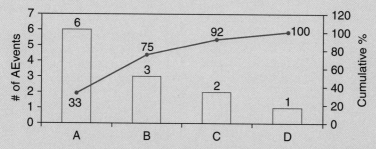

Figure 9-10. Pareto chart of reported adverse drug events for meperidine; $N = 12$. (A) Allergy; (B) central nervous system reactions; (C) renal toxicity; (D) gastrointestinal side effects.

TABLE 9-4. Implementation Strategies

Strategy for Reducing Use of Meperidine	Done
Formulary restrictions to one-time use	✓
Removal from preprinted order forms	✓
Removal of PCA meperidine from the formulary	✓
Computer alert	✓
CPOE order sentences denote alternatives	✓
Active pharmacy intervention	✓
Update of hospital electronic "Pain Card" guidelines	✓
Intranet posting of guideline	✓
Continuing medical education article	✓
"Med Alert" to prescribers	✓

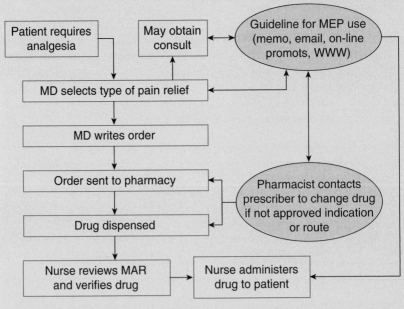

Figure 9-11. Process changes made (see the shaded areas).

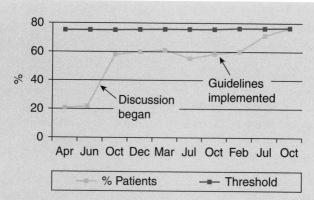

Figure 9-12. Results: percent appropriate meperidine use.

Check the change.

Post-implementation, data demonstrate that the formulary change has been successful. Pharmacy is responsible for the data collection, and data are collected from a combination of purchase and usage records, along with electronic health record (or paper) chart review. Data are collated by physician prescribing service for any outliers that are identified. With the formulary restriction and "no buy" designation, the use of meperidine has declined compared with total opioid, and the use now is in appropriate circumstances over 80% of the time (see Figures 9-12 and 9-13). Work will continue to identify outliers, upkeep the clinical information systems, and new literature.

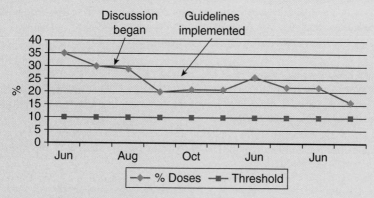

Figure 9-13. Results: percent meperidine versus total opioids.

Act to hold the gains.
The work of the team and the successful limitation for meperidine in the inpatient setting has set the stage for other safety initiatives at the hospital and across the health system. This template of collaboration will be used for identifying additional safety changes and steps needed for success. Continued tracking of the quality indicators will occur monthly, and pharmacists will continue the daily intervention on inappropriate therapy if it occurs. The upcoming CPOE system will not have meperidine CPOE as an orderable formulary choice.

SUMMARY

Measuring the safety and quality of our health care requires a systematic approach using a variety of quality improvement techniques. Which technique is chosen depends on the available resources at an organization along with previous experience, skill, or training in a given technique. The goal of using any CQI technique is to demonstrate that clinical or process outcomes have changed resulting in improved quality of life for our patients.

REFERENCES

1. Bates DW, Cullen DJ, Laird N, et al. Incidence of adverse drug events and potential adverse drug events. *JAMA*. 1995;274:29–34.
2. Institute of Medicine (IOM). *To Err is Human: Building a Safer Health System*. Washington, DC: National Academy Press; 2000.
3. Agency for Healthcare Research and Quality (AHRQ). *Advances in Patient Safety: From Research to Implementation*. Vol 1–4. Rockville, MD: AHRQ; 2005.
4. IOM. *Preventing Medication Errors*. Washington, DC: National Academy Press; 2007.
5. McLaughlin CP, Kaluzny AD. Defining quality improvement. In: McLaughlin CP, Kaluzny AD, eds. *Continuous Quality Improvement in Health Care: Theory, Implementations, and Applications*. Sudbury, MA: Jones and Bartlett Publishers; 2006:3–4.
6. Leape LL, Bates DW, Cullen DJ, et al. Systems analysis of adverse drug events. *JAMA*. 1995;274:35–43.
7. Bates DW, Boyle DL, Vander Vliet MB, Schneider J, Leape L. Relationship between medication errors and adverse drug events. *J Gen Intern Med*. 1995;10:199–205.
8. Gandhi TK, Seger DL, Bates DW. Identifying drug safety issues: from research to practice. *Int J Qual Healthc*. 2000;12:69–76.
9. Brennan TA, Leape LL, Laird NM, et al. Incidence of adverse events and negligence in hospitalized patients: results of the Harvard Medical Practice Study 1. *N Engl J Med*. 1991 Jul 25;325(4):245–251.
10. Allen EL, Barker EN. Fundamentals of medication error research. *Am J Hosp Pharm*. 1990; 47:555–571.
11. Barker KN, Flynn EA, Pepper GA, Bates DW, Mikeal RL. Medication errors observed in 36 healthcare facilities. *Arch Intern Med*. 2002;162:1897–1903.

12. Varadarajan R, Barker KN, Flynn EA, Thomas RE. Comparison of two error-detecting methods in a mail service pharmacy serving healthcare facilities. *J Am Pharm Assoc.* 2008;48:371–378.

13. Cohen MR, Senders, J, Davis NM. Failure mode and effects analysis: a novel approach to avoiding dangerous medication errors and accidents. *Hosp Pharm.* 1994;29:319–324, 326–328, 330.

14. Feldman SE, Roblin DW. Medical accidents in hospital care: applications of failure analysis to hospital quality appraisal. *Jt Comm J Qual Improvement.* 1997;23:567–580.

15. Senders JW. Theory and analysis of typical errors in a medical setting. *Hosp Pharm.* 1993;28:506–508.

16. Skledar SJ. Continuous quality improvement. In: Hagel HP, Rovers JP, eds. *Managing the Patient-centered Pharmacy.* Washington, DC: American Pharmaceutical Association; 2002:217–238.

17. Deming EW. *Out of Crisis.* Cambridge, MA: MIT Center for Advanced Engineering Study Publishing; 1982.

18. Donabedian A. A founder of quality assessment encounters a troubled system firsthand. Interview by Fitzhugh Mullan. *Health Aff (Millwood).* 2001;20:137–141.

19. Donabedian A. The effectiveness of quality assurance. *Int J Qual Health Care.* 1996;8: 401–407.

20. Varkey P, Reller K, Resar RK. Basics of quality improvement in health care. *Mayo Clin Proc.* 2007;82:735–739.

21. Lynn ML, Osborn DP. Deming's quality principles: a health care application. *Hosp Health Serv Admin.* 1991;6:111–120.

22. Donabedian A. The seven pillars of quality. *Arch Pathol Lab Med.* 1990;114:115–118.

23. Donabedian A. *Models of Quality Assurance. Leonard S. Rosenfeld Memorial Lecture, School of Public Health,* University of North Carolina at Chapel Hill, February 26; 1993.

24. Strategos, Inc. *Lean Manufacturing History.* Available at http://www.strategosinc.com/just_in_time.htm. Accessed October 4, 2009.

25. Strategos, Inc. *Lean Manufacturing Principles.* Available at http://www.strategosinc.com/principles.htm. Accessed October 10, 2009.

26. Gross PA, Greenfield S, Cretin S, et al. Optimal methods for guideline implementation – conclusions from Leeds Castle meeting. *Med Care.* 2001;39:85S–92S.

CHAPTER 10

Consumer Assessment of Pharmacy Quality

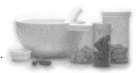

Susan J. Blalock and San Keller

Learning Objectives

At the end of the chapter, the reader will be able to:

1. Discuss the origin, background, and goals of the Consumer Assessment of Healthcare Providers and Systems.
2. List the preliminary domains covered by the Pharmacy Consumer Experience Survey.
3. Identify how the survey can be used to improve patient outcomes with pharmaceuticals.
4. Project the future of the Pharmacy Consumer Experience Survey.

Most people, at one time or another, find themselves in need of ambulatory care pharmacy services. They may need to fill a prescription for a medication, purchase an over-the-counter product, obtain information concerning the medications they are using, or get assistance and advice concerning a broad array of disease prevention and illness self-management issues. In the process of obtaining these services, consumers gain considerable experience-based information concerning the quality of the services they receive. But, other than by word-of-mouth, consumers have had little way of passing this valuable information on to others who may be able to use it. Thus, in most cases, the information relevant to evaluating pharmacy quality that consumers gain through their personal interactions with pharmacies is lost. Quality of care surveys are designed to address this issue by providing a mechanism through which the information that patients gain through personal experiences can be captured, preserved, and summarized.

At the broadest level, one can distinguish between two dimensions of health care quality: (1) the technical or clinical aspects of care and (2) the experiences patients have during the process of seeking and obtaining services.[1] With respect to pharmacy services, technical aspects of care include: whether the patient obtains the correct medication, whether medications are labeled appropriately, and whether the pharmacist checks for potential interactions among the medications that the patient is taking. But, even if these services are provided optimally, the quality of care may be poor from the patient perspective. Pharmacy staff may not give the patient the amount of attention desired or needed, questions may not be answered adequately, or sensitive topics may be discussed without sufficient privacy to prevent embarrassment. These are aspects of health care quality that require consumer input to evaluate.

In this chapter, we discuss recent efforts to develop a standardized survey that can be used to capture consumer assessments of the quality of services they receive during ambulatory care pharmacy encounters. These efforts build on work conducted by the Consumer Assessment of Healthcare Providers and Systems (CAHPS) consortium. Thus, we begin by providing background information about the CAHPS program. Next, we discuss work conducted to develop the Consumer Assessment of Pharmacy Services survey and the instrument that resulted from this work. We then describe how the Consumer Assessment of Pharmacy Services survey might be used in practice to facilitate quality improvement efforts and issues that must be addressed in the interpretation of survey scores. Finally, we discuss directions for future work in this area.

THE CONSUMER ASSESSMENT OF HEALTHCARE PROVIDERS AND SYSTEMS PROGRAM

The CAHPS program was initiated in 1995 by the Agency for Healthcare Research and Quality (AHRQ) and continues to be sponsored and supported by AHRQ.[2,3] Originally launched as the Consumer Assessment of Health Plans Study, the CAHPS program has two interrelated goals. The first goal of the program is to develop a set of standardized questionnaires that assesses the quality of health care services from the perspective of the consumers of those services. The second goal of the program is to develop tools and resources that facilitate use of the instruments by both consumers and health care providers.

To date, CAHPS surveys have been developed to assess the quality of health plans, nursing homes, dialysis centers, physician offices, dental practices, tribal clinics, hospitals, and behavioral health care organizations. Development of all CAHPS surveys is guided by nine overarching principles[4]:

1. CAHPS survey items focus primarily on the experiences consumers have during clinical encounters (e.g., whether a particular service is performed) rather than on more general ratings of satisfaction with care or perceived quality of care. Because general ratings may be influenced by a wide variety of factors, scores may be difficult to interpret and may not suggest the corrective actions needed to remediate deficiencies identified.

2. CAHPS surveys focus on the collection of information that cannot be obtained in a reliable manner from other sources (e.g., medical records). Thus, CAHPS surveys do not include items assessing whether laboratory or diagnostic tests were performed or whether specific medications were prescribed. However, they might contain items concerning whether the patient/consumer was counseled about a particular topic. Because scores on a CAHPS survey should reflect consumer perceptions of the quality of the health care services they receive,

considerable effort is made during the survey development process to identify the range of issues that consumers consider when evaluating service quality and the final survey instrument is designed to capture information concerning those issues.

3. CAHPS survey instruments, administration procedures, and reporting guidelines are standardized. This facilitates comparisons across different providers of the same type of service (e.g., different providers of pharmacy services).

4. During the development of a CAHPS survey instrument, input is sought from all stakeholders (e.g., clinicians, professional organizations, and accrediting bodies). This ensures that all relevant aspects of quality are assessed and that the information resulting from survey administration will be useful to those responsible for developing policies and programs aimed at quality improvement.

5. State-of-the-art methods are used to develop CAHPS instruments. These methods include: focus groups with consumers to better understand the factors they consider important when evaluating the quality of different service providers, cognitive interviewing to assess comprehension and interpretation of survey items, and field testing to develop valid and reliable scales and scoring procedures.

6. CAHPS survey instruments and reports are evaluated by a variety of audiences to ensure that the information they provide is understandable and can be used to facilitate decision making and quality improvement efforts.

7. Efforts are made to ensure that the instruments are useful across heterogeneous populations. Particular attention is given to vulnerable populations where health disparities may exist. This includes people with disabilities or chronic conditions and people for whom English is not their first language.

8. ARHQ provides benchmarking data that can be used by participants to compare their scores with other participants. The National CAHPS Benchmarking Database (NCBD) allows comparisons at the national, regional, and local levels.

9. All surveys, reports, tools, and resources developed as part of the CAHPS program are in the public domain. They are available through the ARHQ website and may be used free of charge. ARHQ also provides technical assistance to facilitate use of the surveys and reports.

CAHPS Kits

To facilitate use of the CAHPS surveys and optimize standardization across users, each survey has been incorporated into a kit with multiple components. Each kit includes a copy of the survey instrument, including both the primary survey and supplemental questions that might be asked for specific population subgroups (e.g., children and people with disabilities). Each kit includes both English- and Spanish-language versions of the survey. The kits also include protocols for sampling respondents, survey administration guidelines, data analysis programs and instructions, and reporting measures and guidelines. The kits can be downloaded from the AHRQ website at *www.cahps.ahrq.gov.*

CAHPS Users

Potential users of CAHPS data include individual consumers and consumer advocacy groups, regulatory and accrediting agencies responsible for monitoring and assuring health care quality, public and private purchasers of health care services, provider organizations, and health plans. Although consumers represent an important target group for CAHPS reports, a review of the literature completed in 2005 found that most consumers were not aware of the availability of this information and that they often had difficulty interpreting this type of information when it was provided.[5] In addition, findings concerning the effects of quality information on consumer decision making were equivocal. At most, availability of quality information appeared to have only a modest effect on consumer decisions. Thus, the 2005 review highlighted the need to: (1) develop strategies to better disseminate quality information to consumers and (2) develop reporting formats that are readily understandable to consumers, engage their interest, and contain a sufficient amount of information to facilitate decision making. Consequently, in the summer of 2007, AHRQ launched the CAHPS III initiative, focused on the development of tools and resources to facilitate use of the CAHPS instruments and the investigation of reporting formats and methods to communicate CAHPS data in a way that facilitates consumer decision making and quality improvement efforts.

DEVELOPMENT OF THE CONSUMER ASSESSMENT OF PHARMACY SERVICES

Work to develop the Consumer Assessment of Pharmacy Services questionnaire was initiated by the Pharmacy Quality Alliance (PQA). The mission of PQA, established in April 2006, is to:

> Improve health care quality and patient safety through a collaborative process in which key stakeholders agree on a strategy for measuring performance at the pharmacy and pharmacist-levels; collecting data in the least burdensome way; and reporting meaningful information to consumers, pharmacists, employers, health insurance plans, and other health care decision-makers to help make informed choices, improve outcomes and stimulate the development of new payment models.[6]

Shortly after PQA was established, a number of cluster groups were formed to work on specific needs identified by the Alliance. The *Patient Satisfaction Cluster Group* was charged with development of a patient satisfaction survey. The group conducted an environmental scan of existing satisfaction instruments and developed a draft instrument. The draft instrument was presented to the PQA membership for endorsement in November 2006. At that time, it was recommended that additional work be conducted to develop the instrument in a manner that would adhere to the CAHPS principles outlined above. In that way, the final instrument could be submitted to CAHPS for inclusion in their family of quality measures and could be used to standardize the assessment of pharmacy services quality.

In response to this recommendation, in the spring of 2007, PQA issued an RFP to identify a contractor to perform the work required. The contract was awarded to

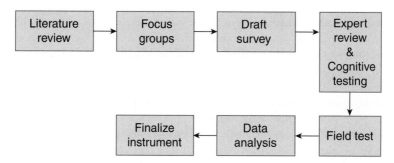

Figure 10-1. Steps in development of the Consumer Assessment of Pharmacy Services survey.

the American Institutes for Research (AIR), where one of the authors of this chapter (San Keller) is a senior investigator. An expert on the CAHPS survey development process, Dr Keller led the development of a similar effort that resulted in a survey that was accepted as an official CAHPS instrument.[7] The research team also included Dr Susan Blalock at the UNC Eshelman School of Pharmacy and support personnel from Synovate and Westat. Synovate is a marketing research organization that is a National Committee for Quality Assurance (NCQA)-certified CAHPS vendor and Westat is a contract research organization that provides support for the CAHPS Consortium and the CAHPS Benchmarking Database.

Development of the Consumer Assessment of Pharmacy Services survey involved several steps. As shown in Figure 10-1, these steps included: (1) performing an extensive review of the literature to identify instruments and items that had been used to assess consumer satisfaction with pharmacy services or consumer evaluations of pharmacy service quality, (2) conducting focus groups to ensure that the final instrument would reflect consumer viewpoints and concerns as they relate to pharmacy service quality, (3) incorporating information from the literature review and focus groups into a draft survey, (4) revising the draft survey based on information obtained via cognitive interviews with consumers and review of the survey by experts in the field, (5) field testing the revised survey, (6) analyzing data obtained from the field test, and (7) revising the survey based on field-test findings. Each of these steps is described in more detail below.

Literature Review

Over the past 30 years, a variety of measures have been developed to assess patient perceptions of the quality of pharmacy services in outpatient settings. Over this same time period, however, the role of outpatient pharmacists (i.e., community pharmacists, ambulatory care pharmacists, and mail-order pharmacists) has expanded considerably, moving beyond the distribution of medications alone toward the provision of comprehensive clinical services.[8] Currently, there is a wide range in the types of services available in different pharmacy settings. Some pharmacies still focus almost exclusively on dispensing functions, whereas others offer a wide variety of disease management and medication therapy management services. This variation in the types of services provided by different pharmacies presents a special challenge to quality assessment efforts.

To identify measures that have been used in the past to assess consumer perceptions of pharmacy services, we conducted a query of the literature published in the past 30 years using the MEDLINE database and the following keywords and keyword combinations: pharmacy OR pharmacist, consumer, satisfaction OR quality, and survey* OR questionnaire*. We retrieved all articles that described items and domains used to assess the quality of pharmacy services based on patient reports. In addition, when the authors of these articles referred to surveys or questionnaires that were presented in previously published work, we also retrieved those cited articles. We reviewed all articles retrieved to identify questionnaires or tabled items. This search strategy yielded 14 item sets including a total of 385 items. In addition, we obtained five more sets of items from unpublished sources. These included two surveys that had been used in peer-reviewed studies of pharmacy service quality and the Medicare prescription drug plan CAHPS survey.

Although satisfaction with pharmacy services has been conceptualized in a variety of ways in past research,[9] most work has used the approach advocated by Ware et al. [10,11] wherein patients are asked to evaluate the quality of services received. Several standardized measures have been developed using this approach. The first such measure was developed in the late 1980s by MacKeigan and Larson.[12] This measure, the Satisfaction with Pharmacy Services Questionnaire (SPSQ), was adapted from the Patient Satisfaction Questionnaire, developed by Ware et al.[10,11] The original SPSQ contained a total of 44 items assessing eight dimensions of quality: interpersonal manner, technical competence, general accessibility, emergency access, financial considerations, medication efficacy, continuity of care, and general satisfaction. Notably, all of these dimensions focus on functions associated with dispensing medications. This focus was retained in a refinement of the instrument published in 1994.[13] Thus, neither the original nor the revised SPSQ assessed the quality of disease management or medication therapy management services that pharmacists provide.

In 2002, a major revision of the SPSQ was published.[14] The revised instrument, the Patient Satisfaction with Pharmaceutical Care (PSPC) scale, focused exclusively on patient perceptions of the quality of pharmaceutical care services. The PSPC contains a total of 20 items, with variability among the items explained by two dimensions: friendly explanation (e.g., *the availability of the pharmacist to answer your questions*) and managing therapy (e.g., *the pharmacist's efforts to help you improve your health or stay healthy*). However, in developing the PSPC, all items from the original instrument that assessed the quality of dispensing functions that pharmacists provide were deleted (e.g., *I am confident that the pharmacist dispenses all prescriptions correctly*). Thus, while the PSPC provides expanded coverage of how pharmacists help patients with their health and medications, it is narrow in breadth with regard to other aspects of pharmacy service quality.

In addition to the PSPC, three other measures that are prominent in the literature assess patient perceptions of the care provided by pharmacists. First, the Purdue Pharmacists Directive Guidance Scale (PPDG) is a short instrument (10 items) designed specifically to address the more intensive care that might be provided by a pharmacist including: helping patients understand their diseases better, helping patients set goals for themselves with respect to taking their medications correctly, and checking periodically with patients to determine whether they are having any problems following their medication regimens.[15] Subsequent research using the PPDG showed these pharmacist behaviors to be positively related to overall patient satisfaction.[16] Second, the Satisfaction with Pharmacist Scale (SPS) is a seven-item questionnaire, available in both English and Spanish, that is similar in content to the PSPC and the PPDG (e.g., "My pharmacist advises me on the proper use of my medicines").[17] Finally, the Pharmaceutical Care Satisfaction Questionnaire (PCSQ) is a 30-item instrument designed to assess patient perceptions of the quality of pharmaceutical care services that are delivered by the pharmacist to community-residing patients/consumers.[18] PCSQ items include: evaluating medication care plans, providing education about health problems, identifying medication problems and working with patients to plan their pharmaceutical care, and discussing medications with the patients' physicians to ensure their appropriateness.

Three other measures assess the quality of pharmacy services more broadly. First, the Pharmacy Encounter Survey (PES),[19] modeled after the Visit-specific Satisfaction Questionnaire developed by Ware et al.,[20] asks about access (convenient location and getting through to the pharmacy by phone), wait time (wait before seeing a pharmacist and wait for prescription to be filled), and the quality of interaction with pharmacy personnel. Second, the Response-oriented Patient Evaluation Survey (ROPES)[21] has 19 items assessing five domains of pharmacy services: the pharmacist, access, availability of written information, handling of complaints, and wait times. Finally, a 14-item survey developed by Kaiser Permanente to assess the quality of outpatient pharmacy services includes items concerning: wait time, patient counseling by the pharmacist, courteousness of pharmacy staff, and overall satisfaction.

Content analysis of yield from literature search.

To provide structure for the Consumer Assessment of Pharmacy Services survey, we sought commonalities among the 385 items identified in the literature review by using the American Society for Health-system Pharmacists (ASHP) minimum standard for pharmaceutical services in ambulatory care as a conceptual framework.[22] The value of using the ASHP standard as a conceptual framework is that it represents a broad consensus among experts and stakeholders regarding factors that are important to the quality of pharmacy services. Two of the ASHP standards are particularly relevant to the quality of pharmacy services that might be reported upon by consumers and patients: (1) *Medication Therapy and Pharmaceutical Care* and (2) *Drug Distribution and Control*. The *Medication Therapy and Pharmaceutical Care* standard addresses comprehensive pharmaceutical care services including rapport, medication therapy, and patient education and counseling. The *Drug Distribution and Control* standard addresses maintaining the availability of medications, the labeling of medications, and processing medication orders. [The remaining ASHP standards involve aspects of quality that are not readily observable to consumers (e.g., whether the pharmacy has adequate drug information resources) or for which consumers lack sufficient knowledge to evaluate (e.g., adequacy of automatic dispensing systems).]

As part of content analysis procedures, we categorized items identified via the literature review according to the quality criteria identified in the ASHP standard (see Table 10-1). We were able to categorize approximately two thirds of the 385 items

TABLE 10-1. Sample from Content Analysis of Items Identified by the Literature Review Using the ASHP Minimum Standard for Pharmaceutical Services in Ambulatory Care as a Conceptual Framework

ASHP Criteria	Example Items from Existing Surveys
ASHP standard: Medication Therapy and Pharmaceutical Care	
Relationship with patients	The pharmacy staff should be more friendly Pharmacist listens to what I have to say
Patient education and counseling	The pharmacist explains how my medications help me The pharmacist explains how to take my medication
Medication therapy management	[The pharmacist] Asked about allergies or previous bad reactions to drugs My pharmacist never asks if I am getting the best results from my medications
ASPH standard: Drug Distribution and Control	
Purchasing and maintaining availability of drug products	The pharmacy can always be relied upon to have my prescription medication My pharmacist works with my insurer concerning my pharmacy needs
Processing prescriptions	I sometimes wonder about the accuracy of the prescriptions that the pharmacist dispenses The pharmacy allows me to phone in refills
Preparing, packaging, labeling	My prescription medications are always clearly labeled Warning labels on prescription bottles are used consistently

identified in this manner. Items that did not fit within this classification system assessed: the physical layout of the pharmacy (e.g., adequacy of space, pleasant appearance, and availability of comfortable chairs in waiting area), convenience for ordering and picking up prescriptions (store location, parking, availability of drive-through, and hours), ease of obtaining prescription medications without having to visit the pharmacy (e.g., phone-in refills and home delivery), easy access to the pharmacy by telephone, cost (e.g., prescription medication prices, copays, and insurance coverage), other health services available (e.g., health screenings and immunizations), and availability of other products (e.g., consumer household items.)

Focus Groups

To better understand how present-day consumers evaluate the quality of pharmacy services, we conducted four consumer focus groups, two with Medicare beneficiaries and two with consumers not receiving Medicare benefits. A total of 30 consumers participated in the focus groups. Use of focus groups during the design phase of a survey helps to ensure that the final instrument will be relevant to consumers and will capture their viewpoints and concerns.[23,24] Thus, the focus groups were used to better understand: (1) what words and phrases consumers use when discussing the quality of pharmacy services, (2) whether consumers distinguish between different aspects of pharmacy services when assessing quality, and (3) whether Medicare beneficiaries evaluate the quality of pharmacy services in qualitatively different ways than other consumers. We also assessed the extent to which consumers differentiate between the quality of services provided by the pharmacy and the quality of services provided by the pharmacists who staff the pharmacy. Some examples of questions asked during the focus groups include:

1. What are some things about your pharmacy that make you want to keep using that pharmacy? Remember, right now we will only talk about the pharmacy, not individual pharmacists who work there.

2. What are some reasons you might stop using a particular pharmacy? If you have stopped using a particular pharmacy, what was the reason?

3. Now let us do the same thing for pharmacists. First, what are some of the things about the pharmacists at your pharmacy that make you want to keep using that particular pharmacist?

4. What are some reasons you might avoid a particular pharmacist? If you have avoided a particular pharmacist, what was the reason?

5. Is there anything you would like a pharmacy or pharmacist to do that they currently are not doing? Are there any services you would like more available or more accessible?

6. Anything you wish a pharmacy or pharmacist would not do?

The focus groups were conducted in two different geographic regions of the country. In both regions, one focus group comprised Medicare beneficiaries and the other group comprised consumers who had some other type of insurance or no insurance. Three groups had 8 participants and the remaining group had 6 for a total of 30 participants across the four groups. Participants included consumers of retail, mail-order, and home-delivery pharmacy services. The groups were also demographically diverse. Participants in the non-Medicare groups ranged in age from 40 to 60 years old and those in the Medicare groups were between the ages of 65 and 75 years. One third of the participants were non-white and approximately two thirds had at least some college education.

Each focus group was conducted by a trained moderator. After all issues concerning the quality of services provided by pharmacies and pharmacists had been elicited, the moderator asked the participants to group the issues into "buckets," with each bucket containing issues that were similar to one another, but different from the issues placed in other "buckets." In this way, distinct quality domains were identified. Discussion then turned to which domains were most important to participants and participants were given stickers to indicate those domains that they considered most important.

Taken together, the four focus groups resulted in the identification of 48 unique attributes of pharmacy quality and 23 unique attributes of pharmacist quality. For ease of interpretation and summary, we generated category labels that represented the content of the attributes. Where possible, we designed the category labels to be similar to those found in other CAHPS surveys. For example, nearly all of the CAHPS surveys include summary measures to tap "provider communication" and "access to timely

TABLE 10-2. Quality Attributes Relevant to Pharmacies and Pharmacists Identified in Focus Group Sessions

ASHP Criteria	Conceptual Quality Domains	Attributes Identified in Focus Groups
Purchasing and maintaining availability of drug products; processing prescriptions; preparing, packaging, labeling	Convenient/prompt prescriptions	• Timely (prescriptions filled quickly, no wait, ready when they are supposed to be) • Adequate staff (enough staff, enough staff so we don't have to wait) • Home delivery (home delivery/ mail delivery options) • General (convenient, no hassle)
	Prescription accuracy and packaging	• Accurate prescription • Accurate dose • Packaging – easy to open • Prescription information clear (good inserts, clear labeling)
Relationship with patients; patient education and counseling	Staff communication	• Language (can speak your language) • Attending to person (pays attention, concerned) • Friendly (knows person's name) Courteous • Personalization (not just a number, genuine) • Helpful (willingness to help, respond to questions) • Can understand you/communicate with you in a way you can understand (layman's terms)

(continued)

TABLE 10-2. (Continued)

ASHP Criteria	Conceptual Quality Domains	Attributes Identified in Focus Groups
Relationship with patients; patient education and counseling	Pharmacist communication	• Style • Personable (approachable, considerate, good people skills) • Friendly (friendly, pleasant/ friendly) • Knowledgeable of patient (knows name, knowledgeable about patient) • Discrete (trustworthy) • Helpful • Takes time with you (spends time with you) • Respectful • Courteous • Able to communicate in layman's terms • Patient • Genuine • Explains medicines to you (provides information, information about medication) • Recommends generics (willing to recommend generics, identify alternate medicines)
Processing prescriptions; medication therapy management	Prescriptions medicine quality/ management	• Accurate prescription (fills prescriptions accurately – dose and medication) • Manages prescriptions (reviews prescriptions, is aware of medical history)

care." To inform development of the draft survey, we then selected attributes that pertained to aspects of pharmacy service quality: (1) for which the consumer is the best or only source of information; (2) for which the consumer is qualified to report; (3) that are relevant to mail-order and home-delivery services as well as traditional community pharmacies to permit comparisons across different pharmacy settings; and (4) that emerged in at least two of the focus groups. The pharmacy and pharmacist attributes that met those criteria are presented in Table 10-2, grouped according to the ASHP criterion to which they correspond and the category label (i.e., *conceptual quality domain*) that we assigned to them.

Creation of Draft Survey

Findings from the literature review and focus groups were used to create a draft survey that adhered to CAHPS principles for item content and survey design. CAHPS surveys must conform to several design principles that facilitate the ease of information processing for respondents. These principles affect the way questions are drafted and formatted. First, questions must be written in a list format with the question written first and the possible responses listed under each question. Usability studies show that, compared to the tabular or grid format often used in surveys, the list format is easier for participants with limited literacy skills to understand.[25] Second, to ensure that instructions are read and remembered, they are incorporated into the numbered part of questions. If the instructions are short (e.g., the instruction to think about the last 12 months when answering the question), they are repeated in each question stem. Third, to enhance readability, surveys use large type and question stems and skip instructions are bolded. In addition, if two adjacent questions are identical with the exception of a single phrase, that phrase is underlined. Finally, as much "white space" as possible is incorporated into the layout of the survey when it is presented in a self-administered format.

With respect to content, most CAHPS items have the following characteristics:

1. *Questions based on observables*: Questions involve behaviors or events that the consumer observes, rather than feelings or opinions. Therefore, most CAHPS questions ask respondents to report on whether the health care provider performed a specific behavior or how frequently a specific behavior was performed.

2. *Answers based on experience*: Respondents are not asked to report on topics about which they have no experience. This requires the use of skip patterns in the survey or inclusion of "Not Applicable" as a response option.

3. *Complex questions avoided*: Each question concerns only one subject. Thus, no questions should contain multiple clauses.

4. *Abstract terms avoided*: The interpretation of each question should be clear and unambiguous. Abstract terms, which often are subject to a variety of interpretations, are avoided.

5. *Plain, simple language*: Questions are written in the simplest language possible to facilitate comprehension by respondents with limited literacy skills.

The first two item characteristics described above are dictated by the purpose of the measure that is to provide information that is based on the consumer's direct experience.[26] The last three characteristics are to minimize the cognitive complexity of the questions.[27]

Our goal in drafting quality items for the survey was to ensure that all of the quality domains that emerged with consistency in the literature review and focus group sessions were included in the survey. However, many of the specific items identified by the literature review did not satisfy the CAHPS criteria for item content. For example, items that asked for opinions about the pharmacist or feelings toward the pharmacy do not conform to the first principle that requires that survey items ask about things that are observable. Other items identified in the literature review referred to very general subjects and could not be rewritten in such a way that they were specific and simple without losing their meaning. Therefore, we created many new items to ensure that the survey would provide a comprehensive assessment of consumer perceptions of the quality of services delivered by pharmacies and pharmacists.

In addition to the quality items described above, CAHPS surveys always include three other types of items: case-mix adjusters, items assessing other sociodemographic characteristics, and overall quality ratings. Case-mix models have been developed and evaluated in multiple studies using different CAHPS surveys from data obtained by the demographic section of the questionnaire. Self-rated health, age, and education have been found to be the most robust case-mix adjusters across quality of care surveys,[28–31] including CAHPS surveys.[32,33] However, whenever a new CAHPS survey is developed, case-mix adjusters particularly relevant to that survey are evaluated.[34] For example, in the draft of the Consumer Assessment of Pharmacy Services survey, we included a question asking about the number of different prescriptions the respondent had filled during the past year, regardless of the pharmacy they used. Other questions often included in the sociodemographic section of a CAHPS survey include: ethnicity, race, and whether someone helped the respondent complete the survey. Finally, in addition to the specific quality questions described above, CAHPS surveys usually include items that ask respondents to provide overall ratings that represent a summary of their experience with regard to a particular quality domain included in the questionnaire. For example, the draft of the Consumer Assessment of Pharmacy Services survey included overall ratings of the quality of the pharmacy staff, the pharmacy services, the pharmacist, and medication information.

Expert Review and Cognitive Testing

To refine the draft survey prior to field testing, we submitted it to a panel of experts for their review and conducted two rounds of cognitive interviews with consumers.[35] Figure 10-2 depicts diagrammatically the processes followed during this stage of survey development.

Expert review.

A total of 50 individuals with expertise in pharmacy practice were invited to serve on an expert panel to review the survey before field testing. Of these, nine agreed, and ultimately served, on the panel. The final panel included individuals from academia, community pharmacy practice, and pharmacy professional associations. Panelists reviewed the draft survey at several stages, both before and after cognitive testing with consumers. At each stage, the survey was revised to incorporate suggestions made by the expert panelists as long as the changes recommended did not violate the CAHPS principles outlined above.

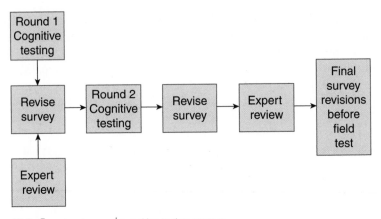

Figure 10-2. Expert review and cognitive testing process.

Cognitive testing.

We conducted two rounds of cognitive interviews with consumers to assess the following issues related to the draft survey.[36,37] First, we assessed the extent to which survey items reflected quality domains that were important to consumers and about which consumers had sufficient experience to be able to provide reliable information. Second, we assessed whether consumers were able to understand the items and whether they interpreted the items as intended. Third, we assessed whether consumers were able to remember events that were queried by survey items in order to report reliably. Fourth, we assessed whether the questions were relevant to consumers who obtained prescriptions from either mail-order or community pharmacies. Finally, we assessed whether respondents had difficulty with the way the questions were sequenced on the survey or with the font and general formatting of the survey and the extent to which consumers were able to navigate the survey when they were required to skip over a number of questions because those questions did not apply to them.

Cognitive interviews were conducted with a total of 12 consumers, evenly divided between two stages of testing. The survey instrument was revised following the first round of testing based on the information obtained and the revised instrument was subjected to a second round of testing. We sought to obtain diversity in respondents by recruiting participants from two different regions of the country and by including both Medicare and non-Medicare patients. We also wanted to include a number of individuals who were most likely to encounter problems responding to the survey: those with less education and those who primarily used mail-order services. Among the participants, three were age 65 years or older, six had no more than a high school education or vocational training, and three obtained prescriptions by mail order.

Each cognitive interview was conducted in an in-person, one-on-one setting. Interviews lasted an average of 2 hours each and used a "think-aloud" approach.[36,37] Participants were given a written copy of the questionnaire and were asked to: (1) read each question, one at a time; (2) give a response verbally; and (3) explain the basis for their response. The interviewer then followed up with probes after each question to identify potential problems. The survey was revised to address all issues identified.

Field Test

The final field-test instrument that emerged from the expert review and cognitive testing process contained a total of 50 items, 28 of which pertained to consumer assessments of the quality of pharmacy services. The remaining items were case-mix adjusters, items assessing other sociodemographic questions, or filter questions designed to facilitate respondent navigation through the questionnaire. The field-test methods and analysis of field-test data are detailed elsewhere,[38] so they are presented only in summary form here.

The survey instrument was field tested in the fall of 2007. The sampling plan for the field test was designed to enable two types of comparisons: (1) comparisons across pharmacies providing different types of services (i.e., community pharmacies, mail-order pharmacies, and pharmacies providing medication management services for consumers on complex drug regimens) and (2) comparisons across different pharmacies providing similar services (e.g., different community pharmacies). To achieve these goals, we recruited participants from: 27 different pharmacies in a community pharmacy chain, a health system mail-order pharmacy, and a pharmacy that specializes in medication therapy management services for people on complex medication regimens. A total of 895 consumers completed the field-test instrument. Participation was limited to adults (age 18 years or older) who had filled at least one prescription on three different dates during the period from June 1, 2006 to May 1, 2007. These criteria were designed to ensure that respondents had multiple pharmacy encounters on which to base their responses to survey questions. Most participants completed the survey in the form of a self-administered mailed questionnaire. However, data were collected from a subsample of participants using a version of the survey suitable for administration via telephone interview.

Data Analysis

The 28 specific quality items included in the field-test instrument are shown in abbreviated form in Table 10-3, grouped according to the conceptual quality domains identified in the literature review and focus groups. Confirmatory factor analysis was used to identify the distinct dimensions of quality that were tapped by the items. This analysis identified a subset of 15 items that formed three distinct subsets. The first subset contained six items that assessed general characteristics of communication with pharmacy staff (e.g., How often the pharmacy staff are easy to understand). The second subset contained five items that addressed staff communication specific to health and medication-related issues (e.g., How often pharmacy staff talk to you about your health). The final subset contained four items related to the quality of written information provided by the pharmacy (e.g., How often instructions on medicine labels are easy to read). Items within each subset were combined to form three composite indicators that we labeled: *General Staff Communication, Health and Medication-focused*

TABLE 10-3. Items in Consumer Assessment of Pharmacy Services Field Survey Instrument

Initial Conceptual Quality Domain	Abbreviated Item Text	Scale in Final Consumer Assessment of Pharmacy Services Survey
Staff communication	Staff easy to understand	
	Staff listen carefully to you	
	Staff show you courtesy and respect	General staff communication
	Staff spend enough time with you	
	Staff show concern for you	
	Able to talk to staff as soon as I wanted	
	Staff talk to you about your health	
	Staff ask me if I had problems with my Rx	
	Staff tell you how to take new Rx	Health and medication-focused communication
	Tell you what to avoid taking with new Rx	
	Tell you what to do if bad reaction to new Rx	
	Staff too busy to answer questions	Deleted from final version of survey
	Didn't ask questions because no privacy	
	Asked staff for advice about OTC Rx	
	Staff ask me if I had questions about my Rx	
Prescription packaging	Medication labels easy to read	
	Medication labels easy to understand	Clarity of written information about medicines
	Written info about meds easy to read	
	Written info about meds easy to understand	
Pharmacist communication	Talk to RPH about how your meds may help	
	Ask RPH how to treat a health problem	
	Talk to RPH about drug interactions	

(continued)

TABLE 10-3. (Continued)

Initial Conceptual Quality Domain	Abbreviated Item Text	Scale in Final Consumer Assessment of Pharmacy Services Survey
Medication access and convenience	Pharmacy have my meds in stock	Deleted from final version of survey
	Pharmacy make mistake with meds	
	Pharmacy ever contact you to refill Rx	
	Staff help with Rx refill problems	
	Meds delivered to your home on time	
	Pharmacy have meds ready on time	

Communication, and *Clarity of Written Information about Medicines*, respectively. Each composite indicator exhibited excellent reliability as assessed by Cronbach's alpha[39] and only minor differences in reliability were observed across the three types of pharmacies included in the sampling frame. In addition, each composite indicator was strongly related to respondents' general rating of pharmacy service quality. The *General Staff Communication* composite demonstrated the strongest correlation ($r = 0.76$), followed by the *Clarity of Written Information about Medicines* ($r = 0.44$) and *Health and Medication-focused Communication* ($r = 0.42$). Statistical analysis supported the reliability and validity of the composite and global scores for the telephone version of the survey as well.

Due to sample size, analyses to identify a subset of respondent background questions to be used as case-mix adjusters were not definitive. For this reason, we retained all of the questions pertaining to respondent characteristics so that they could be used to collect more data for evaluation.

Final Instrument

The final Consumer Assessment of Pharmacy Services survey contains a total of 33 items. The cover of the survey provides space to indicate the name of the pharmacy being assessed and instructions are provided for respondents to answer survey questions only in relation to the pharmacy named. The survey is divided into five sections labeled: *Pharmacy Staff Communication, Information about Medicine, Written Information, New Prescriptions,* and *About You.* All items included in the three composites described above are included in the final instrument. In addition, the final questionnaire includes three items that ask participants to provide more general ratings of pharmacy staff, information about medications, and pharmacy services. These items are:

🔘 Using any number from 0 to 10, where 0 is the worst pharmacy *staff* possible and 10 is the best pharmacy *staff* possible, what number would you use to rate the *staff* at this pharmacy?

◔ Using any number from 0 to 10 where 0 is the worst information possible and 10 is the best information possible, what number would you use to rate the information that you got from this pharmacy about medicines?

◔ Using any number from 0 to 10 where 0 is the worst pharmacy *service* possible and 10 is the best pharmacy *service* possible, what number would you use to rate the *service* that you got from this pharmacy in the last 12 months?

Finally, in the *About You* section of the survey, information is collected concerning participant: health, age, gender, education, and race and ethnicity. This section also includes items that ask about the number of prescriptions the participant has had filled during the previous 3 months, the type of health insurance that the participant has, whether someone helped the participant complete the survey, and, if so, the type of help provided (e.g., reading the questions to the respondent).

The Consumer Assessment of Pharmacy Services survey is formatted using design features to facilitate reading[40] that are incorporated into most CAHPS surveys including:

◔ *List format*: Questions are presented in a list format with the question written first and the possible responses listed under each question.

◔ *Instruction salience*: To ensure that they are read and remembered, instructions are incorporated into the numbered part of the question. If the instructions are short (e.g., the instruction to refer to the last 12 months in answering the questions or the instruction to refer to a particular pharmacy), they are repeated in each question stem.

◔ *Readability enhancements*: Large type is employed. Question stems and skip instructions are bolded. If two questions that follow one another are identical with the exception of a single phrase, that phrase is underlined.

◔ *Question placement*: As much "white space" as possible is incorporated into the layout of the questionnaire when it is presented to the respondent as text.

Following development of the final version of the questionnaire, a Spanish version of the survey was created following standard CAHPS translation procedures: (1) two forward, independent translations, (2) development of a version that reconciled any differences between the translations, and (3) cognitive testing of the translated version. The procedures for cognitive testing were the same as followed for the English version except that native Spanish speakers conducted the interviews and the participants were either Spanish dominant or monolingual in Spanish.[41] The Consumer Assessment of Pharmacy Services survey including English- and Spanish-language versions will be submitted to the CAHPS Consortium to be evaluated for adoption into the CAHPS family of instruments in 2009.

APPROPRIATE USES OF THE CONSUMER ASSESSMENT OF PHARMACY SERVICES SURVEY

As noted at the beginning of this chapter, most people, at one time or another, find themselves in need of ambulatory care pharmacy services. But, when selecting among available pharmacies, they often have little information on which to base their choice. If they use medications to treat a chronic condition, they will acquire information based on personal experience over time. Still, this information will be restricted to the pharmacy (or pharmacies) they use. They may also acquire information based on the anecdotal reports of family and friends or via pharmacy advertisements. However, at the current time, it is impossible for them to obtain objective, standardized information that they could use to compare the quality of services available from different pharmacies in their area. Once the Consumer Assessment of Pharmacy Services survey has been adopted into the CAHPS family of instruments, this situation is very likely to change. Below, we discuss the wide variety of ways in which the survey may be used to facilitate quality improvement efforts and enable consumers to make more informed choices among available pharmacies.

The potential users of the Consumer Assessment of Pharmacy Services survey are similar to those for other CAHPS instruments. First, pharmacy managers can use the instrument to compare the performance of their pharmacy with other pharmacies. The benchmarking database maintained by AHRQ will enable managers to compare the results for their pharmacy (or pharmacies) with regional, state, and national averages. This will enable managers to identify quality deficits and take appropriate action to correct the deficits noted. Because the majority of items in the CAHPS survey assess aspects of pharmacy practice that are directly observable (e.g., how often a particular service is provided) and are important to consumers, CAHPS surveys provide information that can be translated readily into the specific actions needed to improve quality. Second, managers of chain pharmacies can use the Consumer Assessment of Pharmacy Services survey to compare the results across the pharmacies within their chain. In addition to initiating actions to remediate quality deficits, managers might reward the top-performing pharmacies through a variety of mechanisms (e.g., awards that recognize those pharmacies that achieve the best ratings or that surpass previously specified benchmarks, providing financial incentives). Third, pharmacy organizations might encourage pharmacies to participate in the CAHPS program on a voluntary basis. As an incentive for participation, organizations could provide some type of special recognition for participating pharmacies and pharmacies could use this recognition as a marketing tool. Fourth, insurance providers could require that pharmacies collect data using the Consumer Assessment of Pharmacy Services survey and set minimal performance levels required for reimbursement. Fifth, state pharmacy boards could require that pharmacies collect data using the Consumer Assessment of Pharmacy Services survey. They could also require that pharmacies make data from the survey available to consumers. Finally, consumer advocacy groups, such as AARP, could demand that pharmacies use the CAHPS survey. They could then make this information available to their members.

At this point in time, it is too early to know exactly how the Consumer Assessment of Pharmacy Services survey will ultimately be used or how readily it will be adopted by pharmacies across the nation. Demand for the survey is likely to be stimulated by organizations that set standards for quality in health care as well as those that purchase health care and demand accountability. Development of the CAHPS Health Plan survey began in 1995; however, the Balanced Budget Act of 1997 that mandated Medicare to present information on health care quality to beneficiaries created a market for the survey.[42] Widespread dissemination of the CAHPS Health Plan survey was also encouraged when the NCQA began requiring the survey for accreditation reporting.[26] In 1998, construction of the NCBD was initiated by soliciting voluntary contributions of CAHPS Health Plan survey data from survey sponsors.[43] The latest report on the NCBD describes 11 years of data including 3.4 million completed adult and child surveys from commercial and public plans (Medicaid, Medicare, and SCHIP).[44] Availability of this type of evidence base on health care quality is a rich resource for health services research as well.[45] The ability of CAHPS users to compare their CAHPS scores to those of other users is enormously helpful in interpreting the data and stimulates further demand for the survey. Other large users include the Department of Defense's TRICARE, the Federal Employees Health Benefit Program, and the Ford Motor Company, among other commercial entities.[46] Adoption of the CAHPS Health Plan survey continues to grow. In 2008, the Veteran's Administration (VA) began using the survey to assess their ambulatory care divisions. If the Consumer Assessment of Pharmacy Services survey is adopted by an accrediting agency or a large purchaser of pharmacy services (such as CMS), demand for and use of the survey across many different applications will proliferate as well.

The Consumer Assessment of Pharmacy Services survey exists today because of efforts initiated by the PQA. Although development of the survey represents an enormous first step in attempting to capture consumer perceptions of pharmacy quality, much more work is needed to ensure that the instrument is used in a way that facilitates quality improvement efforts and informs consumer decision making. In the next section, we discuss some of the additional work that is needed.

DIRECTIONS FOR FUTURE WORK ON THE CONSUMER ASSESSMENT OF PHARMACY SERVICES SURVEY

Development of any new measure is a complex and ongoing process. Data from the developmental study described in this chapter represent one contribution to the evidence documenting the properties of the Consumer Assessment of Pharmacy Services survey. However, further evaluation of the reliability and validity of survey scores should be conducted in subsequent data collection efforts that include an even broader range of pharmacies than were used in the developmental study. Such analysis would address the robustness of the psychometric properties of the instrument across patient subgroups. For example, individuals with limited literacy skills and those needing complex pharmaceutical care services were included in the developmental data collection, but there was not a sufficient number of these individuals to support subgroup analyses.

To permit valid comparisons across pharmacies, work is also needed to better understand the case-mix adjusters that should be incorporated into scoring procedures. Characteristics of the patient population often differ radically from one pharmacy to another. For example, some pharmacies serve primarily young adults and their families, whereas other pharmacies serve primarily older adults. Similarly, some pharmacies are located in relatively affluent areas and serve patients with the resources needed to meet their health care needs, whereas other pharmacies serve patients with more limited resources and inadequate access to needed health care services. Work involving other CAHPS instruments has found that survey responses can be influenced by patient characteristics, in addition to the quality of services received.[47] Thus, to permit valid comparisons across different providers, it is necessary to adjust provider scores statistically to remove variation caused by differences in the patient population (i.e., case mix) served. As indicated earlier, the patient characteristics that have been shown most consistently to affect patient responses to CAHPS questions are self-reported health, age, and education. However, based on the results of the Consumer Assessment of Pharmacy Services survey developmental analysis, we cannot be certain that adjustment for these characteristics is sufficient to control for differences in case-mix when comparing different pharmacies. Therefore, additional work is needed to determine if other case-mix adjusters (e.g., insurance coverage) are needed.

In addition to developing the survey itself, standardized methods must be developed for data collection. Otherwise, it will not be possible to make valid comparisons across pharmacies.[48] For example, if some pharmacies had patients complete the survey in conjunction with picking up a prescription, while other pharmacies mailed the survey to customers at periodic intervals, the differences in data collection procedures could influence respondent ratings in unknown ways, rendering it impossible to interpret any differences observed. Likewise, data obtained by telephone interview or via the Internet may not be comparable to those obtained via self-administered questionnaires.[49] Previous research comparing data provided by telephone and mail modes shows that reports of care tend to be more favorable when obtained over the telephone.[49,50] Indeed, the CAHPS hospital survey scoring algorithm adjusts for mode of administration.[51] Thus, work is needed to identify the most efficient data collection methods that are feasible to implement across a wide variety of pharmacy settings and that yield a sufficiently high response rate to permit valid comparisons.

Work is also needed to develop formats for reporting information from the Consumer Assessment of Pharmacy Services survey in a way that facilitates comprehension, judgment, and decision making by those in the intended audiences. As noted above, potential audiences for this information include consumers, pharmacy managers, and insurance providers. Work is currently underway to develop a standard reporting format. However, it is unclear if the same format will be optimal for all audiences. For example, research on consumer understanding of health plan quality data suggests that understanding is better when a limited amount of critical information is provided.[52,53]

Finally, the practice of pharmacy continues to evolve. Therefore, it is necessary to plan for evolution of the Consumer Assessment of Pharmacy Services survey. In the process of developing the survey, we attempted to incorporate items that assessed more comprehensive pharmaceutical care services that some pharmacies provide (e.g., disease state management and medication therapy management). However, some of these items fell to the wayside during the focus group sessions and cognitive testing. Others were eliminated from the composite scores in the analysis of the field-test data, but will be available as supplemental item sets. Because most consumers were not familiar with more comprehensive pharmaceutical care services, they were not factors that consumers considered when evaluating the quality of pharmacy services. With the inclusion of medication therapy management services under Medicare Part D, it seems likely that consumer awareness of these services will grow over the next few years. At that time, it may be possible to broaden the scope of the Consumer Assessment of Pharmacy Services survey to better capture the quality of these more comprehensive pharmacy services. The supplemental item set on pharmacist care contains items such as:

- In the last 12 months, how often did you talk to a pharmacist at this pharmacy about how your medicine is supposed to help you?
- In the last 12 months, if you had a new health problem, how often did you ask the pharmacist at this pharmacy for advice about how to treat the problem?
- In the last 12 months, in addition to the prescription medicines that you regularly take, did you have a new prescription filled at this pharmacy?
- Did you talk to the pharmacist about whether it would be safe to take the new prescription medicine along with your regular prescription medicines?

CONCLUSION

Development of the Consumer Assessment of Pharmacy Services survey represents an important step forward in the measurement of consumer perceptions of the quality of pharmacy services. The survey was developed using state-of-the-art methods to ensure that the attributes of pharmacies and pharmacists that consumers consider when evaluating quality would be included in the final instrument. The PQA made development of the survey possible through its vision and financial support. However, development of the survey is the beginning of the story, not the end. Over the next few years, it is our hope that the Consumer Assessment of Pharmacy Services survey will be adopted for widespread use across the United States and that it will serve as a stimulus for quality improvement efforts that ultimately improve the health outcomes experienced by all Americans.

REFERENCES

1. AHRQ. *CAHPS: Assessing Health Care Quality from the Patient's Perspective.* October 2008. https://www.cahps.ahrq.gov/content/cahpsoverview/07-p016.Pdf. Accessed April 6, 2009. AHRQ publication no. 08-PB015.
2. Hays RD, Shaul JA, Williams VS, et al. Psychometric properties of the CAHPS 1.0 survey measures. Consumer assessment of health plans study. *Med Care.* 1999;37(3 suppl):MS22–MS31.
3. AHRQ. *CAHPS: Surveys and Tools to Advance Patient-centered Care.* https://www.cahps. ahrq.gov/default.asp. Accessed April 6, 2009. Last updated on March 31, 2009.
4. AHRQ. *CAHPS Principles.* https://www.cahps.ahrq.gov/content/cahpsOverview/OVER_ Principles.asp?p=101&s=13. Accessed April 6, 2009. Last updated on October 29, 2008.
5. Lake T, Kvam C, Gold M. *Literature Review: Using Quality Information for Health Care Decisions and Quality Improvement.* Cambridge, MA: Mathematica Policy Research, Inc; 2005.
6. *PQA Homepage.* http://www.pqaalliance.org/. Accessed April 6, 2009.
7. Keller S, Martin GC, Evensen CT, Mitton RH. The development and testing of a survey instrument for benchmarking dental plan performance: using insured patients' experiences as a gauge of dental care quality. *J Am Dent Assoc.* 2009;140(2):229–237.

8. Cipolle RJ, Strand LM, Morley PC. *Pharmaceutical Care Practice*. New York: McGraw-Hill; 1998.

9. Schommer JC, Kucukarslan SN. Measuring patient satisfaction with pharmaceutical services. *Am J Health Syst Pharm*. 1997;54(23):2721–2732.

10. Ware J, Snyder M, Wright W. *Development and Validation of Scales to Measure Patient Satisfaction with Medical Care Services. Vol I, Part A: Review of Literature, Overview of Methods and Results Regarding Construction of Scales*. Springfield, VA: National Technical Information Service; 1976. NTIS publication no. PB 288-329.

11. Ware J, Snyder M, Wright W. *Development and Validation of Scales to Measure Patient Satisfaction with Medical Care Services. Vol I, Part B: Results Regarding Scales Constructed from the Patient Satisfaction Questionnaire and Measures of Other Health Care Perceptions*. Springfield, VA: National Technical Information Service; 1976. NTIS publication no. PB 288-329.

12. MacKeigan LD, Larson LJ. Development and validation of an instrument to measure patient satisfaction with pharmacy services. *Med Care*. 1989;27(5):522–536.

13. Larson LJ, MacKeigan LD. Further validation of an instrument to measure patient satisfaction with pharmacy services. *J Pharm Mark Manage*. 1994;8(1):125–139.

14. Larson LJ, Rovers JP, MacKeigan LD. Patient satisfaction with pharmaceutical care: update of a validated instrument. *J Am Pharm Assoc (Wash)*. 2002;42:44–50.

15. Gupchup GV, Wolfgang AP, Thomas J. Development of a scale to measure directive guidance by pharmacists. *Ann Pharmacother*. 1996;30:1369–1375.

16. Singhal PK, Gireesh GV, Raisch DW, Schommer JC, Holdsworth MT. Impact of pharmacists' directive guidance behaviors on patient satisfaction. *J Am Pharm Assoc (Wash)*. 2002;42(3):407–412.

17. Hernandez L, Chang C-H, Cella D, Corona M, Shiomoto G, McGuire DB. Development and validation of the Satisfaction with Pharmacist Scale. *Pharmacotherapy*. 2000;20(7): 837–843.

18. Gourley GK, Gourley DR, La Monica Rigolosi E, Reed P, Solomon DK, Washington E. Development and validation of the Pharmaceutical Care Satisfaction Questionnaire. *Am J Manag Care*. 2001;7(5):461–466.

19. Briesacher B, Corey R. Patient satisfaction with pharmaceutical services at independent and chain pharmacies. *Am J Health Syst Pharm*. 1997;54:531–536.

20. Ware JE, Hays RD. Methods for Measuring Patient Satisfaction with Specific Medical Encounters. *Med Care*. 1988;26:393–402.

21. Kucukarsian S, Pathak DS, Summers K. Response-oriented Patient Evaluation Survey (ROPES): an administrator's tool for identifying opportunities for service quality improvement. *J Manag Care Pharm*. 1998;4:311–320.

22. The American Society of Health-Systems Pharmacists. *ASHP Guidelines: Minimum Standard for Pharmaceutical Services in Ambulatory Care*. http://www.ashp.org/s_ashp/bin. Asp?Cid=1411&did=5456&doc=file.Pdf. Accessed March 12, 2007.

23. Huston SA, Hobson EH. Using focus groups to inform pharmacy research. *Res Soc Adm Pharm*. 2008;4(3):186–205.

24. Jobe JB. Cognitive psychology and self-reports: models and methods. *Qual Life Res*. 2003;12:219–227.

25. Harris-Kojetin LD, Fowler FJ, Brown JA, Schnaier JA, Sweeney, SF. The use of cognitive testing to develop and evaluate CAHPS 1.0 core survey items. *Med Care*. 1999;37(3):MS10–MS21.

26. Crofton C, Lubalin JS, Darby C. Foreword (to special issue on CAHPS). *Med Care.* 1999;37(3):MS1–MS9.

27. Lessler J, Forsyth, B. A coding system for appraising questionnaires. In: Schwartz N, Sudman S, eds. *Answering Questions: Methodology for Determining Cognitive and Communicative Processes in Survey Research.* San Francisco: Jossey-Bass; 1996.

28. Cleary PD, McNeil BJ. Patient satisfaction as an indicator of quality of care. *Inquiry.* 1988;25(1):25–36.

29. Ware JE, Berwick DM. Patient judgments of hospital quality. *Med Care.* 1990;28(9): S39–S44.

30. Hall JA, Dornan MC. Patient sociodemographic characteristics as predictors of satisfaction with medical care: a meta-analysis. *Soc Sci Med.* 1990;30(7):811–818.

31. Woodbury DD, Tracy D, McKnight E. Does considering severity of illness improve interpretation of patient satisfaction data? *J Healthcare Qual.* 1998;20:33–40.

32. Weisman CC, Henderson JT, Schifrin E, Romans M, Clancy CM. Gender and patient satisfaction in managed care plans: analysis of the 1999 HEDIS/CAHPS 2.0H adult survey. *Womens Health Issues.* 2001;11(5):401–415.

33. Zahn C, Sangl J, Meyer GS, Zaslavsky AM. Consumer assessments of care for children and adults in health plans. How do they compare? *Med Care Rev.* 2002;40(2):145–154.

34. O'Malley AJ, Zaslavsky AM, Elliott MN, Zaborski L, Cleary PD. Case-mix adjustment of the CAHPS hospital survey. *Health Serv Res.* 2005;40(6):2162–2181.

35. Fayers P, Hays P. *Assessing Quality of Life in Clinical Trials.* 2nd ed. Oxford: Oxford University Press; 2005.

36. Fowler FJ Jr. *Survey Research Methods.* 3rd ed. Thousand Oaks, CA: Sage Publications; 2002.

37. Willis G. *Cognitive Interviewing: A tool for Improving Questionnaire Design.* Thousand Oaks, CA: Sage Publications; 2004.

38. Keller S. PQA Pharmacy Services Survey Field Test Report, February 28, 2008. Available from PQA upon request at www.PQAalliance.org.

39. Cronbach LJ. Coefficient alpha and the internal structure of tests. *Psychometrika.* 1951;16(3):297–334.

40. Lubalin J, Schnaier J, Forsyth B, et al. *Design of a Survey to Monitor Consumers' Access to Care, Use of Health Services, Health Outcomes, and Patient Satisfaction.* Research Triangle Park, NC: Research Triangle Institute; 1995. NTIS no. PB95-196036INZ.

41. Hurtado MP, Castillo G, Levind R. *Spanish Translation and Cognitive Testing of the PQA Pharmacy Services Survey.* Silver Spring, MD: American Institutes for Research; March 4, 2009. Unpublished report.

42. Goldstein E, Fyock J. Reporting of CAHPS quality information to Medicare beneficiaries. *Health Serv Res.* 2001;36(3):477–488.

43. AHRQ. *Fact Sheet: CAHPS and the National CAHPS Benchmarking Database.* Rockville, MD: Agency for Healthcare Research and Quality (AHRQ); March 2003. the Agency for Healthcare Research & Quality publication no. 03-P001.

44. AHRQ. *What Consumers Say about the Quality of their Health Plans and Medical Care: National CAHPS Benchmarking Database.* 2008 CAHPS health plan survey chartbook. Rockville, MD: Agency for Healthcare Research and Quality (AHRQ); September 2006: 47 pp.

45. Anderson R, Rice TH, Kominski GF. *Changing the U.S. Health Care System.* 3rd ed. Somerset, NJ: John Wiley & Sons; 2007.

46. Committee on Enhancing Federal Healthcare Quality Programs. In: Corrigan JM, Eden J, Smith BM, eds. *Leadership by Example: Coordinating Government Roles in Improving Health Care Quality.* Washington, DC: National Academy of Sciences; 2002.

47. Zaslavsky AM, Zabrorski LB, Cleary PD. Does the effect of respondent characteristics on consumer assessments vary across plans? *Med Care Res Rev.* 2000;57:379–394.

48. Fredrickson DD, Jones TL, Molgaard CA, et al. Optimal design features for surveying low-income populations. *J Health Care Poor Underserved.* 2005;16(4):677–690.

49. de Vries H, Elliott MN, Hepner KA, Keller SD, Hays RD. Equivalence of mail and telephone responses to the CAHPS hospital survey. *Health Serv Res.* 2005;40(6 Pt 2):2120–2139.

50. Fowler F, Gallagher P, Nederend S. Comparing telephone and mail responses to the CAHPS survey instrument. *Med Care.* 1999;37(3):MS41–MS49.

51. Elliott MN, Zaslavsky AM, Goldstein E, et al. Effects of survey mode, patient mix, and non-response on CAHPS hospital survey scores. *Health Serv Res.* 2009;44(2 Pt 1):501–518.

52. Hibbard JH, Peters E. Supporting informed consumer health care decisions: data presentation approaches that facilitate the use of information in choice. *Annu Rev Public Health.* 2003;24:413–433.

53. Peters E, Dieckmann N, Dixon A, Hibbard JH, Mertz CK. Less is more in presenting quality information to consumers. *Med Care Res Rev.* 2007;64(2):169–190.

CHAPTER 11

Risk Management
·····································
Kenneth Baker

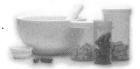

Learning Objectives

At the end of the chapter, the reader will be able to:

1. Understand the risks usually associated with pharmacy dispensing.
2. Explore the relative numbers of mechanical dispensing errors as compared with intellectual pharmacy claims.
3. Review the type of errors often involved in prescribing as they relate to the practice of pharmacy.
4. Discuss how insurance affects pharmacy risks and the decisions to be made by the risk manager.

A STUDY OF RISKS

Pharmacy risk management goes beyond merely putting the right tablets in the bottle with the correct directions on the label. It is even broader than protecting the patient from harm, although that must remain the primary focus of all pharmacists. Risk management means managing a wide spectrum of risks that could affect the practice of pharmacy. It involves protection of the patient, protection of the pharmacists and technicians, and protection of the pharmacy itself.

In this chapter, we look first at identifying some of the most common types of medication errors in pharmacy practice – prescribing, dispensing, administration, and monitoring. For each of these types of medication errors, we will particularly explore the first step in the risk management process, that of identification of the risk. While the risks involved in prescribing errors may usually be more properly described as a medical error, and a mistake in administration may be a nursing error, in the context of pharmacy practice, and the effects on pharmacy patients, the result can be viewed as a pharmacy medication error. The physician may have ordered medication for the wrong patient, and the nurse may have injected the drug IM when it was supposed to be IV, but the problem results in the medication being wrong and the patient injured.

Pharmacy risk management needs to also look beyond medication errors, and explore those risks associated with other quality-related events (QRE) in professional practice. These other risks, while not technically medication errors, have an impact on pharmacy practice and, eventually, how well medication errors are handled and prevented. The other risks we will explore in this chapter are environmental risks, including the environment within the pharmacy or the workplace in general, and financial risks, including insurance coverage for professional liability issues, and exclusions commonly found within professional liability policies.

The first step in risk management is to identify these risks, and to use that information to eventually prevent errors and underlying QREs (plural of QRE) QREs. If we fail to prevent our mistake, we then try to address its consequences and learn from the experience. If we learn from our mistakes, errors, and near misses, we can then identify where the next mistake may be made, thereby preventing future ones. In that regard, we will look at the process by which we record and document, not only errors, but also the near misses, which could have become an error had not there been an intervention somewhere within the system.

Finally, in this chapter, we will look at what may be described as the final step in risk management, dealing with an error once it has occurred. We will look at the consequences of ignoring errors, as well as the consequences of an apology. In that regard, there is one final member of the risk management team that must be considered as part of the solution, the patient. We will explore ways in which the patient can be made a part of the risk management process.

DEALING WITH THE RISKS

Dispensing

While filling a prescription for digoxin 0.1 mg, the pharmacist became distracted by a telephone call from the physician's office.* Instead of finishing the first prescription for digoxin, the pharmacist started working on the called-in prescription from the physician's office. Before he finished with the second prescription, however, he returned to the digoxin order, finishing both prescriptions at about the same time. As a result, the prescription that was supposed to be for digoxin was filled with warfarin. The prescription called in by the doctor's office for warfarin actually contained digoxin tablets. Two prescriptions were filled, and two mechanical dispensing errors occurred. Each of these errors had the potential of causing serious harm to the patients.

According to the Pharmacists Mutual Insurance Company Claims Study, 76% of all claims against pharmacists reported to the insurance company from 1989 to 2009 alleged that either the wrong drug or the wrong strength of the drug was dispensed by error. Throughout the years of the Pharmacists Mutual Claims Study, these statistics for wrong drug and wrong strength have been consistent. This problem, then, filling a prescription with a wrong drug, or with the wrong strength of the correct drug, would

---

*Claim from the file of Pharmacists Mutual Insurance Company. The digoxin patient who received the warfarin was hospitalized, and later filed a claim against the pharmacy and the pharmacist. When the claim was first reported to the pharmacy, an internal investigation discovered the second prescription, called in by the physician's office, had not been picked up. That prescription was still in the "will-call" area. It was labeled as containing warfarin, but actually contained tablets of digoxin.

seem to be the largest risk of mistake in the pharmacy. That conclusion would probably not be correct. While the mistake may be the most likely to result in a professional liability claim, it is probably not the most common dispensing mistake made by pharmacists and pharmacy technicians. It is important to understand, when identifying the risk of a dispensing error, the difference between a claims study, an error study, and a QRE study, which combines errors and near misses.

Just as the claims in the Pharmacists Mutual Claims Study are but a small subset of the total number of errors actually made by the pharmacies insured by the company, the number of errors reaching patients is a subset of the total number of mistakes or QRE actually made in the pharmacy. Each set or subset of this information is useful in identifying the risks of a medication error occurring.

It is important to study claims submitted, as this gives information as to which of the errors are most likely to result in harm to the patient, and thus to result in the patient making a professional liability claim against the pharmacy or pharmacist. By studying the errors that actually reach a patient, we can get an indication of which of our mistakes or QREs are likely to go through the entire dispensing process without being caught. Studying the total number of QREs, which include near misses, errors, and ultimately claims, allows the pharmacist to use information that can prevent mistakes from occurring in the first place without having to wait for a mistake to make it all the way to a patient (Box 11-1).

A study of QREs allows the pharmacy to determine vulnerabilities within the system, which, if not discovered, will eventually result in an error reaching a patient. Once an error reaches a patient, whether it results in an injury, a claim, or a lawsuit may be considered partially a result of luck. While preventing a near miss from becoming an error is a success story that can be pointed to proudly as proof that the quality process worked, a larger success is in designing a process that prevented the mistake from being made in the first place.

BOX 11-1. Medication Error vs. QRE

"Medication error" means any unintended variation from a prescription or drug order. It does not include any variation that is corrected prior to dispensing the medication to the patient or patient's agent, or any variation allowed by law.

"Quality-related event" *or* "QRE" means both:

- a medication error as defined in this section; and
- an occurrence (often called a near miss) during one part of the prescription process that would have resulted in a medication error except that intervention by a pharmacy staff member at another part of the prescription process prevented delivery of the potential medication error to the patient or caregiver.

A Claims Study shows which mistakes may be most likely to result in a professional liability claim. They are probably not the most common dispensing mistake by pharmacists and pharmacy technicians. In a series of reviews of a number of pharmacies that voluntarily recorded all dispensing mistakes or QREs, the results were very different. For more than 5 years, Pharmacists Mutual Insurance Company collected and analyzed such information, consisting of errors that reached a patient, plus near misses caught by the pharmacy staff before they got to the patient. The purpose of collecting and analyzing this information was to alert pharmacists to the risk of prescription errors, and to reduce the number of mistakes, errors, and claims. While these small studies made no claims of scientific validity, they did provide a window into typical community pharmacies, and provided information the pharmacies could use in their quality assurance programs. These reviews, which typically aggregated the data from several pharmacies, were usually analyzed for periods of 30 days, or 6 months. One 30-day review distributed to the pharmacies that participated showed that only 27% of the QREs, combining errors and near misses, were caused by the wrong drug or the wrong strength. This is far different from the 76% shown in the Claims Study. This type of review was performed several times throughout the years, and the percentages of wrong drug and wrong strength were usually close to the range of 25% of all QREs. With this information, the pharmacy staff can narrow its root cause search, and discover vulnerabilities lying within the system in each process.

Pharmacists Mutual's category of mechanical errors – wrong drug, wrong strength, and wrong directions – represents over 80% of all claims reported to the insurance company during the period of time covered by the study. Examining each individual year during the study shows the 80% figure for mechanical errors to be very consistent year to year. This is not surprising for a Claims Study, since the areas covered by the category called "mechanical errors" are most likely to result in harm and, thus, most likely to result in a claim being made against the pharmacy and pharmacist.

The balance of the claims is categorized by Pharmacists Mutual as "intellectual claims," referring to those claims that involve a more cognitive action, such as counseling and drug review. The majority of the remaining claims are for failure to counsel, inadequate counseling, drug review, or failure to properly protect confidential information from unauthorized disclosure. The counseling claims, or failure to counsel claims, have varied over the years of the study from approximately 2% to a high of over 10%, with the average at 3.5% of all claims during the entire time of the study. Because claims are usually made, based on actual injury, and usually involve a more serious injury, it is, perhaps, not surprising to see a low number of counseling-related claims. In order for a plaintiff to make a claim against a pharmacist for failure to adequately counsel, the plaintiff would have to be able to prove causation, including what attorneys generally refer to as a "but for" test. The "but for" test, as the name indicates, would amount to showing that the injuries would not have occurred had the counseling been proper. Since counseling could generally be made up of both oral and written directions and instructions, such claims would be expected to be a lower percentage of total claims. The fact that 2–3% of all claims reported within a given year involve counseling, however, alerts pharmacists that a real risk does exist anytime counseling is not properly performed when required, or is not documented when performed.

The Pharmacists Mutual Claims Study reports an average of 2% of all claims during the period of 1989 through 2009 characterized as "non-bodily injury" claims. The insurance company uses this designation of "non-bodily injury" claims for what its insurance policies refer to as "personal injury." Under most standard property and casualty insurance policies, personal injury is described as libel, slander, release of confidential information, and items such as false arrest or malicious prosecution. With only a few exceptions for claims involving a pharmacist who reports a suspected forged prescription to the police resulting in the arrest of a pharmacy customer, most of the claims in this category are for unauthorized release of confidential records. This area is expected to increase in number, if not percentage of claims, as more attorneys and member of the public become familiar with the Health Insurance Portability and Accountability Act of 1996 (HIPAA) requirements.

Prescribing

Heidi's physician made a mistake. Dr Lorenc's records informed him that his patient was allergic to aspirin, ibuprophen, and acetaminophen. Avoiding these, he prescribed Toradol for her pain. In a later deposition, he admitted he did not know about a possible cross-sensitivity of Toradol and Heidi's aspirin allergy. Heidi suffered a severe allergic reaction but fortunately was rushed to the hospital emergency room in time.[†]

A prescriber's error is a risk management concern for pharmacists. When Heidi had an allergic reaction to Toradol, she sued the physician and the pharmacy. In her deposition, the pharmacist testified she was aware of the potential danger of cross-sensitivity for these drugs. Even though the allergy to aspirin was in the pharmacy's computer system, the pharmacist indicated she was not alerted to the entry. The Court reviewed the pharmacist's testimony:

> If the Toradol information was in the pharmacy's computer, a "drug interaction" warning would have flashed across the screen, halting the prescription process for customers such as Heidi for whom Toradol was contraindicated. At that point, the pharmacist was to call the physician and notify him of the contraindication. [The pharmacist] did not remember calling Dr. Lorenc about Heidi's prescription, nor did she remember seeing any documentation indicating that she made such a call.

The Court described what happened as a result of the physician's error and the pharmacy's failure to catch it:

> There were directions on the bottle that Heidi received from the pharmacy, but there was no warning about contraindications. Heidi took the first dose of Toradol at about 4 p.m. on August 4, and within 40 minutes she began to experience respiratory problems including a tightness in her chest. She began

---

[†] Happel v. Wal-Mart 766 N.E.2d 1118 (Ill. 2002).

a breathing treatment with a nebulizer, and called the pharmacy to ask if she could be having a reaction to Toradol. Her call was disconnected. She called again, and was told that there should be no drug reaction problem. Heidi then called a friend who was a pharmacist and was aware of her allergies. He told her to begin a nebulizer treatment if she had not already done so, and to go to the emergency room if her condition worsened. She went to the emergency room, and was found to be experiencing anaphylactic shock.

While the Court was reluctant to find it a general pharmacist duty to warn, it did so in this case because of the "special circumstances" present. The special circumstances the Court noted in this case were the presence of the allergy in the pharmacy's computer system and the pharmacist's knowledge of the potential reaction regarding Toradol in a patient with an aspirin allergy. The Court said:

> It is undisputed that Wal-Mart had "special knowledge" of Heidi's medical history, that is, her drug allergies. In addition, Wal-Mart knew that Toradol was contraindicated for persons such as Heidi with allergies to aspirin and other NSAIDs. In such limited circumstances, a narrow duty to warn clearly exists.

The Court explained the "narrow duty" in its holding:

> [W]e hold that a narrow duty to warn exists where, as in the instant case, a pharmacy has patient-specific information about drug allergies, and knows that the drug being prescribed is contraindicated for the individual patient. In such instances, a pharmacy has a duty to warn either the prescribing physician or the patient of the potential danger.

The problem for pharmacists is that these "special circumstances" are present in most allergy and contraindication cases. The Illinois Supreme Court is not alone in finding it a duty to warn the patient or the prescriber in some circumstances. Similar "limited" duties are found in state court opinions in Washington,[‡] Arizona,[§] Pennsylvania,[¶] Tennessee,[**] Missouri,[††] and Indiana[‡‡] among others.

Unfortunately, the lack of knowledge regarding allergies demonstrated by Heid's physician was not as uncommon as might be hoped. Mag Mutual is an insurance company that provides malpractice coverage for physicians. In its newsletter it regularly reports selected closed claims in an effort to educate its insured physicians of the risks. In one issue, Mag Mutual reported several pharmacy-related claims against physicians,

---

[‡] McKee v. American Home Products Corp., 113 Wash. 2d 701, 715, 782 P.2d 1045, 1053 (1989) [agreeing that "pharmacists should have a duty to be alert for patent errors in a prescription, (including) *** known contraindications *** and to take corrective measures"].

[§] Lasley v. Shrakes Country Club Pharmacy, 880 P2d 1129 (Ariz. Ct. App. 1994).

[¶] Riff v. Morgan, 353 Pa.Super. 21, 508 A.2d 1247 (1986).

[**] Dooley v. Everett, 805 S.W.2d 380 (Tenn. App. 1990).

[††] Horner v. Spalitto, 1 S.W.3d 519 (Mo. Ct App. Western Dist. 1999).

[‡‡] Hooks SuperX, Inc. v. McLaughlin, 642 N.E. 2d 514 (Ind. 1994).

including a prescription for amoxicillin for a patient with a penicillin allergy, a serious overdose of Alkeran due in part to a pharmacy communication failure, and a 2.5 mg per day dosage of Coumadin inadvertently ordered and filled as 10 mg.[1]

In 1993 the Physician Insurers Association of America conducted a study of medication-related claims against physicians insured by member companies.[2] The study reported that medication errors are the second leading cause of malpractice claims against physicians. This was reaffirmed in a 2006 data sharing study.[§§]

In its medication error study, PIAA reported that physician's medical malpractice claims related to prescribing included the following areas of which pharmacists should be aware. Such prescriber claims could lead to drug review or counseling claims against a pharmacist or pharmacy[2]:

- incorrect dosage (10.9%);
- inappropriate for condition (9.6%);
- failure to monitor (side effects) (7.9%);
- communication failure with patient (6.7%);
- failure to monitor (drug levels) (5.1%);
- lack of knowledge (interactions) (5.1%);
- most appropriate medication not used (5%).

Pharmacists need to be on guard for risks associated with prescribing errors. In the Pharmacists Mutual Claims Study, all claims that are not categorized as mechanical errors are place into a category labeled intellectual claims. The largest category of intellectual claims is what the study refers to as "drug review" claims. Drug review claims include allegations that the pharmacist failed to protect the patient from allergic reactions, interactions, overuse, and underuse problems associated with filled prescriptions. These claims correspond with the Omnibus Budget Reconciliation Act of 1990 (OBRA 90) requirement to perform a prospective drug review prior to filling a new prescription. These claims also correspond to many of the prescriber errors found in the PIAA study.

The Pharmacists Mutual Claims Study started in 1989, when drug review claims were relatively rare. In subsequent years these claims have consistently grown. By 1997, 12% of all claims received by Pharmacists Mutual Insurance Company were within this category. In the years since 1997, the percentage of drug review claims has averaged 8.5% of all claims. A study of drug review claims over the individual years shows that this category is the fastest growing area of claims according to this study. Unlike counseling claims, which tend to be hard to prove and usually result in less significant injuries, drug review claims can be very injurious, and relatively easy to pass the causation test.

The drug review category within the Pharmacists Mutual Claims Study should alert pharmacists to the risks in the DUR part of the dispensing process. Each time the pharmacy is alerted to an error concerning an allergic reaction, or potential interaction, the pharmacy should perform a root cause analysis to determine how the interaction was missed, and if there was any way that the pharmacy could have detected it. Since

---

§§ PIAA Data Sharing Project, June 2006, reported in *2006 Mag Mutual Newsletter*, supra.

most of the drug review claims involve an error made by a prescriber and/or the patient, the root cause analysis also involves non-pharmacy factors. The higher the foreseeability of injury, and the higher the risk of more serious injury, the more likely it is that a court would find a legal duty for drug review on the pharmacist, and the more likely that a claim would be made. Most importantly, when the risk to the patient is higher and more likely, pharmacists can be found to have a higher ethical duty, which is more demanding than even the "legal" duty.

The duly of a pharmacist to be vigilant against the errors of prescribers is not new. As early as 1932 a Maryland court held, "A pharmacist cannot escape liability in compounding and dispensing poisons in deadly and unusual doses even though the physician's prescription called for such dosage."[§§]

Administration

Following the doctor's orders on the chart, the nurse administered Vibramycin to the patient intramuscularly. It should have been administered intravenously. The pharmacy had recognized the error and had changed the doctor's order from IM to IV and marked it such before sending it to the floor. The pharmacist did not, however, contact the doctor or instruct the nurses on the floor to disregard the doctor's notation of IM in the chart. The court in this case held ". . . a pharmacist has a limited duty to inquire or verify from the prescribing physician clear errors or mistakes in the prescription."[***]

Most times when nurses or physicians incorrectly administer medication filled accurately by the pharmacist, there is no liability on the pharmacist. If, however, the pharmacist had a duty to correct a mistake on the face of the prescription, and failed to do so, the pharmacist may be added to the suit or claim. Pharmacists need to be cognizant to these administration risks.

In a Pennsylvania case,[†††] a pharmacist was held liable with the physician when the prescriber's directions on a prescription for Cafergot suppositories read only, "insert one every four hours." The patient was not informed that Cafergot poisoning may result when the dose exceed the recommendation of "no more than 5 suppositories should be taken during any 7-day period." The patient's use greatly exceeded that maximum and the patient was hospitalized. The court held the pharmacist may be sued and share payment of damages with the prescriber when the prescription contains an error on its face, such as, in this case, incomplete directions.

Claims have been made against pharmacists in many instances when the prescription was correctly filled. A patient was changed from a short-acting nitrate to a one-a-day dose, sustained release form of the drug.[‡‡‡] The pharmacist filled the prescription correctly, including the directions of "take one daily." The patient, however, continued to take the new tablets in the same manner as the former prescription – three a day. Neither the physician nor the pharmacist informed the patient the medication had

---

[§§] Peoples Service Drug Stores v. Somerville, 161 Md. 662, 158 A. 12 (1932).
[***] Gassen v. East Jefferson General Hospital, 628 So.2d 256 (La. App. 5th Cir. 1993).
[†††] Riff v. Morgan, 353 Pa.Super. 21, 508 A.2d 1247 (1986).
[‡‡‡] From the claims files of Pharmacists Mutual Insurance Company. Claim was settled prior to suit.

been changed to a long-acting form that required a dosage adjustment. The fact that the elderly patient was also negligent for failing to read the new directions did not fully excuse either the doctor or the pharmacist.

Often pharmacists are not in a position to prevent an administration error, but when they are, there is a risk that the pharmacist will be held at least partially liable for the patient's injuries. By recognizing the risk, pharmacists can avoid a claim and assist the patient to avoid unnecessary harm.

Monitoring Patient Use

It is said that today's pharmacist is the patient's medication risk manager. Pharmacists are in a good position to regularly monitor a patient's use of medication. The pharmacy computer usually contains a record of the patient's compliance with the doctor's directions. As drugs become more powerful and compliance more significant, the role of the pharmacist in assisting patients to take their prescription properly and to its best results becomes more important. When a professional is in a position to help, his or her failure to do so can eventually lead to liability.

By January 1993, almost every state had passed a statute or a board of pharmacy regulation implementing the federal OBRA 90 guidelines. As a part of those regulations, the pharmacist was required to perform a prospective drug review prior to dispensing a prescription. As part of the DUR, the pharmacist was directed to look for, among other items, overuse and underuse of prescribed medication. This mandate may be said to include a duty to monitor patient drug use. In no place is this duty more evident than with controlled substance use.

As a lumberjack in the state of Washington, Patrick McLaughlin injured his back. He returned to his home state of Indiana to recuperate and for treatment of the pain. During treatment he became addicted to propoxyphene. He sued his physician and the pharmacy that filled his prescriptions. Against the pharmacy, McLaughlin alleged, it should not have allowed him to keep filling his prescriptions when the pharmacists should have seen that the amounts he was receiving greatly exceed the prescribed dosage. Prior to the McLaughlin case, Indiana had held pharmacists have only limited duties to warn, but in this case the Indiana Supreme Court saw the duty differently.[§§§] The Court, after reviewing the pharmacy–patient relationship, foreseeability of addiction from overuse of controlled substances, and the public policy concern surrounding addiction, held:

> Where a pharmacy customer is having a prescription for a dangerous drug refilled at an unreasonably faster rate than the rate prescribed, the pharmacist has a duty to cease refilling the prescription pending direct and explicit directions from the prescribing physician.

Criminal enforcement of controlled substance laws raises a different risk for the pharmacist in this particular type of claim. Section 1306.04 of the Federal Code of

---

[§§§] Hooks SuperX, Inc. v. McLaughlin, 642 N.E.2d 514 (Ind. 1994).

Regulations may be said to impose a duty on pharmacists to monitor controlled substance use. The rule, referred to as the corresponding duty rule, says:

> A prescription for a controlled substance to be effective must be issued for a legitimate medical purpose by an individual practitioner acting in the usual course of his professional practice. The responsibility for the proper prescribing and dispensing of controlled substances is on the prescribing practitioner, *but a corresponding responsibility rests with the pharmacist who fills the prescription.* An order purporting to be a prescription issued not in the usual course of professional treatment or in legitimate and authorized research is not a prescription within the meaning and intent of section 309 of the Act (21 U.S.C. 829) and the person knowingly filling such a purported prescription, as well as the person issuing it, shall be subject to the penalties provided for violations of the provisions of law relating to controlled substances. Federal Code of Regulation § 1306.04, (emphasis added)

Often, in order for a pharmacist to know that a particular prescription is for a "legitimate medical purpose," the pharmacist must know how often it has been refilled and whether the patient is taking it in accordance with the prescribed directions. The pharmacist in such cases must monitor his or her patient's usage. The computer software can usually be counted on to alert pharmacists to overuse, but, as in the case of Heidi's allergy, neither the system nor the computer is infallible. Pharmacists need to recognize the risks involved with these types of prescriptions and use procedure to manage those risks.

Too often overlooked is the opposite problem of underuse, which is also a part of the OBRA 90 guidelines. Risk to the patient of underuse of medication or noncompliance is real. The State of Massachusetts publishes a health newsletter on the Internet.[3] In its Winter 2005 issue, it was estimated that "125,000 deaths in the United States each year are attributed to noncompliance with a doctor's prescription." If this number is correct, it is three times the number of people killed in automobile accidents each year. According to the newsletter, the most common types of noncompliance include:

- not having a prescription filled;
- taking an incorrect dose – too much or too little;
- taking the medication at the wrong time;
- forgetting to take one or more doses;
- stopping the medication too soon.

Personal, Non-bodily Injury

When pharmacists consider medication errors and pharmacy liability risks, they naturally tend to think of some form of injury to the body of the patient. There is, however, another risk associated with medication use and the practice of pharmacy – personal or non-bodily injury. As we shall see when we discuss insurance, patients may be harmed even if the prescription is filled correctly and the medication works as intended with no noticeable side effects.

Marie was 15 years old and a freshman in high school.⁵⁵⁵ Marie's doctor prescribed low-dose hormonal therapy to treat Marie's acne. Her parents filled the prescription, which was more commonly associated with birth control, at the local pharmacy. The cashier at the pharmacy was a female student in Marie's class and when she rang up the charge for Marie's prescription on the cash register, she recognized the packaging and soon the fact that Marie was taking birth control pills was a source of gossip throughout the school. Marie was a shy girl and the talk of her medication use and the implications she was sure accompanied it was, according to her parents, devastating. The effect on the pharmacy's reputation was also bad and far outweighed the dollars paid for the malpractice claim.

Jack was a divorced male nurse who lived with and was the sole support of his 12-year-old son.⁵⁵⁵⁵ Jack worked at a local hospital in a small town. At a time when much less was known about AIDS and HIV, Jack had engaged in risky, sexual behavior, but he had been able to keep his HIV status and his occasional homosexual activity a closely guarded secret, particularly from his employer and his son.

Jack purposefully had his prescriptions for HIV filled at a pharmacy in a neighboring, larger city. He consulted freely with the pharmacist who, over time, he came to trust and whose advice he relied upon. When a refill was needed, Jack called and made sure his pharmacist would be on duty. The pharmacist understood the need for confidentiality and took steps to safeguard the information trusted to him. He made only one exception.

The pharmacist's nephew was a nursing student and at the family's annual Thanksgiving dinner the nephew told his uncle about his upcoming training schedule, which included time at the facility where Jack worked as a nurse. Swearing his nephew to absolute secrecy, the pharmacist confided in his nephew that a nurse named Jack worked in that hospital and warned that it was possible to transfer HIV via accidental syringe punctures. The nephew's pledge of secrecy lasted only through the weekend. The nephew told several student nurses in his class and soon everyone in the hospital knew about Jack's problem. Shortly thereafter everyone who attended junior high school with Jack's son also knew. A lawsuit followed that was quickly followed with a monetary settlement. The pharmacist was fired.

Mrs Jenkins began having pain and while at her son's basketball game complained to a dentist who was attending the game. Mrs Jenkins and the dentist did not know each other well, but the dentist wrote a prescription for a pain medication containing hydrocodone. He told her to call the office in the morning to make an appointment if she could not get a hold of her regular dentist. The dentist wrote the prescription on a prescription blank he carried in his billfold. The blank was a little worn and wrinkled, but the information was clearly visible.

---

⁵⁵⁵ Claim from the files of Pharmacists Mutual Insurance Company. The names have been changed. It is presented here, as all such examples, as a warning to pharmacists of the potential of claims and patient injury.
⁵⁵⁵⁵ Claim from the files of Pharmacists Mutual Insurance Company. The names have been changed.

Mrs Jenkins did not fill the prescription that night, but instead took it to a pharmacy the next day. It was not her regular pharmacy and the pharmacist became suspicious because of the condition of the prescription blank on which it was written. The pharmacist called the dentist's office and was told Mrs Jenkins was not one of their patients. The receptionist checked with the dentist, who did not remember writing the prescription and had not made a record of it. While Mrs Jenkins waited, the pharmacist called the police to report the facts as he understood them. The police came to the pharmacy and arrested Mrs Jenkins, who spent a few hours in custody until the police finally called the dentist who confirmed that he indeed had written the prescription. Mrs Jenkins sued the pharmacy, but the claim was dismissed after a few months because the pharmacy has only relayed the facts as they knew them to the police. It was the police who decided to arrest Mrs Jenkins. The pharmacy did not have to pay any damages, but its insurance company did incur almost $2000 in attorney fees.

In each of the above claims there was no bodily damage to the patient. Release of confidential information, libel, slander, false arrest, and malicious prosecution are all examples of personal injury. In some cases non-bodily injury to the patient may be just as painful as damage to the body, and may take longer to heal. All of these claims are reported in the Pharmacists Mutual Claims Study under the category of personal injury. From 1989 through 2009, personal injury averaged 2% of all claims against pharmacists received by Pharmacists Mutual Insurance Company.

Claims, lawsuits, and loss of reputation are not the only risks associated with the unauthorized release of confidential patient information. The pharmacist risk manager must also protect the pharmacy, hospital, or enterprise against civil fines and criminal prosecutions related to possible violations of federal HIPAA laws and regulations.

In 2002 the U.S. Department of Health and Human Services issued its Privacy Rule implementing the requirements of HIPAA. Under these rules the Office of Civil Rights has the power to enforce patient privacy with civil fines. The website HG.org reported, "As of October 31, 2005, HHS' Office of Civil Rights ('OCR'), the agency charged with HIPAA Privacy Rule enforcement had received and initiated reviews of over 16,000 privacy complaints from health care consumers and others across the country."[4] The risks are real and the penalties can be high. In 2008, a Seattle-based not-for-profit health system paid $100,000 to settle a HIPAA complaint.[5]

Reducing the risk of personal, non-bodily injury begins with well-considered policies and procedures and ends with staff training. Consider each of the examples above as a potential risk to the pharmacy and develop a policy for avoiding or mitigating each and then write a procedure of how employees are to handle each. Good policies and procedures usually do not involve a spark of brilliance, but the glow of common sense.

A good place to start reducing the risk of personal injury is in developing and enforcing a rule that all laws must be obeyed to the letter. In personal injury, obeying the law means not only HIPAA regulations, but also confidentiality statutes and rules in force at the state level. While HIPAA preempts any state legislation or rules that contradict it, or that are less strict, in cases where the state law goes beyond the requirements of HIPAA, the state law is enforced. Not only must each employee be trained in HIPAA, but they should also be well versed in state rules. In addition, pharmacy staff should be educated in examples of appropriate responses in all cases. Training not only may involve giving these appropriate responses in a series of situations, but should also include a program in ethics and simple customer relations. The pharmacist who was faced with the dilemma regarding Jack, the male nurse, and his nephew would have been better able to deal with the situation if he had studied how difficult choices between two unsatisfactory ethical choices may be made before the actual problem arose (Box 11-2).

For many situations, simply instructing the staff that they are not to release any information regarding prescriptions is sufficient, but occasionally, more difficult questions arise. In the situation with the pharmacy clerk and the high school student's birth control prescription, the training needs to go beyond pharmacy staff to include all employees. Developing methods that would eliminate the risk of other employees knowing or guessing the contents of a patient's prescription may go a long way in solving such a problem in the future.

A staff-training manual, which would include instructions to avoid personal injury liability, should include scenarios on libel and slander, as well as other personal injury

---

BOX 11-2. Possible Appropriate Responses on Discovery of an Error

- Technician: "Mrs. Jones, I am sorry you had to come back. I am sure the pharmacist will want to deal with this personally. I am going to interrupt him/her and he/she will be here as soon as he/she can."
- (Obvious error involving the wrong drug in the bottle.) Pharmacist: "Mrs. Jones, we made a mistake. I am so sorry. We are going to correct this immediately (and, if acceptable under pharmacy policy) we are going to refund what you paid for this prescription. We are certainly human and can make errors, but we do not make many mistakes like this. I do not yet know how this happened, but we will find out. We are going to completely review every step taken in filling this prescription and we will find out what caused this mistake. I cannot guarantee we will never make another mistake, but we will take whatever steps are necessary to try to make sure this does not happen again. I will call you when we figure this out." (The pharmacist must then make sure the patient is called and told what happened and what changes were instituted.)
- (Not an obvious error.) Pharmacist: "Mrs. Jones, I am sorry you had a problem. I do not yet know what happened or if it is our mistake or not, but we are going to find out. We are certainly human and can make a mistake and if so, we need to figure that out. I will tell you that we will take this very seriously. If it turns out it is our error, I will tell you that and what we are going to do to correct any situation we discover. If it is not our mistake, I will let you know that, too." (The pharmacist must carry through with any promises.)

areas. Dealing with situations in which illegal activity is suspected should begin with the rule that some questions or situations are "pharmacist-only questions." Not only must the pharmacist be trained to deal with such situations, but the staff must also be trained that, with each situation, confidentiality remains a part of their duty, even in cases where illegality is suspected. A mention over the dinner table that "Mrs. Jenkins tried to pass a phony prescription" could end with a situation almost as traumatic as an arrest.

A part of the training in this area needs to also include lessons as to when police should be called, and that the fear of "getting involved" may be a failure of legal duty, as well as a risk equal to making the phone call. Training as to the words to be used in the phone call, and that only the facts should be given, rather than opinions stated as if they were facts, should be provided.

Identifying Environmental Risks

Perhaps the best indicator of risk in a pharmacy can be summed up in the word "environment." A counter with clutter provides a special risk, particularly if some of the clutter involves stock bottles of medication that have not been reshelved. Prescriptions that have been filled but not yet bagged and completed may also provide a special danger. One unscientific but illuminating study was performed by a Pharmacists Mutual attorney who was viewing 100 consecutive errors at a small chain. The resulting chart showed that of the 100 errors, 8 involved prescriptions that were filled correctly but given to the wrong patient. In some of these cases, the wrong prescription was put into the sack with a different receipt; in some cases, it was handed to the wrong patient; and, in some cases, they were delivered to the wrong house. It seems a simple rule in risk management that if pharmacists fill prescriptions correctly, with the correct label and the correct drug, it should be easy to make sure it is given to the right person. In many of these situations, a part of the problem was a messy prescription counter.

One of the first jobs of a risk manager is to stand back and survey the area in which the prescription work-flow is occurring. Before trying to identify risks of errors and mistakes, as part of the work-flow, the risk manager should look at the surrounding area itself. The risk manager should not only look at the area, but should listen to it as well. Loud or inappropriate sounds can cause increased stress as much as a cluttered workspace or a suddenly large workload. Inappropriate visiting among staff, as well as other sounds, can increase the noise clutter in the pharmacy.

The workspace should be clean and open with sufficient room for each process of the work-flow, or work-flow stations. In addition to open space, lighting should also be bright enough for the job to be performed without producing a glare that would be distracting. Often these surrounding environmental factors will differ according to the personnel involved, so it may be difficult to design a "one-size-fits-all" background.

The environment may also include tools that can assist the pharmacy staff. A magnifying glass available for reading prescriptions may be considered an environmental tool, as well as a tilted tray designed to hold a prescription at a comfortable level while it is read and entered into the computer. Scanning and image technology may serve the same purpose, and also could be considered environmental tools.

In one pharmacy that was having a problem of too many errors addressed it by emphasizing the pharmacist's quality review station. The environment within the pharmacy was altered to mark off a section of the prescription counter that was used only for the pharmacist's final quality check. In one pharmacy, an additional monitor was placed at the pharmacist's quality check station to allow the pharmacist to review patient profiles, and computer-generated DUR warnings.

When considering environmental risks, the risk manager should think beyond questions of noise, lighting, and neatness to include all parts of the pharmacy environment. This may include how drugs are arranged on the shelves, and the convenience or inconvenience of retrieving a certain drug. For example, when one pharmacy noted that a disproportionate number of errors involved incorrectly giving Coumadin 5 mg, the pharmacy placed all bottles of Coumadin 5 mg in the narcotic drawer. This forced any staff member using Coumadin 5 mg to give additional thought, along with additional effort, to use that particular drug. The results were so dramatic that all members of the staff decided to make that situation permanent within their pharmacy.

FINANCIAL – TRANSFER OR RETENTION OF RISK

If a risk manager were able to successfully identify every potential mistake and prevent them all before they were able to pose a problem for the hospital, pharmacy, or enterprise, insurance would still be necessary. Insurance pays not merely for the damages caused by errors, but also for the attorney fees to defend the cases in which errors are made, and the cases in which no error existed. Winning a lawsuit, or defending a claim to zero payment, may often be more expensive than paying to settle a doubtful claim.

One of the risks that a risk manager must consider is the financial risk to the pharmacy, hospital, or enterprise. There are several ways to handle financial risks, including retention of risk by setting aside an amount of dollars to be able to defend and pay claims when appropriate. Many large hospitals, and most large pharmacy chains, will retain from twenty-five thousand dollars to 1 million dollars of each claim throughout the year. These self-insured retentions may be less expensive in the long run than purchasing insurance. Even in these cases, however, the large chain pharmacies, or large hospitals, will purchase insurance for catastrophic losses or as a stop for annual payouts for a number of small claims within a year. Regardless of the size of the enterprise, the manager should consider the financial risk of medication errors, and develop either a method for retention of the risk or a transfer of the risk. To transfer a financial risk usually involves the purchase of insurance.

Insurance is a contract. Like all contracts, insurance contains terms, exclusions, conditions, and limitations. Unlike many contracts, however, the insurance contract is written in fairly straightforward English. Since insurance is regulated by state insurance departments, in most cases, the language has been reviewed and usually tested for its "readability quotient." Most insurance contracts are designed to be read at sixth-grade reading levels. This does not mean that the terms are simple, but rather means that the word choice and the length of sentences are understandable for most people. Insurance contracts look formidable because of length of most insurance policies, and the details concerned with coverage, exclusions, and conditions.

Professional Liability Insurance

A risk manager may have to consider several types and forms of insurance, including Workers' Compensation policies, general liability coverage, property loss protection, and product liability coverage, but in this chapter we will limit the discussions to professional malpractice coverage issues. Pharmacy malpractice differs from other health care insurance issues because of the central focus of the product or medication. Until recent decades, "products liability and completed works operations" coverage was the primary focus of pharmacy malpractice insurance. As pharmacy practice has changed to encompass more duties, however, the pharmacy malpractice insurance policy has moved away from strictly product coverage to a more traditional health care malpractice model. While products and completed works operations coverage are still important in pharmacy, the subject is beyond the scope of this chapter, so we will limit the discussion to the professional acts.

For large hospitals or large pharmacy chains, it may be possible for a risk manager to negotiate terms and price with the insurance company. In this way, the insurance can be tailored like any contract to the needs and wants of the parties engaged in the negotiations. In most cases, however, insurance policies act as "adhesion contracts." Although not technically contracts of adhesion, insurance policies are sometimes referred to in that manner because the purchaser is "stuck with what coverage the company offers" in its standard contract. Within competitive contracts, however, there are often differences between coverages and terms offered by various companies. A risk manager should review several options with competing insurance companies concentrating on the terms and insuring language before thought is given to the price. A cheap price for an insurance policy that does not cover losses may result in an expensive alternative. When reading an insurance contract, the risk manager should try to answer several questions:

- *Who* is covered under the policy?
- *What* acts are covered under the policy?
- *When* does the policy cover?
- *Where* does the policy cover?

A malpractice policy for a pharmacy or pharmacist may often be part of a larger insurance contract. In a hospital, the pharmacist insurance is usually a part of the medical malpractice policy, and the pharmacy terms may be ill-defined. The pharmacy risk manager may have to ask for clarification as to what acts are covered and how some terms are defined. Within community pharmacy, the pharmacy malpractice coverage may be within the larger, general liability provisions of the contract, with special endorsements to cover pharmacy malpractice. Many of the terms of the general contract will be important, and will be necessary to answering some of the questions raised when reviewing the policies. Since hospital policies tend to be less standard, in this chapter we will use examples from community pharmacy commercial policies and the accompanying pharmacy malpractice endorsements attached to them.

Who?

There are two types of pharmacy professional liability policies. One is the corporate or enterprise policy, which should cover all persons involved in a potential claim, but may not. The other policy is an individual pharmacist professional liability policy, which, as the term implies, covers only a single individual pharmacist. In medical malpractice, the individual physician's policy is normally the primary policy, and nurses or physicians agents will be covered under the language of that individual policy. In pharmacy, however, the individual policy is considered and written as an excess or secondary policy, which comes into play only if the primary, commercial policy fails to respond in some way. Because the individual pharmacy professional policy tends to be excess or secondary, the price is relatively low, as compared to the primary policy. Each pharmacist should read their individual policy to determine when it comes into play and if it is clearly a secondary policy. By protecting the secondary or excess nature of the individual policy, the pharmacist can keep the premiums for that policy low, while relying upon the employer's commercial policy for initial coverage. Because pharmacy claims tend to involve more than one individual, it is often important that the commercial policy responds first so that all staff involved in a claim can be defended in a coordinated manner. If an individual pharmacist feels that his or her situation is different from the rest of the staff, he or she may then ask that his or her secondary policy come into play.

Under the commercial policy, there will be language indicating who is covered by that policy. The pharmacy, hospital, or enterprise will be covered as a named insured, and each staff member, including pharmacists and pharmacy technicians, should then be covered as additional insureds, within the definitional language of the policy. While the named insured will be shown on the declarations page of the policy, in order to find who is included as an additional insureds, the risk manager should turn to the definition section.

Under the definition of "additional insureds," there will usually be a clause stating "your employees" are insured when acting within the scope of their employment. Occasionally, because it is built upon what is basically a standard commercial policy, there will be an exclusion within the definition that the risk manager will have to address. In some policies, the definition of "additional insured" may contain the following language: "however, none of your employees is insured if they perform or fail to perform professional healthcare services." Unless coverage for the pharmacist and pharmacy technicians is added back in a special, professional liability endorsement, there will be no coverage for these professionals. In that case, the risk manager needs to renegotiate or look at other policies and options. The other thing to note is that only the employees are covered, usually not independent contractors. Under the definition section, however, temporary or replacement workers, even though they are independent contractors, may be included in the definition.

The concept of coordinated coverage is important in pharmacy because often the question does not involve whether a mistake was made, but what damages were caused by a mechanical error. Who made the mistake may not be an issue unless the pharmacy staff raises it. If this is allowed to degrade into finger pointing, the amount of damages will usually increase, not because of the injuries, but because the situation is made to appear as grossly negligent or sloppy and without regard to the safety of the patient.

What?

Pharmacists generally give little thought to the question of what is covered under a pharmacy professional liability policy because "everyone knows what a pharmacist does." At one time that answer would have been correct, but pharmacy and the duties of pharmacists have changed dramatically in the last few years. Pharmacists today are involved in drug reviews, immunizations, counseling in the use of medications, and many other activities, which may appear foreign to many insurance professionals who make the initial determination as to whether a particular allegation or claim is included in coverage. The risk manager would be advised to list all activities of the pharmacists within a particular practice setting, and compare that list with the definition in the policy. If there is a question as to whether an activity is clearly included, an inquiry is warranted and clarification needed before decisions are made.

A commercial policy will generally have two types of liability coverage, bodily injury liability coverage and personal injury liability coverage. The risk manager should be certain that both coverages exist and apply to the pharmacy malpractice coverages. It was not uncommon for professional pharmacy coverages to contain only bodily injury coverage. Bodily injury coverage, as the name implies, covers injury to a person's body. Over 95% of all pharmacy liability claims are for bodily injury. The wrong tablet in the bottle, the wrong directions on the label, lack of counseling, or failure to properly perform a drug review all lead to bodily injury, or at least the allegation of bodily injury. At one time, insurance companies did not consider the possibility of a claim being made against a pharmacist or pharmacy that did not involve bodily injury. Such is no longer the case. The risk manager should look for personal injury protection, which will usually be defined as "personal and advertising injury." Commercial policies typically define "personal and advertising injury" as:

1. oral or written publication, including electronic publication, of material that:
   a. slanders or libels a person or organization,
   b. disparages a person's or an organization's goods, products, or services, or
   c. violates a person's right of privacy;
2. false arrest, detention, or imprisonment;
3. malicious prosecution;
4. misappropriation of advertising ideas of another in your advertisement;
5. infringement of a copyright slogan or trade dress of another in your advertisement; or
6. wrongful entry into, wrongful eviction from, or invasion of the right of private occupancy of a room, dwelling, or premises that a person occupies.

While some of these coverages are more important in the general liability portion of the commercial policy, some are critical in professional pharmacy coverage. In particular, the right of privacy, malicious prosecution, false arrest, and libel or slander have become more common in pharmacy claims in the last two decades. Personal and advertising injury will include HIPAA-type violations, in most cases, but may not include fines or actions instituted by the Office of Civil Rights, the organization that enforces

HIPAA on a federal level. These are not covered because fines and punishments are neither personal injuries, nor bodily injury, and are usually specifically excluded under other portions of the policy.

When?

Professional health care malpractice policies are either "occurrence policies" or "claims made policies." All insurance policies will contain language indicating that the action leading to the claim must have occurred during the period in which the policy was in effect. This is called a "trigger" because it determines which and when a policy responds. In some policies, called "claims made policies," in addition to this "occurrence trigger," there is a second trigger that also must be in play. This second trigger involves when the claim is first presented. In a "claims made" policy, the act must occur when the policy is in effect, *and* the claim must be made when the policy is in effect. In the single trigger "occurrence policy," it does not matter when the claim is made, and whether the policy is still in effect; so long as the policy was in effect at the time of the action that led to the claim, the claim is covered. Under the "claims made policy," however, the policy will not respond unless the notice of the claim is made while the policy is still in effect. The exception to this rule is that the insurance company will usually provide an extended reporting period after the policy has expired or has been terminated. This extended reporting period may be from 6 months to 3 years, and additional reporting periods can usually be purchased. The risk manager must know whether they are purchasing an "occurrence policy," or a "claims made policy." While a "claims made policy" may be less expensive initially, the cost of extending the reporting period at the end of the policy may be as expensive as the policy itself. Generally, there is no concern, so long as the "claims made policy" is renewed, since renewal will extend the time for reports, or the time during which a claim may be made. It is only in the final year of the policy that the extension must be purchased.

The other question involved in answering the question of "when" a policy is in effect involves the activities that lead to the claim. Usually a commercial policy is in effect only when the employee is acting within the scope of their employment, meaning that they must be on company business. A pharmacist giving advice outside of the business of the hospital or pharmacy will generally have no coverage under the commercial policy. Individual professional liability policies, on the other hand, are usually 24-hour/7-day per week coverage. Such policies would be primary when the pharmacists' actions are outside of employment, and secondary when the actions are within the employment period.

Where?

Most policies will have restrictions as to where the actions or the claim must be brought in order for coverage to be in effect. Most policies, by their terms, are limited to coverage within the United States, its possessions, and Canada. Foreign travel, even to Mexico, and even if on company business, may not be covered, absent a special clause.

Exclusions.

It is generally true that no policy covers everything, and if it did, you could not afford it. Every policy has exclusions and conditions, which change the basic coverage of the policy. Out of a typical 40-page commercial policy, about 4 pages will be spent telling what is covered, with the balance taking away some of that coverage. This process of taking away is usually by exclusions, terms and conditions within the policies. Typical exclusions within commercial policies include pollution, bodily injury to an employee during the course of his or her employment, refusal to employ a person, termination of employment, discrimination, and discipline. The professional liability exclusions include the willful violation of a statute or regulation, a criminal act, or the process of manufacturing as differentiated from compounding. The pharmacy risk manager needs to carefully read and understand all exclusions within the policy, particularly as they apply to the practice of pharmacy.

There are many conditions within a policy that may not amount to an exclusion. Typically, the insured is required to cooperate with the insurance company in the defense or investigation of a claim. Coverage may be denied if an insured fails to report a claim within a reasonable period of time, or if the insured makes any volunteer payments without the consent of the insurance company. In addition, generally, an insured may not make a payment or assume a liability without the insurance company's permission. Most policies contain a clause indicating that an insured shall not "admit liability." This restriction, typically, does not include a prohibition against an apology, or an admission of an error when the error is obvious. Prior to entering into an insurance contract, however, the pharmacy risk manager should be certain as to how the insurance company expects questions of obvious error to be approached. Most insurance companies now realize that an apology made at an appropriate time, including the admission of an obvious error, may result in lower claims being paid. In addition, many states now have apology laws, which limit how an apology may be used in court.

Matching the Insurance Policy to the Need

The explanation of insurance in this section is extremely limited, and should not be used as the sole guide to purchasing insurance. The risk manager should read and understand the policy, and should deal with insurance professionals in making certain that the policy fits the needs of the pharmacy. Besides professional malpractice coverage, general commercial coverage is also necessary, and the risk in some of these areas may be greater than the risk involving pharmacy malpractice. In some areas, such as unemployment compensation insurance, and Worker's Compensation, purchase of insurance may be mandatory, with considerable fines and penalties for not doing so.

IMPORTANCE OF A SYSTEM TO IDENTIFY AND PREVENT ERRORS

Risk management is about recognizing and dealing with risks, hopefully before they actually occur. Sentinel events warn us when something is wrong. The Joint Commission defines a sentinel event as:

> A sentinel event is an unexpected occurrence involving death or serious physical or psychological injury, or the risk thereof. Serious injury

specifically includes loss of limb or function. The phrase, "or the risk thereof" includes any process variation for which a recurrence would carry a significant chance of a serious adverse outcome. Such events are called "sentinel" because they signal the need for immediate investigation and response. (http://www.jointcommission.org/SentinelEvents/)

If a risk manager cannot properly identify risks, he or she stands little chance of avoiding or controlling them. In order to identify the risks, the risk manager must study the organization's sentinel events. In order to study the sentinel events, they must be recognized and recorded. *We are able to prevent errors, including medication errors, because we understand the vulnerabilities within our own system. Not all systems contain the same vulnerabilities.* While knowledge of general vulnerabilities that affect other systems is valuable, in order to truly be effective, we must understand the system in which we work, and the particular vulnerabilities that are inherent to it. We can then change those inherent problems, and, over time, reduce the risk of QRE and thus errors occurring.

While the goal is to reduce errors, the best way to reduce errors is to reduce the mistakes that led to the error initially. The vulnerabilities within the system are most readily apparent when studying all mistakes that are made within the system, not just that small portion of our mistakes that were able to survive our entire system to reach the patient.

The Pharmacists Mutual Claims Study shows that approximately 9% of all claims are caused by incorrect directions appearing on the label. Incorrect directions may be caused in many ways, including entry at the computer system, incorrect labels being applied to the bottle, or misunderstanding the prescriber in a telephone communication.

In a separate study looking at all QREs in a group of pharmacies who agreed to record their mistakes, the percentage of wrong direction cases was considerably higher. Whether the information was scientifically valid, it was interesting as it showed the mistakes (or QREs) in each position within the work-flow. For example, 17.9% of all of the mistakes (errors plus near misses, or QREs) were made by entering the wrong directions during data entry. This indicates that, within this collection of pharmacies, a significant vulnerability, which needed to be addressed, was the preparation of the label during computer entry. Based on this information, the recommendation to each of the participating pharmacies was for 1 month to concentrate on checking the directions entered on the label. This was to be done in three places. The first place was during computer entry; the second place was during the filling process to check all labels prior to filling the prescription; and the third was for the pharmacist at the pharmacist's quality check area to specifically note the directions on a new prescription compared with the directions on the label.

By collecting information of all near misses and errors, a pharmacy can select an area of concentration. By being able to demonstrate vulnerabilities by posting charts, management can emphasize the importance of the area in which it has decided to concentrate for the next few days. Such information allows management to select and emphasize specific techniques to answer specific vulnerabilities. It is difficult for staff members to work on several areas of concern at one time, but by selecting the most obvious vulnerability, at a specific time, the pharmacy and its pharmacists and technicians can focus their attention in one particular area. It also allows management to compare results at the beginning to results after specific vulnerabilities have been targeted.

Encouraging Reporting

Without information telling us where we make mistakes, when we make mistakes, the type of mistakes we make, and how we discover those mistakes, it is difficult to improve our system of quality within a pharmacy. The weakness of any system of continuous quality improvement is the inability to receive accurate information. It is human nature to avoid reporting of our own mistakes. Every pharmacy must have a system that overcomes this tendency and encourages its pharmacists and pharmacy technicians to report all mistakes.

The surest way to discourage pharmacy staff members from reporting is to institute a system of blame and punishment for reported errors. While failure to report may result in consequences, reporting should have associated with it only positive consequences.

One way in which to encourage pharmacists and pharmacy technicians to report is to design a system that removes identification of the person who makes the mistake. The collected information should then be used in a visible manner, which allows staff to see the results of their efforts. If we collect all QREs, including near misses and errors, and compare those numbers with the total number of prescriptions filled during a period of time, visible results showing "how we are doing" can be posted within the pharmacy. Collecting the information concerning a comparison between the total number of prescriptions filled and the total number of errors allows the pharmacy to post an error rate. Staff should be encouraged to work to reduce that error rate each month. This can be demonstrated on a simple chart that is posted in the pharmacy where staff members, but not patients, can see the information. By then comparing the number of near misses to the number of errors, the pharmacy can also post a success rate, showing the percentage of mistakes that resulted in errors, compared with the total number of mistakes made for a given period. By showing this in positive terms of a success rate (the number of mistakes that did not reach a patient), the staff can see the rewards of their efforts. A final graph of the total number of QREs (errors plus near misses) compared to the number of total prescriptions for the period will give the staff a full picture of their continuous quality improvement program, and how well it is working.

In order to judge the effectiveness of the reporting system, the pharmacy must have some way in which it can know whether the information is accurate, in other words, how effective the staff is at capturing all QRE information. By looking at national statistics, a pharmacy can compare what would be expected with the information received. For example, based on information collected by PMC Quality Commitment Inc. for QREs in selected reporting pharmacies over a period of 3 years, pharmacies were able to judge the value of the numbers reported in their pharmacy. The information collected indicated that pharmacies reporting more than 2% QRE statistics had a potential problem within their system. Every time there is a QRE, whether the mistake is caught or not, the efficiency of the pharmacy is decreased because of the amount of rework required to correct each mistake. Greater than 2% QRE rate would indicate that the amount of rework would greatly affect efficiency. This figure can also be compared to error reports published elsewhere. On the other hand, a pharmacy reporting less than 0.5% QRE rate may have an indication that their staff are not reporting all QREs. While this range of 0.5–2% may not be entirely accurate for a particular pharmacy, it does give an indication of when management may need to make specific efforts to address the question of reporting. While these numbers do not provide answers, they do provide questions for management, and suggest potential problems.

In this chapter, we have looked at risk management in a broader perspective, and particularly, have looked at risks associated with pharmacy practice. The first step in risk management is to identify the risks. Identifying the risks is, however, only the beginning of the risk management process. Through other parts of this book, the pharmacist will look at specifics of quality-based interventions, quality management, and quality improvement in a more specific and focused method.

HOW TO DEAL WITH AN ERROR WHEN ONE OCCURS

In all human endeavors, errors are inevitable. The final test of our quality program is how we deal with an error that, in spite of our best efforts, reached a patient. The specific steps we take in a given situation will depend on the facts of the situation. Whether the patient took the wrong drug, whether the patient was injured, and whether the patient discovered the error or we did will determine our next step. There are, however, some basic rules that may be developed and incorporated into a training program. The best guide is usually the Golden Rule – how would you want to be treated if someone you trusted made a mistake? This is not only a reasonable ethical approach, but usually also a good business decision.

Every person in the pharmacy should be trained in how to respond to a patient or a prescriber when they announce there has been an error. Usually this kind of problem will involve a mechanical error – wrong drug, wrong strength, or wrong directions. First the pharmacy must decide who can handle such a call. This is normally a "pharmacist-only question" and technicians are taught to perform a first response only. The technician can show empathy and concern and say, "I will get the pharmacist immediately."

The pharmacist then must communicate to the patient how seriously the pharmacy takes the question. Often just showing empathy can change the tenor of the conversation from one of belligerence to relief that someone cares and is going to help. Next the pharmacist must gather information to discover what happened and whether there really is an error. While a patient's concern about the color and shape of the tablet changing is more likely to be a generic brand change, the rule is "It's an error until proven otherwise." Other questions will include discovering if the patient took the medication and, if so, is there any injury or is some remedial medical action necessary.

The pharmacist must follow the company's policy and procedures when handling an error, but generally, the patient may be given a refund or a special offer designed by the company, but may not be offered a settlement or any form of payment. Usually, if the pharmacist is convinced the pharmacy has made an obvious error, an apology can be given and a genuine "I'm sorry." The pharmacist should not admit liability however, which is to acknowledge the results of an error. There is usually not enough information known at the time of the initial conversation and it could violate the insurance policy and probably company policy as well. Even if there is not an obvious error, the pharmacy should express empathy for any suffering the patient believes he or she has suffered.

Most states have apology laws that do not permit any apology in any form being used against the health care professional. In most states these apology laws cover the pharmacy and pharmacist as well as physicians. Even without these laws a sincere "I am sorry" may prove valuable and will generally not harm the defense of a claim or lawsuit.

Practicing such conversations before they are required for real errors will be very valuable. Questions can be raised and discussed during training. While what to do in case of an error is the last step in risk management, it should be the first part of training for all staff members.

A FINAL THOUGHT

Everyone should be considered a part of the risk management team. Everyone has a role in preventing medication errors and providing information to improve the quality system. The one person we usually forget is the patient.

Making the patient a part of the system is not easy because in entails admitting to the patient we can make a mistake. We may have to explain what kind of mistakes we make and that some may become errors that get to the patient.

Consider a guide for patients explaining the pharmacy's commitment to quality and that in spite of every safeguard we are all human and we can make a mistake. Tell the patient they are a part of our entire system of preventing medication errors. Then explain how they as patient can help and what to look for and finally what to do if they suspect an error has occurred. If a pharmacist wants an example of how this can be done, visit Mayo clinics in Phoenix. In the physician's offices and in the area around the pharmacy is a pamphlet for patients that starts with, "We are human. . . ."

REFERENCES

1. Samaritan G, Austin CA, eds. *Mag Mutual Newsletter, Health Care Risk Manager.* Vol 12. Number 31; 2006.
2. Physician Insurers Association of America. *Medication Error Study,* Washington, DC: June 1993.
3. Massachusetts Commonwealth Group Insurance Commission, Benefit Newsletter, page 1, Winter 2005, http://www.mass.gov/gic/healthartdrugcompliance.htm.
4. World Service Group, HG Newsletter, *How will HIPAA Privacy or Security Rules be Enforced?* March 2006. http://www.hg.org/articles/article_1450.html.
5. Krauss S. *Privacy Law Blog;* August 2008. http://privacylaw.proskauer.com/2008/08/articles/medical-privacy/hhs-enters-into-first-monetary-settlement-under-hipaa/.

Part IV
Quality-based Interventions
and Incentives

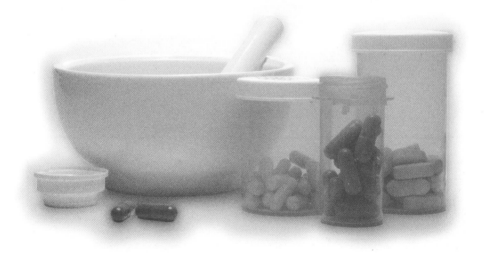

CHAPTER 12

Implementing Change to Enhance Quality

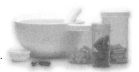

Ana C. Quiñones-Boex and
Thomas J. Reutzel

Learning Objectives

At the end of the chapter, the reader will be able to:

1. Compare and contrast reengineering and incremental approaches to quality improvement implementation.
2. Briefly describe several factors that help determine the selection of the best quality improvement strategy.
3. Discuss potential barriers to change.
4. Apply change concepts to the dispensing process to enhance quality.
5. Briefly describe examples of models used to facilitate and maintain change and how they can be applied to pharmacy practice.

APPROACHES TO QUALITY IMPROVEMENT IMPLEMENTATION

The overall objective of this book is to make the case for the use of quality improvement strategies in pharmacy settings and processes. At the core of any quality improvement implementation lies change. Thus, this chapter explores the challenges and opportunities of implementing organizational change to enhance quality. This chapter will discuss major types of change implementation (reengineering versus incremental techniques), resistance to change, and strategies for facilitating and maintaining change. Finally, the chapter will address how change can enhance the quality of pharmacy services.

Some of these concepts are examined in other chapters, so, to minimize redundancy, we provide truncated explanations of them.

Reengineering versus Incremental Changes

Changes aimed at improving the quality of any organizational process could be classified as belonging to two major groups: reengineering and incremental models. In general, reengineering suggests the complete overhaul of a process while incremental models are characterized by gradual change. Reengineering and incremental techniques [such as total quality management (TQM) and Six Sigma] have been explored widely in the business world and applied to health care relatively recently. Both concepts represent innovative business management models characterized by an "orientation toward change and creativity."[1] These models differ from more traditional business management techniques in that they allow organizations to better respond to health care's dynamic environment, characterized simultaneously by the pursuit of quality and the containment of costs. They "are more complex and more difficult to implement . . . but have the potential for producing major improvements in quality, service and cost."[1]

The concept of reengineering, one of the American business buzzwords of the 1990s, has been defined as "the fundamental rethinking and radical redesign of process to achieve dramatic improvements in critical, contemporary measure of performance, such as cost, quality, service, and speed."[2] Also known as business process reengineering (BPR), this model is cross-functional in nature and recommends the reorganization of staff by processes (e.g., reorganizing health care teams by disease state rather than functional departments). These process-based teams would be in charge of redesigning the structure of their process "from start to finish" rather than improving upon existing methods.[1,3] BPR is a radical change process that requires upper management commitment and leadership.[4]

Though popular when first originated, reengineering has acquired a negative image because its implementation often focused on downsizing, at least in certain industries.[3] The data on reengineering's use in the hospital setting are limited and mixed.[1] Health care's complex business nature (i.e., taking care of patients) makes the implementation of a radical model such as BPR especially difficult. Reengineering processes within a hospital would entail an organizational culture overhaul and potentially several years for complete implementation.[1] The extended implementation time required in health care is in contrast with the faster changes embraced by BPR. Moreover, "any complex change process must be regarded as temporary and likely to have a maximum top management attention span of no more than two years."[3]

TQM, an example of an incremental change technique, is a quality improvement model that gained popularity in the United States in the mid-1980s, though some trace its origins to Deming's work in Japan in the 1950s and onward. "TQM can be broadly defined as a management system for improving performance throughout an organization by maximizing customer satisfaction, making continuous improvements and promoting expanded employee involvement."[1] At the core of TQM is the notion that management must ensure quality through adequate systems and effective leadership.[1] Since employee training and empowerment are essential to performance improvement under TQM, this model requires team-based, participative management.[1] Some consider TQM the "foundation upon which other improvements approaches are based."[3] These approaches include reengineering and Six Sigma.[3,5]

TQM appears to have had more acceptance than reengineering within the health care sector. Some types of TQM models had been adopted by most American and Canadian hospitals as of 1995[6] despite the fact that transitioning into a TQM model may take up to 5 years or longer in more complex institutions with strong corporate cultures such as teaching hospitals.[1] Yet, there is evidence of high failure rates for hospital TQM programs.[1] Failures are considered to be implementation breakdowns rather than flaws within the concept of TQM. Some of the shortcomings of TQM include: no method of quantifying financial gains, no top management buy-in, not dealing with the root cause of errors, and lack of evidence of improved patient outcomes.[5]

Six Sigma, another incremental change model, was conceived at Motorola in the mid-1980s.[3] Considered superior to TQM by some, Six Sigma relies heavily on statistical methods and a five-step process consisting of problem: definition, measurement, analysis, improvement, and control.[3] The goal is to decrease variation and errors within a system, quantify results in dollar figures, and improve customer satisfaction.[5,7] Six Sigma has become a popular quality improvement model in health care because of its "near-zero tolerance for mistakes."[8]

Six Sigma's limitations include its complexity and lack of "standard solutions to common problems."[9] This method requires significant employee training and the use of root cause analysis and other metrics to analyze every process under consideration.

Reengineering and incremental changes share several commonalities: quality improvement, need for upper management commitment and support, process improvement, customer satisfaction, teamwork and training, and cultural change in the organization.[4] It is important to note that a study completed in the 1990s found that most companies using BPR were also using TQM.[10] This suggests that reengineering and incremental changes can be approached as components of a process rather than as a discrete dichotomy.

The basic differences between BPR and incremental techniques include the structural and radical changes inherent in reengineering and the narrow scope of the incremental changes. Interestingly, BPR and Six Sigma embrace rapid change while TQM follows a slower paced implementation. Reengineering and Six Sigma also share more "top-down hierarchical" leadership styles, more amenable to American managers.[3] Thus, one can view Six Sigma as an intermediate model between BPR and TQM (Box 12-1).

It has been proposed that selecting the best improvement model for an organization depends on two factors: its key operating parameters and key personnel turnover rate.[3] If a company is doing poorly and has considerable room for quality improvement,

---

BOX 12-1. Which Type of Change Is Best?

Having reviewed the strengths and weaknesses of radical and incremental improvement models, one could argue that the combined approach is the best solution. For instance, a study suggested that change efforts utilizing TQM followed by BPR were more successful for companies.[10] Ultimately, the decision to select a change model should be based on organization-specific considerations.

then perhaps a model, such as TQM, that allows every employee to be involved in the process might be the best approach to follow. If an organization experiences a high turnover of key personnel, then a faster-paced change model, such as BPR or Six Sigma, might be more suitable. Top management would be faced with a difficult choice if their organizations fall somewhere in the middle regarding their operating parameters and personnel turnover. Organizations can choose to excel in certain areas, such as quality, and select a change model "that best suits their history culture and business environment."[3]

REASONS FOR RESISTING CHANGE

Change is a phenomenon that encompasses all aspects of life. It is inevitable, yet the ability of a particular organization to properly manage change can determine whether that organization fails or thrives. Change within an organization can be defined as a continuous process of improvement, which involves the introduction of adjustments to current policies and procedures to achieve new objectives.[11,12] Change can be driven by countless reasons, including new technology, new opportunities, emerging obstacles, and an organization's need to stay competitive within its market.[12] Organizations are dynamic entities, illustrating the importance of change to facilitate this constant dynamic and to encourage progress.

Examining the nature of human beings elucidates their behavior when confronted with change. Overall, humans have a conservative disposition.[11] This can be inferred from several change models that, although they may differ in their representation of the stages of change, agree that humans have an aversion to change. For example, the transtheoretical model of change, which examines behavioral change for the purpose of optimizing health, delineates three stages that an individual experiences prior to the "action stage."[13] In this model, the most ardent change resisters reside in the "pre-contemplation stage," and they may deny that change is necessary or may simply be unmotivated.[13] Another model that can be applied to organizational change is Kübler-Ross's model, first described in her book *On Death and Dying*.[14] The intent of this model was to describe the human response to grief and tragedy. However, simply considering the classifications of the stages – denial, anger, bargaining, depression, and acceptance – allows one to realize the parallels between the grief response and the response to any major life change, including change within an organization.[15] The critical point in both models is that there is a resistance stage prior to implementation of change. Moreover, closer inspection uncovers the individual barriers to change (complacency, fear, anger, and pessimism) in either model.

Resistance to change within the organizational setting has been specifically noted and studied. Such analyses often make use of psychological, sociological, and even political science frameworks to understand resistance to organizational change. Some of the more general approaches to barriers to organizational change and policy implementation follow.

Organizations can be loosely defined as collections of people.[16] This means that an organization must take into account the complexities of how people react to change.

To many, change can be a frustrating and disruptive force. Those who seek to implement change must realize that it is a process that requires planning to address employee concerns and to assist employees during the transitioning process. This recognition is essential if a change effort is to be successful.[17] Many organizations cannot seem to find equilibrium between successfully implementing a change and accommodating employees to facilitate a smooth transition. Research from the *Harvard Business Review* found that only 15% of the workforce willingly embraces a new change initiative, 60% are uncertain, and 25% heavily resist change initiatives.[18] Ensuring that a change initiative is successfully embraced requires leaders to motivate and coach employees, in addition to listening to concerns and encouraging employees to voice those concerns.[18] An unwillingness to involve and inform employees of changes will ultimately result in failure.[16,17] In addition, for an organization to successfully implement a change, it must first understand the concept of change and the barriers that may hinder its effectiveness.

Barriers to Change

One of the most pressing challenges faced by organizations is how to address the barriers to change, which, despite the voluminous literature, can be generally described as the behavior of people reacting to change.[19] Change management authors have succinctly described these undesirable behaviors as complacency, fear, anger, and pessimism.[19] Complacency is characterized by the refusal of employees to challenge the status quo, whose perpetuation is a key factor in change resistance.[11,19] Fear, as a mechanism of self-protection, foments inertia, which blocks change.[19] Anger often manifests when employees feel that change is being forced upon them, and this may provoke a stubborn repudiation of the organization's new vision.[19] Pessimism precludes change, because pessimistic employees tend to doubt the validity of the new vision.[19]

Other barriers to change identified in the literature include: (1) inherent human resistance to change; (2) lack of commitment, fear, and poor understanding of the change; (3) poor leadership, including lack of trust between management and employees, lack of support from management, failure to implement effective change techniques, lack of resources to support change, and lack of vision; (4) lack of a payoff for change; and (5) lack of consequences for poor performance.[16]

Other scholars of organizational change have developed similar points of view. One paper with a psychological bent[20] states that resistance is a natural part of the change process and occurs, because ". . . change involves going from the known to the unknown," making some individuals uncomfortable.[21–24] Managers often neglect these human factors and focus, instead, on technicalities (e.g., quantifying profit goals). They often give little attention to training, communication, and follow-up. They might request and then ignore staff input into change efforts, resulting in disillusionment among employees. For organizational change to be successful, people must change themselves. These authors further dichotomize resistance into unconscious (anxiety) and conscious (behavioral intention) processes.[20]

In an analysis aimed specifically at health care organizations, barriers to change are classified into three categories: input related [inputs (patients) are difficult to control and experiment with], process related (processes are complex, critical, and difficult to standardize), and output related (outputs are difficult to measure, control, and relate back to causes). These barriers stem from health care providers typically considering their work to be "sacred" and not fully incorporating patients into the system.[25]

CASE EXAMPLE 1

A consultant once worked with a pharmacy organization on a quality improvement project. The effort was promoted company-wide. In the middle of the planning stage, a staff pharmacist refused to fill a prescription for a controlled substance, because he was quite certain that the patient in question was a drug abuser. The patient complained, and the pharmacist was chastised. This case illustrates the pitfalls when goals are not congruent (i.e., the pharmacist's definition of quality patient care versus the company's definition of quality customer service). Also, it shows the importance of establishing a trust relationship between management and employees.

The policy implementation literature also has a long history of exploring obstacles to change. It is worthwhile to segment these obstacles into two categories. The first occurs when there is a lack of agreement on goals, or on what the policy/change actually should be. Policy implementation problems are often due to lack of agreement on goals because: each level of the organization has its own goals and policies, authority is never total, and interested parties try to influence policy at all levels.[26]

The second category of problems includes barriers of a more technical nature. That is, even when goal consensus exists, implementation problems may still occur in the form of technical obstacles that arise as the policy makes its way through the organization. Table 12-1 summarizes two articles from the policy literature that identify barriers to policy implementation. Each barrier is categorized as a "different goals" or "technical" problem.

Relating our discussion to the incremental quality improvement model of Six Sigma, we find that even though it is a relatively new and innovative process, barriers to its success are similar to those identified in the previous discussion. These include ambivalence of management, lack of broad participation, dependence on consensus, initiatives that are too broad or too narrow, failure to attack cultural obstacles, and, finally, lack of understanding of the principles of Six Sigma.[7]

PRACTICES THAT FACILITATE AND MAINTAIN CHANGE

The importance of addressing barriers to change cannot be overstated, as the consequences of change resistance are quite severe and include noncompliance with the new

TABLE 12-1. Implementation Barrier Types Identified in the Policy Literature

	Type
Kaufman: barriers to implementation include	
(1) Communications – people do not know what they are supposed to do. This requires clear, accurate, and consistent communication of standards, objectives, and instructions	Technical
(2) Capability – people are not capable of doing what they are supposed to do. Three resources are required to ensure capability: staff competence, information, and authority	Technical
(3) Disposition – people refuse to do what they are supposed to do	Different goals
Van Meter and Van Horn: implementation depends on	
(1) The identification of performance indicators to assess the extent to which standards and objectives are realized	Technical
(2) The availability of resources to pursue objectives	Either
(3) Interorganizational communication and enforcement activities, which relate to the need for standards and objectives to be communicated clearly accurately, and consistently; and the fact that the extent of authority relates to the likelihood that policy will be followed	Technical; different goals
(4) Characteristics of implementing agencies, which include	
• Competence and size of staff	Either
• Degree of hierarchical control of subunit decisions and processes	Different goals
• Political resources	Different goals
• Vitality	Either
• The degree of open communications within the organization	Either
• Formal and informal linkages with the source of the policy	Different goals
(5) Economic, social, and political conditions, which relate mainly to the fact that policies will continue to be influenced by those with a stake in them and that not all parties agree on a given policy	Different goals
(6) The disposition of implementers	Different goals

Data from Refs.[27,28]

vision, apathy, and negative attitudes.[11,29] In fact, those that resist change might even overcome their normal inhibitions and go so far as to sabotage the organization.[11] For example, if the company's change involved a new procedure, a disgruntled employee may deviate in a manner that would ensure disruption. Other employees might act with increased malice and sabotage an organization's products or services.[11]

Even the less severe implications of change resistance are significant as they represent stagnation, a waste of energy, and perhaps, more importantly, time, which to the many subscribers of a famous adage is equal to money.[11] Thus, change resistance minimally yields inertia, and at its worst may lead to wanton sabotage, with a propensity for wasted energy, time, and money.[11,19,29] The consequences of the change barriers and related resistance underscore the pertinence of change management, which when carried out properly can improve the chances of success. This poignantly reminds us that the level of change achieved is dictated by the response of those who are directly affected by it.[11]

Six Sigma attempts to align patient goals with the organization's strategic goals, and this is reminiscent of the barriers to policy implementation literature's concern with lack of agreement on goals. The prospect of lack of convergence on goals is especially germane to the pharmacy setting. Most pharmacies are for-profit entities dedicated to increasing the wealth of their proprietors or stockholders, whereas the typical pharmacist employee has been socialized in professional school to take care of their patients at any cost. As the article by Zimmerer et al.[25] notes, health care professionals often consider their work to be "sacred" and the welfare of patients to take precedence over the goals of the organization. Even though there is a strong bureaucratic hierarchy in corporate pharmacy organizations, pharmacists at the counter still have some leeway to follow their own – versus their employers' – policies. Hopefully, the cry to rally around improved quality can be seen to satisfy both organizational and health care goals. If so, tackling technical impediments to change carries a much higher probability of success.

CASE EXAMPLE 2

A consultant once worked with a pharmacy corporation on a project aimed at a full-blown attempt to implement clinical pharmacy services in the community setting. These services included a complete drug utilization review accompanied by counseling for each patient. A private counseling room was even constructed to facilitate the process. All actors involved accurately perceived that this was a genuine attempt by management to upgrade the quality of pharmacy services. A pharmacy school faculty member was placed in the store to facilitate the process. The initiative was continually frustrated during the first year of implementation, though, because the existing pharmacy staff had neither the will nor the knowledge to provide the services. Eventually, a training program was implemented to overcome these obstacles, but progress on the project had been slowed considerably. Also, project participants were surprised to see that, for the most part, patients did not admire or demand the new services. Most wanted their prescriptions filled quickly with minimal interaction with the pharmacist. This case illustrates how important it is for management to address the topics of training, communication, and follow-up often and early. Also, it shows that health care providers must remember to incorporate patients' experiences and expectations into their change effort.

Kotter[30] and Reger et al.[31] have elaborated two formal approaches to overcoming barriers to change. Kotter[30] examined companies that embarked on change efforts and looked at the reason that some succeeded while others failed. He synthesized a framework of reasons for failure. If we look at these from a positive point of view, we can identify strategies that organizations can use to increase the likelihood of success when undergoing change. First, such organizations should establish a sense of urgency. Over half of the companies that he observed failed when executives did not communicate the importance of the change effort broadly and dramatically. Second, a powerful guiding coalition should be formed. For small, and even some large, organizations, the coalition may consist of only three to five people. This group should grow, though, to 20–50 before an organization can truly advance. Companies that fail to create a robust guiding coalition do so simply because they overlook the relevance of this group. Third, a vision should be created. Kotter states that companies who fail at this step often obfuscate the vision with superfluous information in their handouts and presentations. He goes on to suggest that if a vision cannot generate interest in 5 minutes, then it needs to be amended until it does so.

According to Kotter, others should be empowered to act on the vision. He implores organizations to zealously communicate the vision to their employees, because even sound visions languish in the absence of genuine enthusiasm. Then, planning for and creating short-term wins should be done. This is necessary because the urgency driving change fades when it becomes evident that the benefits of change will not be realized overnight. Next, improvements should be consolidated and even more change should be produced. This is essential, because without new change, organizations will likely be preoccupied with early successes and may again become complacent. Finally, new approaches should be institutionalized. This is accomplished by proving to the organization that the change was responsible for new successes and by ensuring that the next cadre of management embraces the change (Table 12-2).[30]

Reger et al.[31] provide a different framework for overcoming barriers to change, but the overlap with Kotter is obvious. They suggest that an organizational identity audit be conducted. This includes interviewing employees, listening to their concerns, and observing the daily work habits of employees at all levels affected by the change. By performing periodic organizational identity audits, top management can obtain an idea of employees' beliefs and views of what the current identity or character of the organization is as well as its ideal characteristics. If the changes stray too far from current or ideal organizational characteristics or are perceived as unattainable, resistance will be more likely. Next, the change should be tailored to fit the organization. Since

TABLE 12-2. Two Models that Facilitate and Maintain Change

Kotter	Reger et al.
Establish a sense of urgency	Conduct organizational identity audit
Form a powerful guiding coalition	Tailor change to fit the organization
Create a vision	Present the change as significant while tying it to valued aspects of organizational identity
Empower others to act on the vision	Introduce change in a series of midrange steps
Plan for and create short-term wins	Take the path of least resistance
Consolidate improvements and produce still more change	Know how much change your organization can handle
Institutionalize new approaches	

Data from Refs. [30,31]

every organization has its own distinct identity, it would be wise to customize changes to encompass the valued elements of that organization.

Third, the change should be presented as significant while simultaneously being tied to valued aspects of organizational identity. If employees view change as unnecessary or change efforts as merely a fine-tuning of existing practices, organizational inertia will prevent successful change implementation. In addition, the change must incorporate components of the current or ideal identity of the organization in order to keep employees motivated to sustain change.

The change should be introduced in a series of midrange steps. This creates opportunities for management to assess progress, evaluate target goals, and adjust current efforts. A stepwise approach also enables management to introduce a sufficient (but not excessive) amount of change and, therefore, further enhance the motivation to change. Eventually, parts of the change initiative will be integrated into the current identity of the organization. Ensuring success at each step increases the chance that the changes will be solidified.

Also, the path of least resistance should be taken. It can be assumed that within an organization, employees in different divisions or departments will have differing views on organizational identity. These differences can be a barrier to the implementation of change. Managers can overcome this barrier, though, by first initiating change efforts in those that are more willing to embrace the change. Success with these groups may encourage employees who are opposed to the change to reevaluate their own perception of the ideal organizational identity.

Finally, change agents should know just how much change their organization can handle. The range of change acceptance varies among organizations. It is important to continuously evaluate employee acceptance and understanding of the change in order to facilitate a successful change initiative.[31]

CASE EXAMPLE 3

A consultant once worked with an organization while it was revamping its strategic plan. The plan called for both short-term and long-term (10 years out) goals. The plan was guided by the overarching goal of improving the quality of all services performed by the organization. Senior- and middle-level management were responsible for translating overall plan objectives along these lines into actionable steps that could be taken in the next year. When the final plan was distributed to members of the organization, there was a widespread view that the action steps were not consistent with the quality-guided objectives and, in some cases, even undermined the objectives. This case illustrates the importance of incorporating employee input into the change effort early in the process. Conducting an organizational audit and forming guiding coalitions comprising employees from all levels of the organization are good ways to do this.

CHANGING PHARMACY PROCESSES TO ENHANCE QUALITY

Having discussed quality improvement change models and the challenges and possibilities inherent in change, how can we change the medication use process in a way that enhances quality? Strategies to facilitate and maintain such change and, therefore, to overcome technical impediments to change, spring directly from the barriers to change that have been identified over the years. These are seemingly simple and obvious management responsibilities, but they are often overlooked.

First, we must decide what we mean by improved quality. Is it a reduction in the number of dispensing errors? This is an attractive concept, because it lends itself to measurement, and it is relatively easy to achieve goal consensus around this objective. Unfortunately, we know that improving quality in the drug therapy context is more complicated. The concept of rational drug therapy (RDT) is a useful way to capture the complexity of quality in drug therapy in an efficient conceptual fashion.[32] To put it simply, RDT occurs when prescribing, dispensing, and ingestion take place in a way that maximizes patient health status, minimizes adverse drug reactions and risk, and achieves these goals at the lowest possible social cost.[32] As individuals interested in improving quality at the pharmacy level, we must focus on dispensing, but this process cannot be divorced from the physician (prescribing) and the patient or caregiver (administration).

Over the last several decades, pharmacy has embraced several paradigms aimed at achieving RDT. These include clinical pharmacy, pharmaceutical care, and, the present rage: medication therapy management (MTM). These strategies vary in their particulars, but they overlap more than diverge. The essence of all of them can be captured by the drug utilization review (DUR) concept. The DUR approach has three components: prospective, concurrent, and retrospective. During prospective DUR, the pharmacist reviews the prescription in the context of an evidence-based therapeutic formulary, a patient-specific database, and other relevant drug information sources prior to dispensing the medication. If the prescription is deemed suboptimal, the pharmacist contacts the prescriber to have the therapy changed to an optimal status. Once this goal is achieved, the pharmacist must counsel the patient and/or caregiver in an attempt to ensure that this optimal therapy is operationalized properly at the ingestion level. Concurrent DUR occurs when the pharmacist continues to monitor the patient while they are undergoing their optimal therapy, because untoward events can still occur (e.g., unanticipated adverse reactions and pregnancy). If such events do occur, the pharmacist again contacts the prescriber to move the therapy in a better direction and, again, talks to the patient and caregiver to ensure adherence.

While prospective and concurrent DUR are patient-specific, retrospective DUR makes use of aggregate patient databases and reviews them over time to look for suboptimum prescribing, dispensing, and ingestion trends. Because pharmacists lie at the intersection of the prescriber and the patient, they are in an excellent position to also perform this function. The principles underlying DUR apply to the hospital setting even though the phrase drug use evaluation (DUE) or other such terms may be used instead. It is our view that this DUR model, easy to describe but difficult to implement, carries the essence of the previous paradigms that have evolved since the emergence of prepackaged dosage forms and that seek to define the pharmacist as the drug therapy manager.

Unfortunately, achieving goal alignment around the concepts of RDT and DUR is a much more daunting challenge than agreeing on the need to reduce dispensing errors. As long as pharmacy lies at the crossroads of the market ethos and the health care ethos, some goal conflict seems inevitable. Also, as long as market factors (e.g., reimbursement schemes, cost containment goals, and profit objectives) prevent us from developing comprehensive evidence-based formularies and patient medical records, we will have a built-in excuse for not pursuing these types of goals. Thus, for true quality improvement to occur in the dispensing process, decision-makers must sincerely buy into the RDT concept of quality and believe that, in the long run, it will further shareholder or proprietor goals. If the pursuit of a better dispensing process that seeks to optimize drug therapy is merely lip service, it will soon become obvious, and the pharmacy will likely be worse off on both counts. This relates to the discussion of participation that follows.

Once genuine goal alignment has been obtained, management should give attention to several important processes that can be gleaned from the study of change and its impediments. First, they must communicate the reason for the change and the specific activities that everyone needs to undertake to achieve it. During this communication phase, care should be taken to anticipate employees' psychological resistance and ensure them that the change will help – not hinder – their job satisfaction. Also, participation must be widespread and genuine. Nothing is more likely to undermine a change effort than a disingenuous invitation to staff to provide input. True participation will also go a long way toward relieving the anxiety that the prospect of change is likely to engender in staff. If participation and communication are handled properly, then support for the change effort will follow. In a more technical sense, changes to the dispending process can also be pilot tested before actual full-scale implementation, and an evalu-

TABLE 12-3. Essential Components of a Pharmacy Quality Improvement Model

Define meaning of improved quality
Achieve goal alignment
Communicate reason for change
Encourage participation
Foster support for the change effort
Pilot test on a small scale
Evaluate

ation component should always be built into the change. This requires specifying the objectives of the change effort and identifying aspects of those objectives that can be measured (Table 12-3).

A reduction in dispensing errors and an improvement in drug therapy can both be considered outcome measures of quality. Measuring dispensing error outcomes is relatively much easier than improvements in drug therapy outcomes. Dispensing errors are tangible and can be attributed directly to the pharmacy's activities. Improvements in drug therapy depend on forces often outside of the pharmacist's control (e.g., prescriber, patient, and caregiver behavior; the idiosyncratic nature of disease; etc.). Still, there are more tractable ways to address quality improvement other than outcomes: namely, structure and process.[33,34] In terms of our DUR model, structure refers to the hardware, software, data, drug information sources, pharmacist credentials, and other raw materials that we need to enact the model. Process refers to pharmacists routinely making use of the software, databases, and drug information to ensure optimal therapy and, also, intervening with prescribers, patients, and caregivers as necessary. The beauty of the DUR model is that it should also reduce dispensing errors, because the pharmacist's interaction with the patient includes taking a look at the medication before the patient leaves the pharmacy. This gives both the pharmacist and the patient an additional opportunity to identify a mistake.

Can We Completely Reengineer Pharmacy Processes?

A review of the literature was performed to address which change model would be most effective in improving the quality of pharmacy processes. The pharmacy literature includes some articles dealing with pharmacy-related quality improvement via reengineering, continuous improvement, and Six Sigma.[8,35–38]

An article on reengineering the medication error-reporting process at Yale-New Haven Hospital portrays some of the concepts presented in this chapter.[38] True to the concept of reengineering, an interdisciplinary team was created to completely redesign the error-reporting process within the hospital. Moreover, the program was rapidly and successfully launched hospital-wide and fully implemented within 4 months. As suggested in our discussion on change implementation, resistance ensued when the organization culture was challenged during the pilot testing phase of the project. Ultimately, the new concept of anonymous nonpunitive reporting won over the belief on accountability and a new error-reporting culture has been created.[38] The author concludes by suggesting that an ongoing quest is necessary to keep this new program thriving. Stump makes a good case for reengineering specific pharmacy processes, but this notion would not be considered "true" reengineering by purists.

The introduction of Six Sigma as a pharmacy quality improvement method appears to be a recent trend. Six Sigma can build upon existing quality techniques at use in an organization, such as TQM.[8] Six Sigma appears to be particularly well suited for the analysis of medication errors.[8,35,36] It allows for benchmarking and strives for zero errors.

It seems to combine the best characteristics of BPR and TQM, yet it requires extensive staff training for successful implementation. There is evidence that even newer models are being considered as better choices to tackle pharmacy-related quality concerns.[9]

Besides choosing a quality improvement model, those seeking to improve pharmacy processes need to remember the importance of change management. Practices that facilitate and maintain change relating to pharmacy are no different than those in any type of organization and addressed throughout this chapter. Change improvement processes usually become unpredictable a year after their implementation, and the outcomes of quality improvement efforts might not be those originally intended.[3] Therefore, although it can be argued that a complete reengineering of the medication use system is possible, it is our contention that such an undertaking is not preferred. Based on this discussion of operating parameters, goal-driven and technical barriers, personnel turnover, and corporate culture, it is easier to make the case for incremental quality changes. Examples of quality-focused changes in pharmacy processes include: "redesigning" portions of the process (e.g., error-reporting), improving prospective DUR, providing better counseling, and increasing the use of technology (e.g., bar codes and automation).

A very recent study of quality improvement efforts at community health centers supports our analytical conclusion. It was found that, in order to maintain morale and reduce burnout during the implementation period, it was important to provide adequate staffing, leadership, and fair task distribution. Also, employees were more positive when they recognized that the new skills required of them would contribute to potential career advancement (Graber et al., 2008).[39] This supports our notion that, while preoccupation with reengineering, TQM, Six Sigma, and quality improvement models in general is important, the success of any change ultimately depends on the ongoing commitment of all individuals involved in the change effort.

ACKNOWLEDGMENTS

The authors would like to acknowledge the invaluable assistance of four pharmacy students from the Midwestern University Chicago College of Pharmacy: Ms Rachel Pullin, Ms Stefanie Stulgin, Ms Christina Leav, and Mr Derek Griffing.

REFERENCES

1. Trisolini MG. Applying business management models in health care. *Int J Health Plann Manag*. 2002;17(4):295–314.
2. Ginter P, Swayne L, Duncan W. *Strategic Management of Health Care Organizations*. Malden, MA: Blackwell; 1998 [as cited in Ref.[1]].
3. Van der Wiele T, Van Iwaarden J, Dale BG, Williams R. (2006). A comparison of five modern improvement approaches. *Int J Productivity Qual Manag*. 2006;1(4):363–378.
4. Selladurai R. An organizational profitability, productivity, performance (PPP) model: going beyond TQM and BPR. *Total Qual Manag*. 2002;13(5):613–619.
5. Black K, Revere L. Six Sigma arises from the ashes of TQM with a twist. *Int J Health Care Qual Assur*. 2006;19(3): 259–266.
6. Ho S, Chan L, Kidwell R. The implantation of business process reengineering in American and Canadian hospitals. *Health Care Manage Rev*. 1999;24(2):19–31 [as cited in Ref.[1]].
7. Lazarus IR, Stamps B. The promise of Six Sigma. *Manag Health Care Executive*. 2002;12(1):27–30.
8. Revere L, Black K. Integrating Six Sigma with total quality management: a case example for measuring medication errors. *J Health Care Manag*. 2003;48(6):377–391.
9. De Koning H, Verer JPS, van den Heuvel J, Bisgaard S, Does RJMM. Lean Six Sigma in health care. *Natl Assoc Health Care Qual*. 2006;28(2):4–11.
10. Edwards C, Peppard JW. Business process redesign: hype, hope, or hypocrisy? *J Inf Tech*. 1994;9:251–266 [as cited in Ref.[4]].
11. Carr DK, Hard KJ, Trahant WJ. *Managing the Change Process: A Field Book for Change Agents, Consultants, Team Leaders, and Reengineering Managers*. New York: McGraw-Hill; 1996.
12. Certo SC, Certo ST. *Modern Management*. 10th ed. New Jersey: Pearson-Prentice Hall; 2006.
13. Prochaska JO, Norcross JC, Diclemente CC. *Changing for Good: The Revolutionary Program that Explains the Six Stages of Change and Teaches You how to Free Yourself from Bad Habits*. New York: W. Morrow; 1994.
14. Kübler-Ross, E. *On Death and Dying*. New York: Macmillan; 1969.
15. Conner DR. *Managing at the Speed of Change*. Villard Books; New York; 1992.
16. Gilley A. *The Manager as Change Leader*. Westport, CT: Praeger Publishers; 2005.
17. Olson ML. Controlling the perils of change. *Training Dev*. 2008;62(9):38–43.
18. Mirza B. Organizational change starts with individual employees. *HR Mag*. 2009;53:31–34.
19. Kotter JP, Cohen DS. *The Heart of Change: Real-life Stories of how People Change their Organizations*. Boston, MA: Harvard Business School Press; 2002.
20. Bovey WH, Hede A. Resistance to organizational change: the role of defence mechanisms. *J Managerial Psychol*. 2001;16(7):534–548.
21. Coghlan D. A person-centered approach to dealing with resistance to change. *Leadership Organ Dev J*. 1993;14(4):10–14 [as cited in Ref.[20]].
22. Myers L, Robbins M. 10 rules for change. *Executive Excellence*. 1991;8(5):9–10 [as cited in Ref.[20]].
23. Nadler DA. Managing organizational change: an integrative perspective. *J Appl Behav Sci*. 1981;17(2):191–211 [as cited in Ref.[20]].
24. Steinburg C. Taking charge of change. *Training Dev*. 1992;46(3):26–32 [as cited in Ref.[20]].

25. Zimmerer LW, Zimmerer TW, Yasan MM. Overcoming barriers to effectiveness in a health care operational environment: building on the lessons of American industry. *Health Marketing Q.* 1999;17(1):59–81.

26. Hyman D, Miller JA. *Community Systems and Human Services: An Ecological Approach to Policy, Planning, and Management.* Dubuque, IA: Kendall/Hunt; 1985.

27. Kaufman H. *The Limits of Organizational Change.* University of Alabama Press; Tuscaloosa; 1971.

28. Van Meter DS, Van Horn CE. The policy implementation process: a conceptual framework. *Adm Soc.* 1975;6(4):445–488.

29. Senge PM. *The Fifth Discipline: The Art and Practice of the Learning Organization.* New York: Doubleday; 1990.

30. Kotter JP. Why transformation efforts fail. *Harvard Business Review.* March–April 1995.

31. Reger RK, Mullane JV, Gustafson LT, DeMarie SM. Creating earthquakes to change organizational mindsets. *Acad Manag Executive.* 1994;8(4):31–43.

32. Rucker TD. Pursuing rational drug therapy: a macro view a la the USA. *J Soc Administrative Pharm.* 1988;5(3/4):78–86.

33. Donabedian A. Quality assurance: structure, process, and outcome. *Nurs Stand.* 1992;7(11 Suppl QA) :4–5.

34. Warholak TL. Ensuring quality in pharmacy operations. In: Desselle, SP Zgarrick, DP eds. *Pharmacy Management: Essentials for All Practice Settings.* New York: McGraw Hill Medical; 2009.

35. Castle L, Franzblau-Isaac E, Paulsen J. Using Six Sigma to reduce medication errors in a home-delivery pharmacy service. *Jt Comm J Qual Patient Serv.* 2005;31(6): 319–324.

36. Chan A. Use of Six Sigma to improve pharmacist dispensing errors at an outpatient clinic. *Am J Med Qual.* 2004;19(3):128–131.

37. Goldspiel BR, DeChristoforo R, Daniels CE. A continuous-improvement approach for reducing the number of chemotherapy-related medication errors. *Am J Health Syst Pharm.* 2000;57(suppl 4):S4–S9.

38. Stump LS. Re-engineering the medication error-reporting process: removing the blame and improving the system. *Am J Health Syst Pharm.* 2000;57(suppl 4):S510–S517.

39. Graber JE, Huang ES, Drum ML, Chin MH, Walters AE, Heuer L, Tang H, Schaefer CT, Quinn MT. Predicting changes in staff morale and burnout at community health centers participating in the health disparities collaboratives. *Health Serv Res.* 2008;43(4):1403–1423.

CHAPTER 13

Using Technology in the Quality Improvement Process

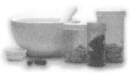

Elizabeth A. Flynn

Learning Objectives

At the end of the chapter, the reader will be able to:

1. Explain how pharmacists can use technology in the quality improvement process.
2. Describe three different technologies that can be used to improve quality in pharmacy.
3. List two challenges to the adoption of technology in the quality improvement process.

INTRODUCTION

Medication errors and adverse drug events (ADEs) are the indicators of choice for the quality of medication distribution in inpatient and outpatient settings. Medication errors are typically defined as any deviation from a prescriber's order, while ADEs are defined as an injury resulting from medical intervention related to a drug.[1,2] Inpatients experience one medication error every day in the hospital,[1] and rates of ADEs have been measured between 2.4 and 52 per 100 inpatients.[2-6] Medication dispensing errors in community pharmacies occur on 2–22 prescriptions out of every 100.[7,8] A systematic review of the literature on ADEs in ambulatory patients found 14.9 ADEs per month out of every 1000 patients.[9] All of these quality results are based on observation or manual chart review, which can be time-consuming. What are the prospects for expanding the collection of such quality indicators using technology and accelerating progress toward error-free systems?

Technology is being used to distribute medications in a variety of settings because it replaces the need for human involvement when the tasks are repetitive, tiring, or require memory-intensive record-keeping. The health care provider's ultimate goal is to close the loop and make it possible to technologically oversee the accuracy of the entire medication distribution process. This oversight would start with prescriber ordering and continue to the patient receiving the intended medication, ending with feedback on the effectiveness of the therapy provided via laboratory tests and physical monitoring. Until this ideal is reached, pharmacists need to monitor the performance of medication distribution technology in terms of quality control measures for each step of the process involving humans or automation.

Chaudhry described one of the important benefits of health information technology (HIT) on the quality of medical care as enhanced surveillance and monitoring of ADEs, which could ultimately lead to fewer ADEs and medication errors. Examples of HIT include:

- electronic health records;
- Computer physician order entry (CPOE);
- decision support (stand-alone systems);
- electronic results reporting;
- electronic prescribing;
- consumer health informatics/patient decision support (DS);
- mobile computing;
- telemedicine;
- electronic health communication;
- administration;
- data exchange networks;
- knowledge retrieval systems.[10]

Some of the above-mentioned technologies have the potential to contribute quality monitoring data and should be designed and used to take advantage of this potential. Computerized surveillance of ADEs has been described since 1991.[11–18] This chapter will describe state-of-the-art electronic quality monitoring systems for medication distribution technologies.

QUALITY IMPROVEMENT INDICATORS MEASURABLE WITH TECHNOLOGY

Clinical event monitoring systems can continuously assess patient data for triggers that may indicate a medication-related problem. Clinical event monitors are automatic and typically programmed into the hospital's information system. They provide feedback to clinicians using alerts and reminders related to medication problems, and are faster than manual methods of ADE detection, such as chart review. Such systems can warn users when there are abnormal laboratory results for patients taking certain medications.[19] Orders for the following drugs are examples of triggers that may indicate an ADE: antidotes, reversal agents such as naloxone, flumazenil, acetylcysteine, vitamin K, Digibind, D50, glucagon, Kayexalate, STAT insulin, and hyaluronidase. Allergic reactions to medications may stimulate orders for diphenhydramine, IV/IM steroids, or code cart drugs.[20]

Handler et al. conducted a systematic review of clinical event monitoring systems to detect ADEs in hospitals and their effectiveness based on positive predictive values (PPVs).[21] They identified 12 studies describing 36 unique ADE signals that appeared in two or more publications. Seven signals were antidotes that were administered to patients: vitamin K (PPV: 0.02–0.30), activated charcoal (positive predictive value (PPV): 0.08–0.45), antihistamine (PPV: 0.03–0.14), oral metronidazole or vancomycin (PPV: 0.07–0.16), antidiarrheal (PPV: 0–0.11), sodium polystyrene (PPV: 0.06–0.12), and oral or topical steroids (PPV: 0.04–0.09). Ten signals were related to supratherapeutic medication levels that may have been the result of a wrong dose error:

	PPV
Quinidine	0.43–0.60
Phenobarbital	0–1.0
Theophylline trough	0.25–1.0
Vancomycin peak or trough levels	0.18–0.33
Procainamide	0–0.42
Lidocaine	0.17–0.50
Aminoglycoside	0.04–1.0
Digoxin	0.08–1.0
Phenytoin	0.07–1.0
Cyclosporine	0–0.04

Nineteen abnormal laboratory test results were found to be signals – PPV ranges for each are available in the report. The goal of the use of triggers is to maximize ADE detection while minimizing false positives, which are equivalent to false alarms that distract pharmacists needlessly. In order to assist with the interpretation of PPVs, consider that fecal occult blood testing to detect colon cancer in adults over 50 years old has a PPV of 0.02–0.18 and is considered a routine test.

Manual chart review uses laboratory result triggers as one indication of ADEs.[2] These laboratory test triggers can now be programmed into the computer, and clinicians alerted when normal values are exceeded via text message or page. Table 13-1 lists examples of laboratory result triggers for medication-related problems.

Laboratory–pharmacy computer links for improved care were proposed by Schiff et al.[19] Two of the suggestions were related to quality improvement: surveillance of drug toxicities and quality oversight. The computer can detect signals of adverse reactions such as hepatotoxicity that were not documented before. With respect to quality oversight, the computer can monitor the time interval between abnormal laboratory results and medication order change or a new order for a medication in response to the abnormal result, for example, time to first dose of an antibiotic in response to a positive blood culture.

TABLE 13-1. Laboratory Value Drug-related Problem Triggers

Elevated blood urea nitrogen (BUN)/Creatine (Cr): example – patient on aminoglycoside with rising BUN/Crs levels (doubled or more). Creatinine: ≥ 2 mg/dl if baseline value is <1.5 or 1 mg/dl increase if the baseline is ≥ 1.5 mg/dl. Note the patient's age
Liver function tests (LFTs): doubled and greater than upper limit of normal
Elevated drug level: aminoglycosides, phenytoin, theophylline, phenobarbital, digoxin (doubled or more)
Decreasing or increasing hematocrit (HCT): 6-point change in the absence of other explanation
Sudden drop or increase in blood glucose for patient receiving insulin or oral hypoglycemic. Glucose <40 or >400
Heme-positive stool
Positive *C. difficile* culture
Serum potassium (K^+): <2.5 or >6.0
White blood cells (WBC); <500 neutrophil count (if differential available)
Platelets: 50% drop and <100,000
International normalized ratio (INR): >4 (upper limit of normal) – for patients receiving warfarin
Partial thromboplastin time (PTT): 5-point increase and greater than normal – for patients receiving warfarin
Prothrombin time (PT): 2-point increase and greater than normal – for patients receiving warfarin
Creatine phosphokinase (CPK) > 500

Drug Triggers

In a study that monitored laboratory values to detect drug-related hazardous conditions, Kane-Gill et al.[22] found that 444 of 590 surgical intensive care unit patients in 3 months had abnormal laboratory values. Laboratory values were compared for serum electrolytes, platelet, creatinine, glucose, magnesium, and liver enzymes to standards. Drug-related hazardous conditions were detected in 22% of patients with abnormal laboratory values, with hypermagnesemia, and hyper- and hypokalemia being most common.[22]

A study to determine the value of using a decentralized automated dispensing machine (ADM) to detect ADEs was conducted by Romero and Malone in two hospitals.[23] Whenever a nurse retrieved a trigger or tracer drug from the automated device, he or she was prompted to enter a reason for drug removal, such as "side effects of narcotic" for naloxone. The tracer drugs at Hospital 1 were dextrose 50% and naloxone, and at Hospital 2, dextrose 50%, naloxone, diphenhydramine, epinephrine, hydroxyzine, vitamin K, protamine, methylprednisolone, and flumazenil. Did the ADM detect more potential ADEs than spontaneous reports? At Hospital 1, there were 19 spontaneous reports (any medication, hospital-wide), while the 2 tracer drugs helped detect 87 ADEs on nursing units using the ADM prompt. Hospital 2 had 1–2 spontaneous reports per month, while the ADM documented 10–15 ADEs per day (extrapolates to 300–450 ADEs per month). Monitoring the frequency of ADEs electronically is an efficient and effective method for identifying drug-related issues and implementing system improvements to decrease such ADEs.

Hwang et al.[24] evaluated a computer-based ADE monitor retrospectively in Seoul, Korea. Two intensive care units and five general wards were studied and 598 patients were included. ADE signals integrated four sets used in previous studies: Latter Day Saints Hospital, Brigam and Women's Hospital, Veterans Health Administration, and Raschke et al.[25] Forty-six ADE signals were used in the study in a computer-based ADE monitor that generated a list of possible ADEs. A pharmacist trained to verify ADEs conducted a targeted chart review to determine whether an ADE had actually occurred. Chart reviews were also conducted on a random sample of patients for whom there were no computer signals to determine if the computer missed ADEs. The computer monitor detected 148 of 187 ADEs (79% sensitivity), while chart review identified 39 additional ADEs that the computer did not detect. The computer recognized more severe ADEs, but all other characteristics were the same. The computer monitor's PPV was 21%, based on 148 ADEs from 718 ADE triggers. The number of alerts and PPV for each trigger are provided in the report.[24]

Signals for adverse drug reaction (ADR) detection in nursing homes have been developed by a consensus process.[26] Experts in geriatrics agreed on 40 signals, including 15 laboratory–medication combinations, 12 medication concentrations, 10 antidotes, and 3 resident assessment protocols.

MONITORING MEDICATION DISTRIBUTION QUALITY IN HOSPITALS

An automated medication system is defined as a mechanical system that performs operations involving the storage, packaging, dispensing, or distribution of medications while enabling control of the operation and electronic documentation of transactions.[27] Systems typically incorporate bar code technology to verify the accuracy of medication, strength, and form and to verify patient identity.[28]

Some hospitals currently employ bar code verification technology to double-check dispensing accuracy in the pharmacy. A recent study of pharmacy dispensing accuracy found that 0.75% of 140,755 doses checked by pharmacists contained an error.[29,30]

A study of the effects of bar code systems on pharmacy dispensing accuracy found an 85% decrease in target dispensing errors from a rate of 0.37% to 0.06%. Target dispensing errors are those that a bar code verification system can prevent.[31]

Bar Code Medication Administration Verification Monitoring

Nine percent of hospitals employ bar code verification technology to double-check administration accuracy at the patient's bedside prior to nurse administration of the medication.[32]

Cummings et al. of the University HealthSystem Consortium (UHC) published recommendations for the use of bar code systems in the medication process. They recommended the use of an ongoing noncompliance or exception report to maximize scanning, determining problem areas, and improving the overall process.[33] These noncompliance reports can reveal the potential for errors. Nurses performed overrides of warnings received when using bar code systems on 23 of 445 BCMA related errors in the MedMarx database.[5] There were also 34 instances of errors because the bar code on the medication was not scanned – medication administration was documented manually.[5] However, Patterson et al.[34] found that electronic reports cannot capture all noncompliance with bar code procedures and documented workarounds using observation that can be employed to circumvent safety-related tasks.[34]

Paoletti et al. described the use of two reports to monitor the bar code medication administration system (BCMA) in their hospital: the Prevented Medication Error Report and Possible Medication Error Report. The Prevented Medication Error Report describes warnings provided to the nurse during medication administration. This aids identification of areas for improvement in the system as well as bar code scanning compliance. The Possible Medication Error Report identifies nurses who are not using the BCMA system correctly and unit nurse managers discuss the findings with the nurses on a daily basis and discuss corrective actions.[35]

Monitoring Overrides

A safety system override is typically necessary in emergencies for removal of a medication from an ADM by a nurse before the pharmacist's review and approval of the prescriber's order. The Joint Commission states that overrides can be performed if delay would harm the patient, and includes sudden change in clinical status.

Override monitoring can be performed by following up on alerts received in pharmacy from decentralized automated drug dispensing cabinets when a nurse retrieves a drug by overriding the system warning that a pharmacist review has not taken place.

Oren et al.[36] studied antimicrobial overrides and found 10 medication errors per day associated with overrides and 21% of overrides resulted in errors. No ADEs were detected in this study. The most commonly encountered categories of overrides were:

1. override occurs despite previous drug entry in computer: 342 (27.5%);
2. override occurs before order entered into pharmacy computer: 334 (26.8%);
3. override occurs with no documented entry in the pharmacy computer and an order has been written: 171 (13.7%);

4. override occurs after drug has been discontinued: 227 (18.2%);

5. override occurs after drug has been inappropriately discontinued in the pharmacy computer: 30 (2.4%);

6. override occurs before MD order: 44 (3.5%);

7. drug is entered in pharmacy computer at a different strength than that obtained from ADM: 70 (5.6%).

Continuous monitoring of overrides and limiting access to drugs using overrides has the potential to decrease drug costs, based in particular on the frequency of continued retrieval of medication after it has been discontinued.[36]

Override management recommendations were reported by Kowiatek et al.[37] after finding that 34 overrides led to errors in a 6-month period in 2001, including 2 serious errors and 13 errors that required additional patient monitoring. Appropriate override requirements were developed and implemented, so that a nurse had to verify that all of the following conditions were present:

1. documentation of urgent need based on nurse's clinical judgment;

2. physician order in chart;

3. medication administration record (MAR) documentation of dose administration;

4. patient not allergic to medication;

5. drug and dose ordered match what nurse gave;

6. medication order not on pharmacy profile and nurse removed it via override.

Compliance with these override criteria ranged from 51% to 90%, and then dropped to 57% and ended at 78%. The reasons for noncompliance with the override criteria included nurses forgetting to chart emergency drug use, and using the override function instead of checking the medication profile first.[37]

Kowiatek et al.[37] recommended the following "Guide for Review Process of Override Medications" when selecting medications that are available to nurses on override at an ADM:

1. Assess types and frequencies of overrides.

2. Focus on drug classes with safety concerns.

3. Expert committee to develop override criteria.

4. Determine if override status will be safe and appropriate.

5. Develop monitoring process to assess appropriateness of overrides.

6. Educate clinicians about process and changes.

7. Measure change in override compliance for high-alert drugs.

8. Establish formal process for adding/deleting overrides.

9. Continue to monitor override access for appropriateness.[37]

Overrides in the ambulatory setting were studied by Isaac et al.[38] who found that 6.6% of e-prescriptions generated alerts. Clinicians accepted 9.2% of drug interaction alerts (high-severity interactions = 61.6% of alerts), 2–43% of high-severity alerts accepted depending on drug classes involved, and 23% of allergy alerts.[38]

INTEGRATED INFORMATION SYSTEMS AND MEDICATION SAFETY

Effects of an integrated clinical information system on medication safety were studied by Mahoney et al.[39] The integrated system included computerized physician order entry (Siemens) interfaced to the pharmacy information system, clinical decision support, electronic drug dispensing systems, bar code point of care medication verification (BPOC), and electronic charting. The rate of intercepted medication errors per 1000 patient days and per 100,000 charted doses was used as an indicator of BPOC effectiveness. Electronic error record reports can be reviewed for details and system improvements made to minimize the risk of such errors. Quality reports are monitored by nursing leadership to verify that the BPOC system is being used appropriately (e.g., explore overrides of BPOC system alerts to ensure appropriateness). The BPOC intercepted 73 medication administration errors every 100,000 charted doses. Fifty-five of the errors were wrong time, 12 intercepted errors were wrong patient, and 6 errors were wrong drug, dose, or route. Most of the wrong time errors were due to the attempted administration of an as-needed dose before the prescribed time interval had passed. The electronic identification and documentation of medication administration errors is a promising area for the use of technology.[39]

SUMMARY

As each part of the medication use system incorporates information technology, it is becoming possible to monitor quality electronically. This capability should be built into information technology (IT) systems in order to save time and labor expenses. An accurate automated description of the quality of medication use in all settings is within reach.

REFERENCES

1. Barker KN, Flynn EA, Pepper GA, Bates DW, Mikeal RL. Medication errors observed in 36 health care facilities. *Arch Intern Med.* 2002;162(16):1897–1903.
2. Bates DW, Cullen DJ, Laird N, et al. Incidence of adverse drug events and potential adverse drug events. Implications for prevention. ADE Prevention Study Group [see comment]. *JAMA.* 1995;274(1):29–34.
3. Senst BL, Achusim LE, Genest RP, et al. Practical approach to determining costs and frequency of adverse drug events in a health care network. *Am J Health-Syst Pharm,* 2001;58(12):1126–1132.
4. Classen DC, Pestotnik SL, Evans RS, Lloyd JF, & Burke JP. Adverse drug events in hospitalized patients. Excess length of stay, extra costs, and attributable mortality. *JAMA* 1997; 277(4):301–306.
5. Cochrane GL, Jones KJ, Brockman J, Skinner A, Hicks RW. Errors prevented by and associated with bar-code medication administration systems. *Jt Comm J Qual Patient Saf.* 2007;33(5):293–301.
6. Nebeker JR, Hoffman JM, Weir CR, Bennett CL, Hurdle JF. High rates of adverse drug events in a highly computerized hospital. [Comparative StudyResearch Support, U.S. Gov't, Non-P.H.S.]. *Arch Intern Med,* 2005;165(10):1111–1116.

7. Flynn EA, Barker KN, Berger BA, Braxton Lloyd K, Brackett PD. Dispensing errors and counseling quality in 100 pharmacies. *JAPhA.* 2009;49(2):48–57.

8. Flynn EA, Barker KN, Carnahan BJ. National observational study of prescription dispensing accuracy and safety in 50 pharmacies. *J Am Pharm Assoc.* 2003;43(2):191–200.

9. Thomsen LA, Winterstein AG, Sondergaard B, Haugbolle LS, Melander A. Systematic review of the incidence and characteristics of preventable adverse drug events in ambulatory care [see comment]. *Ann Pharmacother.* 2007;41(9):1411–1426.

10. Chaudhry B, Wang J, Wu S, et al. Systematic review: impact of health information technology on quality, efficiency, and costs of medical care [see comment]. *Ann Intern Med.* 2006;144(10):742–752.

11. Bates DW, EvansRS, Murff H, Stetson PD, Pizziferri L, Hripcsak G. Detecting adverse events using information technology [see comment]. *J Am Med Inform Assoc.* 2003;10(2):115–128.

12. Classen DC, Pestotnik SL, Evans RS, Burke JP. Computerized surveillance of adverse drug events in hospital patients. *JAMA.* 1991;266(November):2847–2851.

13. Ferranti J, Horvath MM, Cozart H, Whitehurst J, Eckstrand J. Reevaluating the safety profile of pediatrics: a comparison of computerized adverse drug event surveillance and voluntary reporting in the pediatric environment. *Pediatrics.* 2008;121(5):e1201–e1207.

14. Honigman B, Lee J, Rothschild J, et al. Using computerized data to identify adverse drug events in outpatients. *J Am Med Inform Assoc.* 2001;8(3):254–266.

15. Jha AK, Kuperman GJ, Teich JM, et al. Identifying adverse drug events: development of a computer-based monitor and comparison with chart review and stimulated voluntary report. *J Am Med Inform Assoc.* 1998;5(3):305–314.

16. Kilbridge PM, Campbell UC, Cozart HB, Mojarrad MG. Automated surveillance for adverse drug events at a community hospital and an academic medical center. *J Am Med Inform Assoc.* 2006;13(4):372–377.

17. Levy M, Azaz-Livshits T, Sadan B, Shalit M, Geisslinger G, Brune K. Computerized surveillance of adverse drug reactions in hospital: implementation. *Eur J Clin Pharmacol.* 1999;54(11):887–892.

18. Szekendi MK, Sullivan C, Bobb A, et al. Active surveillance using electronic triggers to detect adverse events in hospitalized patients [see comment]. *Qual Saf Health Care.* 2006;15(3):184–190.

19. Schiff GD, Klass D, Peterson J, Shah G, Bates DW. Linking laboratory and pharmacy: opportunities for reducing errors and improving care. *Arch Intern Med.* 2003;163(8): 893–900.

20. Dalton-Bunnow MF, Halvachs FJ. Computer-assisted use of tracer antidote drugs to increase detection of adverse drug reactions: retrospective and concurrent trial. *Hosp Pharm.* 1993;28(August):746–749, 752–755.

21. Handler SM, Altman RL, Perera S, et al. A systematic review of the performance characteristics of clinical event monitor signals used to detect adverse drug events in the hospital setting [erratum appears in *J Am Med Inform Assoc.* 2007;14(5):686]. *J Am Med Inform Assoc.* 2007;14(4):451–458.

22. Kane-Gill SL, Dasta JF, Schneider PJ, Cook CH. Monitoring abnormal laboratory values as antecedents to drug-induced injury. *J Trauma Inj Infect Crit Care.* 2005;59(6):1457–1462.

23. Romero AV, Malone DC. Accuracy of adverse-drug-event reports collected using an automated dispensing system. *Am J Health Syst Pharm.* 2005;62(13):1375–1380.

24. Hwang S-H, Lee S, Koo H-K, Kim Y. Evaluation of a computer-based adverse-drug-event monitor. *Am J Health Syst Pharm.* 2008;65(23):2265–2272.

25. Raschke RA, Gollihare B, Wunderlich TA, et al. A computer alert system to prevent injury from adverse drug events: development and evaluation in a community teaching hospital. *JAMA.*1998;280:1317–1320. [Erratum, *JAMA.*1999;281:420.]

26. Handler SM, Hanlon JT, Perera S, et al. Consensus list of signals to detect potential adverse drug reactions in nursing homes. *J Am Geriatr Soc.* 2008;56(5):808–815.

27. Barker KN, Felkey BG, Flynn EA, Carper JL. White paper on automation in pharmacy. *Consultant Pharm* 1998;13(March): 256, 261, 265–266, 268, 274–276, 279, 283–284, 286, 289–290, 293.

28. Rough S, Temple J. Automation in practice. In: Brown TR, ed. *Handbook of Institutional Pharmacy Practice.* 4th ed. Bethesda, MD: American Society of Health-System Pharmacists, 2006; 329–352.

29. Cina J, Fanikos J, Mitton P, McCrea M, Churchill W. Medication errors in a pharmacy-based bar-code-repackaging center. *Am J Health Syst Pharm.* 2006;63(2):165–168.

30. Cina JL, Gandhi TK, Churchill W, et al. How many hospital pharmacy medication dispensing errors go undetected? *Jt Comm J Qual Patient Saf.* 2006;32(2):73–80.

31. Poon EG, Cina JL, Churchill W, et al. Medication dispensing errors and potential adverse drug events before and after implementing bar code technology in the pharmacy. *Ann Intern Med.* 2006;145(6):426–434.

32. Pedersen CA, Schneider PJ, Scheckelhoff DJ. ASHP national survey of pharmacy practice in hospital settings: dispensing and administration – 2005. *Am J Health Syst Pharm.* 2006;63(4):327–345.

33. Cummings J, Bush P, Smith D, Matuszewski K, on behalf of the UHC Bar-coding Task Force. Bar-coding medication administration overview and consensus recommendations. *Am J Health Syst Pharm.* 2005;62(24):2626–2629.

34. Patterson ES, Rogers ML, Chapman RJ, Render ML. Compliance with intended use of bar code medication administration in acute and long-term care: an observational study. *Hum Factors.* 2006;48(1):15–22.

35. Paoletti RD, Suess TM, Lesko MG, et al. Using bar-code technology and medication observation methodology for safer medication administration. *Am J Health Syst Pharm.* 2007;64(5):536–543.

36. Oren E, Griffiths LP, Guglielmo BJ. Characteristics of antimicrobial overrides associated with automated dispensing machines. *Am J Health Syst Pharm.* 2002;59(15):1445–1448.

37. Kowiatek JG, Weber RJ, Skledar SJ, Frank S, DeVita M. Assessing and monitoring override medications in automated dispensing devices. *Jt Comm J Qual Patient Saf.* 2006;32(6):309–317.

38. Isaac T, Weissman JS, Davis RB, et al. Overrides of medication alerts in ambulatory care. *Arch Intern Med.* 2009;169(3):305–311.

39. Mahoney CD, Berard-Collins CM, Coleman R, Amaral JF, Cotter CM. Effects of an integrated clinical information system on medication safety in a multi-hospital setting. *Am J Health Syst Pharm.* 2007;64(18):1969–1977.

CHAPTER 14

Reporting on Health Care Quality

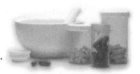

Terri Moore and David P. Nau

Learning Objectives

At the end of the chapter, the reader will be able to:

1. Describe a health care report card.
2. List three reasons why report cards are used in the health care system.
3. List three principles of reporting quality in pharmacy as outlined by the Pharmacy Quality Alliance.
4. Discuss the advantages and disadvantages of reporting quality in pharmacy.

One of the cornerstones of value-driven health care is transparency.[1] It has become common to see public reports on the quality of hospitals, long-term care facilities, and health plans. The Joint Commission and the Centers for Medicare and Medicaid Services (CMS) have both created websites to provide easy access to report cards on hospitals and other institutional providers.[2,3] The National Committee for Quality Assurance (NCQA) has been reporting on the quality of health plans for over a decade using its HEDIS set of performance measures as well as composite ratings of plans.[4] CMS has also begun to report on the quality of prescription drug plans in the Medicare program. This has included "star ratings" of plans based on several dimensions of quality (including drug safety), as well as a website unveiled in November 2009 to provide more detailed information on the quality of each plan.

Within the past few years, a growing number of physician report cards have also become available. While most of these reports are at the clinic or group level, there is a growing demand for information about individual physicians.[5,6] In early 2007, the CMS launched a new pilot project to promote the use of information on physician performance to drive improvement in the quality of care.[7] This project included a set of measures for public reporting of physician performance and was launched by the AQA (formerly known as the Ambulatory Care Quality Alliance) – a national coalition working with a broad group of stakeholders, including CMS, to select measures for public reporting of physician performance. Six "pilots" were selected for testing locally led, collaborative approaches to performance measurement and reporting. Although AQA had selected more than 24 measures of clinical performance suitable for public reporting, many questions remained about how to coordinate data collection and reporting, as well as how to promote the use of the measures among consumers, payers, and providers.

Known as the "Better Quality Information to Improve Care for Medicare Beneficiaries" (or "BQI") project, the project's goals were to test data collection strategies and to promote the use of quality improvement information. These projects began to scratch the surface of the challenges and successes of public reporting of performance data. Using a starter set of clinical measures selected by AQA, the pilot sites generated reports for Medicare beneficiaries and providers, while experimenting with reporting at the individual physician, group, and systems levels in order to explore what types of information and what approaches to information sharing are most effective.

Also in 2007, the Robert Wood Johnson Foundation launched a national project to promote quality improvement through reporting and information exchange.[8] Ideally, these programs set forth to explore a national, coordinated approach to physician measurement that involved the leadership of local, multistakeholder collaborative and that allows for customization to local market conditions. There is clearly significance in the model for coordinating performance measurement at the local levels. These are models that provide some guidance to the efforts to bring public reporting of performance into the pharmacy world.

The discussion of public performance reporting raises several important questions: What are the guiding principles for performance reporting? What are the challenges to public reporting? What should be reported? What should performance reports look like? What is the status and future of performance reporting in the pharmacy arena? Who are the users of performance reports? These are some of the questions discussed in this chapter.

WHAT ARE THE GUIDING PRINCIPLES FOR PERFORMANCE REPORTING?

1. Performance measurement and information exchange are critical in driving quality improvement. In other words, performance reports should focus on areas that have the greatest opportunities to improve quality by making care safe, timely, effective, efficient, equitable, and patient centered.

2. Each type of performance reporting users – consumers, health care providers, payers, etc. – has a role in driving quality improvement and each may have different information needs. Consumers should be involved in the design of reports; the appropriateness of report design and display should be verified through consumer testing. Pharmacists, other providers, and other stakeholders should be able to review and comment on the methodology for data collection and analysis.

3. The use of nationally adopted standard measures and coordinated data collection will reduce "noise" in the marketplace, sending stronger signals to providers about how to drive improvement, while reducing unnecessary administrative burden related to reporting.

4. Performance reports should rely on standard performance and patient experience measures that are valid and reliable, evidence-based, and relevant to patient outcomes.

5. Local communities differ and should have input into selecting measures and in using the information in ways that best suit their needs. Performance reports should be considerate of practice setting and acknowledge that measures of process, outcomes, and structure may need to be tailored when appropriate.

6. Report design and usability reflects the accounting for the differences in the user audiences (e.g., cultural and literacy differences), as well as having performance reports assessable through various media.

7. Performance data should, when available, reflect trend data over time rather than periodic snapshots.

8. Measures, methods, and data specifications should be as transparent and available as possible. Transparency in reporting requires complete and accurate details to be included, with little or no significant information being withheld.

9. The content of reports should include appropriate, contextual information to frame the purpose of the report.

THE CHALLENGES OF REPORTING ON QUALITY

The previously mentioned projects were evidence of the myriad of challenges involved in performance reporting. Some of these challenges in reporting quality stem around the preference of some to protect the confidentiality of participants, to not identify individual facilities or organizations, and to not compare facilities or organizations. Overcoming these challenges requires allowing time to gain acceptance and trust from providers before making such information public. In addition to providing information that is usable and meaningful to the end user, because performance and quality reports also can drive meaningful and measurable quality improvement, they need to focus on promoting knowledge diffusion and provide actionable feedback to health care providers.

Other challenges are more methodological and operational in nature, such as the use of consistent definitions, calculations, and reporting formats. Once data are collected and aggregated, the results need to be reviewed and validated. Some of these challenges will be diminished with more coordination at the national level resulting in the identification of salient measures for performance improvement and reporting.

Challenges also exist around whether or not the user of performance reports, for example, consumers, providers, and payers, will view the information as credible and will be provided with information to understand how the ratings were calculated. This links to some of the previously raised issues of data availability, and other data and measurement issues. Then there is the question of whether or not providers, payers, or consumers will use performance reports. Will public performance reporting stimulate improvement in care, or increase competition, or will it have a negative impact on practice (e.g., provider would not care for the sickest patients, or avoid noncompliant patients)? Is it even feasible to produce performance report cards?

WHAT IS THE STATUS AND FUTURE OF PERFORMANCE REPORTING IN PHARMACY?

Public reporting on physician performance, health plans, hospitals, and other health care providers is not terribly new. Refinements and modifications to such reporting are ongoing. However, what is still embryonic in its development is public reporting of pharmacy performance. Similar to other provider report cards, pharmacy report cards would be used for the following purposes:

● to encourage continuous performance improvement;
● to provide benchmarks as a basis for comparisons with other pharmacies, therefore motivating performance improvement;
● to generate external pressure to have performance meet or exceed that of competitors or peers;
● to identify best practices as outstanding performance is recognized.

WHAT SHOULD BE REPORTED?

Public disclosure of the comparative performance of health care providers is seen as one mechanism for improving quality of care and potentially controlling health care costs. When measures are available, performance reports should include composite (i.e., overall) assessments of practice performance as well as assessments of the individual measures used for the composite assessment. Ideally, both process and outcome measures of quality should be reported.

Organizations such as the Pharmacy Quality Alliance (PQA) are working toward the establishment of reporting tools for individual pharmacies and pharmacists (www.pqaalliance.org). The PQA is spearheading efforts in the development of pharmacy performance scorecards that will serve as the source for information about the quality of retail and mail pharmacies. This reporting is based on a pharmacy's performance on several quantifiable measures reflective of the pharmaceutical care and related services provided by the pharmacy and pharmacists. Some of the measures focus on specific diseases or conditions, such as asthma, diabetes, or cardiovascular diseases; and reflect care issues such as adherence to prescribed medication therapy, the appropriateness of medication therapy, and the effectiveness of medication therapy. Some aspect of medication therapy is frequently included in performance reports. The starter set of clinical measures for the AQA pilot projects previously discussed included 10 measures dealing with medications and medication use.

In addition to assessments of individual pharmacist or pharmacy practice performance, reports should include appropriate contextual information to frame the purpose of the report, descriptions of the measures, identification of the sponsors of the report and the source(s) of the information, and guidance on how to use the report appropriately. Performance reports should include a glossary of terms.

WHAT SHOULD A PERFORMANCE REPORT CARD FOR PHARMACIES LOOK LIKE?

It would be valuable to have a consistent, universal report card for pharmacies so that data collection and comparisons would be done in a consistent manner. A performance report card for pharmacy should:

⬤ include various performance measures or indicators;

⬤ include an explanation of each measurement;

⬤ provide previous results obtained for the organization;

⬤ provide benchmarks based on peer groups.

Having report cards generated with a consistent format and layout, and including consistent data elements, would make the use of pharmacy report cards more meaningful to its users. The creators of reports cards should also be mindful of the reading level of the end users (e.g., consumers) and avoid technical jargon that could be confusing. Simple graphs and pictures can also be useful to show the user when a pharmacy is performing above average or well below average.

A useful resource for information on the use of report cards is the Agency for Healthcare Research and Quality (AHRQ). This agency maintains a compendium of health care report cards that is available at http://www.talkingquality.gov/compendium/. This compendium contains numerous examples of report cards that have been used to provide information to the public about the quality of hospitals, physician groups, clinics, and health plans. However, the AHRQ compendium does not contain report cards for pharmacy services.

Two other organizations have produced reports that allow a comparison between pharmacies. Outcomes Pharmaceutical Health Care has a report that allows the public to compare pharmacies on various parameters including a composite rating. The report card is available at www.getoutcomes.com, but only provides ratings of pharmacies that participate in the Outcomes network. JD Powers recently created a consumer rating program for retail and mail-service pharmacies; however, independent pharmacies are not included in the report (http://www.jdpower.com/healthcare/ratings/retail_pharmacy/).

A report card used by the Australian Quality Care Pharmacy Program appears to be the most similar to the type of report card that could be developed from the PQA quality metrics and provides a comparison between pharmacies on four quality metrics. The metrics are derived from a consumer assessment of service quality (SERVPERF), extent of directive guidance and counseling provided to patients, and the extent of medication nonadherence. More information can be found at http://beta.guild.org.au/qcpp/.

AND WHO ARE THE USERS OF PERFORMANCE DATA?

The government (federal and state) may use performance data as a basis for meeting eligibility criteria for participation in a government-sponsored program, or for payment for performance in a care delivery program. Nongovernmental purchasers and payers, such as business coalitions and large employer companies, similarly may use performance data in determining which service organization and health care provider to contract with. It has been suggested that public reporting and pay for performance be used together to accelerate improvements in care, although research indicates that public reporting and pay for performance, combined, only achieve modestly greater improvements in quality that did the use of only public reporting. Competing providers (e.g., other pharmacies) may use a report card to compare themselves to other organizations and providers.

Ultimately, the average consumer may use performance data in making selection decisions when more than one option for services and care is offered. With the varied array of users of performance data, the details of performance report cards are quite challenging; however, consistency in format and content will help make performance report cards useful to many audiences. Despite many efforts, public reporting has not been shown to be conclusively effective in stimulating consumers to choose their health care provider based on performance information. This may be due, in part, to the numerous barriers to the use of quality information by consumers. Such barriers include lack of awareness, lack of trust, and lack of understanding of the information.

SUMMARY

Public reporting on health care quality will continue to grow as health care purchasers and consumers seek the best value. CMS is rapidly increasing the number of performance measures that it publicly reports about prescription drug plans that serve Medicare enrollees. As the transparency of medication safety grows, it is anticipated that individual pharmacies will soon be seeing public reports about the quality of care of pharmacies. If consumers begin to use the reports to select pharmacies, then it is imperative that pharmacies initiate quality improvement programs to enhance their scores on these report cards.

REFERENCES

1. Department of Health and Human Services. *Building a Value-based Health Care System*. Available at http://www.hhs.gov/valuedriven/. Accessed October 11, 2009.
2. Department of Health and Human Services. *Hospital Compare*. Available at http://hospital-compare2.com/. Accessed October 11, 2009.
3. Department of Health and Human Services. *Nursing Home Compare*. Available at http://www.medicare.gov/NHCompare/. Accessed October 11, 2009.
4. NCQA. *Health Plan Report Card*. Available at http://reportcard.ncqa.org/plan/external/plansearch.aspx. Accessed October 11, 2009.
5. Massachusetts Health Quality Partners. Available at http://www.mhqp.org/. Accessed October 11, 2009.
6. Health Grades. Available at http://www.healthgrades.com/. Accessed October 11, 2009.
7. Better Quality Information to Improve Care for Medicare Beneficiaries. Available at http://www.cms.hhs.gov/BQI/. Accessed November 3, 2009.
8. Aligning Forces for Quality (AF4Q). Available at http://www.rwjf.org/qualityequality/af4q/index.jsp. Accessed November 3, 2009.

RECOMMENDED READING

Bradley EH, Holmboe ES, Mattera JA, et al. Data feedback efforts in quality improvement: lessons learned from U.S. hospitals. *Qual Saf Health Care.* 2004;13:26–31.

Gandhi TK, Cook EF, Puopolo AL, et al. Inconsistent report cards: assessing the comparability of various measures of the quality of ambulatory care. *Med Care.* 2002;40:155–165.

Greenfield S, Kaplan SH, Kahn R, Ninomaya J, Griffith JL. Profiling care provided by different groups of physicians: effects of patient case-mix (bias) and physician-level clustering on quality assessment results. *Ann Intern Med.* 2002;136:111–121.

Hibbard JH, Jewett JJ. What type of quality information do consumers want in a health care report card? *Med Care Res Rev.* 1996;53:28–47.

Hibbard JH, Jewett JJ. Will quality reports help consumers? *Health Aff.* 1997;16:218–228.

Hibbard JH, Sofaer S, Jewett JJ. Condition-specific performance information: assessing salience, comprehension, and approaches for communicating quality. *Health Care Financing Rev.* 1996;18:95–110.

Jewett JJ, Hibbard JH. Comprehension of quality care indicators: differences among privately insured, publicly insured, and uninsured. *Health Care Financing Rev.* 1996;18:75–94.

Hochhauser M. Designing readable report cards. *Manag Healthcare.* 1998;(May);8:15–22.

McCaffrey KJ, MacKinnon NJ. Health care report cards: why should community pharmacists care? *Can Pharm J.* 2005;138:36–43.

McGee J, Knutson D. Health care report cards: what about consumers' perspectives? *J Ambul Care Manag.* 1994;17:1–14.

Schneider EC, Epstein AM. Use of public performance reports. *JAMA.* 1998;279:1638–1642.

Silverman JE, Rosen TR. The case for pharmacy report cards. *J Manag Care Pharm.* 1999;5:176–182.

Van Hoof TJ, Pearson DA, Sherwin TE, et al. Lessons learned from performance feedback by a quality improvement organization. *J Healthcare Qual.* 2006; 28:20–31.

CHAPTER 15

Aligning Financial Incentives for Quality

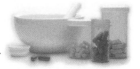

David P. Nau

Learning Objectives

At the end of the chapter, the reader will be able to:
1. Define pay for performance.
2. Describe the rationale for pay for performance in pharmacy.
3. Describe how pay-for-performance programs for pharmacies may be designed.

The use of financial incentives to boost the quality of care is often implemented as pay for performance (P4P).[1] In a P4P system, providers are rewarded financially for achieving high levels of quality or for significantly improving quality of care. To date, hundreds of P4P programs have been implemented within the U.S. health care system with hospitals and physicians being the primary targets of these incentive programs. However, nursing homes and home health providers have also seen rapid growth in P4P and a small number of programs for pharmacies have also been implemented.

A BRIEF HISTORY OF P4P

A 2005 survey of health maintenance organizations (HMOs) found that over half of the HMOs used P4P incentives in their provider contracts.[2] Of those that used P4P, 90% had programs for physicians and 38% included hospitals. In some states, the majority of physicians may be enrolled in a P4P system. For example, Blue Cross Blue Shield of Hawaii has operated a Physician Quality and Service Recognition program since 1998. This program, run through the Hawaii Medical Service Association's preferred provider organization (PPO) network, grew from 50.4% physician participation in 1998 to 77.7% in 2003. A 6-year review of the impact of the financial incentive component of the program indicated that patients who visited one of the participating physicians were more likely to receive recommended care.[3]

Another early adopter of P4P is the Integrated Healthcare Association (IHA) in California. The IHA P4P program began in 2003 and now includes eight health plans and over 35,000 physicians in California. The program was associated with significant improvements in quality during the first 2 years of the financial incentives.[4] A recent evaluation of the P4P program shows that the program continues to drive improvements in clinical quality although significant geographic variation still exists.[5] In 2007, IHA paid out over $65 million in P4P incentives to physician groups although this amounted to less than 2% of physician compensation. The IHA estimates that at least 5%, and preferably 10%, of physician compensation should be based on performance in order to drive significant change in practice.

Although P4P was initiated by employer coalitions and private insurance companies, the federal government has also begun to shift toward a value-based purchasing paradigm that includes P4P.[6] The first step for the federal government is to require providers to report information on quality and efficiency of care (i.e., pay for reporting). For hospitals and physicians, this has meant an incentive payment of up to 2% of reimbursement. For home health providers, the failure to report on quality measures will result in a 2% reduction in payment.

The Centers for Medicare and Medicaid Services (CMS) has initiated demonstration projects related to P4P in recent years. Notably, the Premier Hospital Quality Incentive Demonstration began in 2003 with about 280 hospitals.[7] Hospital quality was assessed using 34 measures across five clinical conditions (acute myocardial infarction, coronary artery bypass graft surgery, pneumonia, heart failure, and hip and knee replacement). The top 50% of hospitals in each condition were recognized on the CMS website, and the top 20% received a financial bonus equal to 1–2% of their reimbursement for those conditions. Hospitals performing in the lowest two deciles were at risk for a reduction in payment of 1–2%. A subsequent analysis showed that the median quality scores across all hospitals increased after the incentive program began; however, the hospitals that began in the lowest deciles experienced the greatest improvement.[8] The hospitals that participated in the P4P program also had greater improvement in quality than a control group of hospitals that only engaged in public reporting on quality.

The CMS is also testing P4P systems for physicians and intends to provide a report to Congress in 2010 regarding the creation of a physician value-based purchasing program. In 2005, CMS began a 5-year P4P demonstration involving 10 large multispecialty physician group practices (known as the PGP demonstration).[6] In the first year, physician groups can receive a payment for up to 80% of the cost savings they achieve. As quality measures are added to the performance scores, physicians will be able to receive payments that are based equally on cost-efficiency and quality. At the end of year 2 of the demonstration, all participating physician groups had achieved benchmark levels for quality and had improved quality for Medicare beneficiaries within diabetes, coronary artery disease, and heart failure. The 10 groups shared the $16.7 million incentive payment.

A home health agency (HHA) demonstration project is also underway to assess the value of incentive payments to HHAs. This project began in January 2008 and continued through December 2009. HHAs who volunteered to participate were randomly assigned to an intervention or control group, and the intervention group is eligible for incentive payments. The incentive pool will be derived from the estimated savings from more costly forms of health care (e.g., hospitalization) with 75% of the pool being distributed to the HHAs within the top two deciles of quality and 25% going to the HHAs with the largest improvement in quality. Since quality scores are based on the existing OASIS database, the HHAs will not have to collect or report any new data. However, if it is determined that no savings occurred through the use of HHAs, no incentive payments will be made.

A nursing home value-based purchasing demonstration is also in progress. As with the HHA demonstration, the nursing home demonstration is required to be budget neutral to Medicare. The incentive pool will be derived from the estimated savings to Medicare from avoided hospitalizations and subsequent skilled nursing facility stays. The quality of the nursing facilities will be measured across four domains: staffing (turnover and staffing levels), hospitalizations (rates of avoidable hospitalizations), minimum data set (MDS) outcomes, and survey deficiencies (from state inspections). Facilities that score in the top 20% of performance and top 20% of improvement will be eligible for incentive payments.

PAYMENT MODELS IN P4P

A plethora of P4P models have been implemented in recent years, but the Institute of Medicine has recommended that an ideal model should reward providers who attain high levels of performance at a given point in time and also reward providers who greatly improve performance over time.[1] Models that reward current performance are important to recognize the top performers; however, these models may be deflating to the lowest performers if they perceive that they are unlikely to ever become a top performer. Thus, the providers in the lowest deciles of performance may not attempt to make improvements. Models that reward improvement in quality may be highly motivating to providers that begin in the lowest deciles of performance because these providers have the biggest opportunity for improvement. For providers who are currently in the top deciles of performance, the improvement model holds little appeal since they have less room for improvement. This is especially true if the overall level of performance is near the maximum value for a particular measure. Thus, it is important to recognize current performance as well as improvement over time.

Rewarding Current Performance

For models of P4P that reward current performance, the threshold for the performance payment may be based on a predefined threshold or based on performance relative to the other providers in the program. The latter approach is sometimes called a tournament model.[9] When using a predefined threshold, a payer usually sets the threshold at a level that is slightly higher than the current average for performance, but not so high as to appear unattainable. Thus, most providers have an incentive to improve. An example would be to reward any provider who had at least 90% of his diabetic patients receive an A1c test during the past year. This level is just slightly higher than the current national average of 88.1%.[10] A variation on this model is to base the payout on the percentage of members who received appropriate care. For example, if a provider had 85% of diabetic patients receive an A1c, the provider would receive 85% of the total payout for which it is eligible. Another variation is to reward the provider a fixed amount per patient multiplied by the number of patients that are provided ideal care. For example, the pharmacist could receive a payment of $10 per patient for every patient who maintains a high level of adherence to target medications. These "current performance" models may be appealing to providers who like the predictability of payment if they reach the threshold. The downside for the payer is the possibility of nearly all providers reaching the threshold and the payer needing to make an extraordinary payout. This risk could be minimized by establishing an incentive pool and dividing the pool among all the providers who achieve the threshold.

A more common approach to rewarding current performance is to reward the top proportion of performers. In this approach, the providers are ranked according to their performance on a set of measures and then divided into deciles of performance (e.g., providers are divided into 10 equally sized groups based on relative performance). Generally, the top decile will receive the largest payment (e.g., 2% bonus) followed by the second decile (e.g., 1% bonus). The other 80% of providers would receive no incentive payment. In some instances, the payers have heightened the stakes by adding a payment decrease for providers in the bottom two deciles of performance. This is sometimes implemented by initially withholding 2% of payments to all providers throughout the year. At the year's end, the providers in the bottom decile receive no additional payment while the providers in the top decile receive 4% additional compensation. The providers in the middle deciles receive 2%. There have been numerous variations on this theme. The appeal of this model for the payers is that the overall payout is fixed.

Rewarding Improvement over Time

As with the model for current performance, the thresholds for rewarding improvement can be a fixed amount or relative to other providers. Some P4P programs set fixed targets for a percentage improvement from period to period, but may vary the targets based on the starting point of the provider. For example, a health plan may set targets for a percentage improvement of generic dispensing rate (GDR) in its pharmacy network; however, the target varies by the starting point of the pharmacy. A pharmacy that starts with a baseline GDR of 50% may have a target improvement of 3% in the following 6-month period but a pharmacy with a baseline GDR of 70% may have a target of only 1% improvement. The lower target for improvement in the pharmacy with higher current performance is based on the assumption that lower performing pharmacy has greater capacity for improvement.

In some "improvement models" of P4P, the payer provides the incentive payment to the providers that have improved the most. Thus, the top 10–20% of providers will receive an additional payment. Some payers prefer this approach since it provides predictability in the amount of incentive payments. This approach is also appealing to providers that may start with the lowest baseline score on a measure. These providers can still achieve significant improvement even if their resulting performance is still well below their peer average.

One challenge is that the payouts for this model cannot begin until enough time has lapsed to measure the change in performance. Thus, even when a mixed-model approach is used, the first round of payment is usually based on current performance and improvement is not a factor until the second round.

How much Is Enough?

Another consideration of P4P is whether the incentive for good performance (or penalty for bad performance) is sufficient to motivate providers to improve performance. A P4P program is unlikely to stimulate improvement if the costs or hassles of improvement outweigh the potential monetary reward. However, payers also want to limit their financial risk and may face budgetary constraints in the amount that can be paid. Some may also believe that they should not have to pay "extra" just to get providers to deliver good care.

There is no clear evidence on the amount of financial incentive that is minimally necessary to drive improved performance. The amount of incentive required to drive behavior may also differ between providers. The CMS incentives for hospitals are typically 1–2% of Medicare-related revenues for the top hospitals; however, this percentage may equate to several million dollars. Results from the Premier Hospital Demonstration indicate that the 1–2% incentive may lead to improved performance across all hospitals. In the IHA of California P4P program for physicians, the average incentive payment in the second year of the program was approximately 1.5% of total physician group compensation.[4] Modest improvements in care were noted following the implementation of the P4P program, but it is not clear whether the payments were the main stimulus for improvement. The IHA estimates that P4P payments may need to exceed 5% of physician compensation to produce substantial improvements in care.[5]

The majority of P4P programs have focused on awarding bonuses for high performance or improved performance. However, some programs may include a financial *penalty* if a provider fails to achieve minimal thresholds on performance measures or is ranked in the bottom one to two deciles relative to other providers.[1,11] Theoretically, this should heighten the stakes for participants in the P4P program and should encourage the lowest performing providers to dramatically improve performance to move out of the bottom deciles. However, if the poorest performing providers are also the poorest financial performers (as is the case with some hospitals that provide a disproportionate share of indigent care), there is also a risk that the penalties will divert needed funds away from the providers that may need it the most.

Which Model Is Best?

Werner and Dudley conducted a simulation of various P4P strategies for hospitals using data from Medicare for 2005. They concluded that no single P4P model was ideal for simultaneously achieving the goals of rewarding high quality, giving all providers an incentive to improve, and creating a payment gradient between high-performing and low-performing hospitals. The model should be selected based on the goals of the P4P program, the baseline data for the targeted providers, and the availability of funds for incentive payments.

CHOOSING THE RIGHT MEASURES

Regardless of the payment model, it is imperative that appropriate measures of performance be selected. Ideal measures will be relevant and important, scientifically sound, feasible, and usable for quality improvement.[12] All of these properties are important to ensure the credibility of the P4P program and provider engagement in the program. Above all, the providers must perceive that they can have an impact on the performance scores. If a performance measure is affected greatly by factors that are unrelated to the quality of the provider's care, it is unlikely that significant improvements will occur through P4P and providers may be discontented. This may especially be true in the case of the "current performance" model of P4P combined with the use of measures that are perceived as being outside of the provider's control. In this situation, the P4P model may actually have unintended consequences for provider behavior. For example, if providers were rewarded based on their relative performance to other providers on a measure of patients' adherence to medication regimens, and if the adherence scores are driven heavily by patient socioeconomic characteristics, then providers have a disincentive to provide care to patients that are deemed likely to be non-adherent. An extreme response would be for providers to move out of geographic areas that are populated by poorly adherent patients.

PAY FOR PERFORMANCE IN PHARMACY

There are two levels at which P4P can be implemented for driving improvements in the pharmacy sector. One level is that of the Pharmacy Benefit Manager (PBM) and/or prescription drug program, and the second level is that of the community pharmacy. Within the Medicare Part D benefit, the drug benefit is provided through private drug plans (as either standalone prescription drug plans or Medicare Advantage plans). Thus, the CMS could expand its value-driven health care initiatives to include rewards to top-performing drug plans. The CMS currently lacks the statutory authority to implement P4P for drug plans, but it can provide public reports on drug plan quality to the public.

If drug plans undergo increased scrutiny of the quality of medication use by their enrollees, this should prompt multifaceted efforts to enhance quality. If a plan identified a performance deficit on a quality measure, it could "drill down" its analyses to the pharmacy level and determine which pharmacies were contributing positively to quality and which ones were not. Plans could pursue a "carrot" or "stick" approach to improving quality within its pharmacy network. A stick approach by a plan could be to eliminate a poorly performing pharmacy from its network, but this approach could create difficulties in access for members and increase complaints from members and employers. Nonetheless, the threat of being removed from a pharmacy network based on poor quality may result in heightened attention by pharmacies to the quality of their services.

A more positive strategy for drug plans is to implement a P4P program that rewards pharmacies that achieve high levels of quality or that significantly improve quality over time. This carrot approach may help to facilitate improved quality while maintaining broad access to pharmacy services for members. The reward could involve higher payment for MTM services for high-performance pharmacies, or a bonus for top performers. Unfortunately, a major impediment to this approach is a lack of funds available within drug plans to create a reward pool. Although Medicare Advantage drug plans could reap the benefits of improved medication utilization through fewer hospitalizations of members with chronic diseases, the standalone drug plans do not directly benefit from efforts to boost medication adherence or to identify patients with under-treatment of their diseases. Thus, they are less likely to create P4P programs that are focused on improving the quality of drug therapy. This could be addressed directly by employers and public payers creating an incentive pool that could be used to reward pharmacies that boost quality.

There are only a few examples of P4P programs for pharmacies. Humana implemented a P4P program for its pharmacy network with the goal of rewarding pharmacies that help to increase the utilization of generic drugs. In this program, the generic drug rate (GDR) at each network pharmacy is tracked on a semiannual basis. Based on the pharmacy's GDR within each 6-month period, a target for increase in GDR is established for the following 6 months. The targets for improvement are set on a sliding scale such that pharmacies with low GDR have higher targets for the percentage increase in GDR. Pharmacies that are above the network average for GDR have smaller targets for increase in GDR. If a pharmacy achieves its target level of increase in GDR, the pharmacy receives an increase in their reimbursement for drugs for the following 6 months.

THE FUTURE FOR COMMUNITY PHARMACY P4P

As employers and CMS continue their movement toward value-based purchasing, there will be heightened demands for transparency in the quality of care being provided. Although community pharmacies have been immune to many of these demands, it is likely that we will soon see reports on the quality of care provided by community pharmacists. Several demonstration projects sponsored by the Pharmacy Quality Alliance (PQA) have shown that the creation of pharmacy report cards is feasible. Although these report cards have only been used by pharmacies for quality improvement, there will inevitably be a call for public reporting of the report card results. Drug plans may use the reports to inform their members about the relative quality of pharmacies within their plan's network. Consumer advocacy groups may also call for the release of the report cards to better inform the public about safety issues in pharmacy.

If the quality of medication utilization is an important factor in the overall value of health care, it makes sense to incentivize all providers who can impact the use of medications. Physicians have been participating in P4P programs wherein medication measures are used to determine the physician's payment. If pharmacists can affect the quality of medication use, then it stands to reason that pharmacists or pharmacies be included in P4P systems. The inclusion of pharmacists in P4P programs can signal the recognition of the profession as an important component of safe and effective care.

As with physician P4P programs, it will be important for pharmacy P4P to be based on appropriate measures of quality. The PQA has tested numerous potential measures of pharmacy quality and a few of the measures appear to have some of the properties of ideal performance evaluation.[13] The measures related to medication adherence reveal that patients' adherence to key chronic medications has substantial room for improvement and that there is variation between pharmacies. Although PQA has not yet tested the ability of community pharmacists to drive improvements in adherence, there have been studies that demonstrated the ability of pharmacists to increase patients' adherence to medications.[14,15] There is also evidence that providing feedback to physicians on their patients' adherence can lead to improvements in adherence.[16] PQA is planning to support research to assess whether feedback to pharmacists on their patients' adherence to medications can facilitate improved adherence by patients.

One concern with using adherence measures for P4P is that patients are ultimately in control of whether they refill a prescription or take the medication. However, this criticism could be levied at almost any performance measure. Patients choose whether they get a flu shot, have their A1c checked, or fill their beta-blocker prescription after a heart attack. Pharmacists and physicians may not control their patients, but they can influence them. The difference between control and influence should be considered when designing the P4P model.

If a pharmacy P4P model is implemented with adherence measures, it may be best to structure the model to reward improvement in adherence rather than current levels of adherence. It would also be wise not to use a penalty to withhold payment to pharmacies that have a patient population with low levels of adherence. The pharmacy does not control the patients' adherence, and it may be unreasonable to punish the pharmacy for serving a population with poor adherence rates. However, if we assume that the pharmacists can influence adherence, then we may want to reward pharmacies that are able to dramatically improve the adherence of their patients to key medications.

There are several other types of measures that could be incorporated into a P4P system for pharmacies. PQA has worked with NCQA to test measures related to the safety of drug therapy and one of these measures is also being used by CMS to evaluate safety within Medicare drug plans. This CMS-adopted measure addresses the use of high-risk drugs in the elderly. Drug plans that have fewer elderly patients on the high-risk drugs receive a higher safety rating from CMS. Thus, it is likely that some drug plans will ask their network pharmacies to help in curtailing the use of these drugs and may integrate this measure into a P4P system. Other measures tested by PQA and NCQA include the appropriateness of drug use in selected subpopulations. For example, one measure assesses the proportion of diabetic patients with hypertension who are receiving an angiotensin-converting enzyme (ACE) inhibitor or angiotensin receptor blocker (ARB).

The amount of payment tied to performance is another important consideration for pharmacies as is the distribution of the incentive payments to the pharmacy staff. The economic premise that underlies P4P is the notion that providers will seek to maximize their revenue and will take actions that are in their best financial interest. The incentive should outweigh the costs to improve performance. Thus, if a pharmacy had to hire an additional technician to free up the pharmacist to spend more time on patient counseling, then the incentive should be sufficient to offset the cost. However,

TABLE 15-1. Example of Pharmacy P4P Based on Current Performance

	Medication Adherence	Medication Safety	Appropriateness: Asthma/Diabetes
No. of patients	200	300	100
No. of quality measures	4	3	4
Composite quality score	60% (120 adherent patients)	90% (270 patients meet criteria)	93% (93 patients meet criteria)
Incentive	$10 per patients	$2 per patients	$3 per patients
Bonus payment	$10 × 120 = $1200	$4 × 270 = $1080	$3 × 93 = $279

the pharmacy should also consider that there is an indirect cost to poor performance when pharmacy report cards are made public. If the public perceives the pharmacy to be a low-quality pharmacy relative to others in the community, the pharmacy may lose business. Thus, the addition of the technician may be warranted to offset the loss of business regardless of the P4P payments.

It is also important for the pharmacy to consider rewarding the individuals within the pharmacy who help to generate the improved performance. This may motivate the staff to strive for improvement since they will anticipate a financial reward for their achievement of improved performance. It is difficult to estimate how large a reward is required to stimulate greater attentiveness to a patient's adherence since no studies have examined this type of P4P model. However, it is likely that drug plans will begin experimenting with these incentives as more pressure is brought to bear on the plans to improve quality while controlling long-term costs.

Two examples of P4P models are shown in Tables 15-1 and 15-2. Both models incorporate three categories of measures and each category contains multiple measures. In most P4P models, the individual measures within a category are combined into a composite score (perhaps by taking the average of the scores on individual measures). The current performance model rewards the pharmacy by giving a fixed amount for each patient that conforms to the desired parameter of performance (e.g., the number of patients on a target drug that have a medication possession ratio ≥80%). The improvement model rewards the pharmacy based on improvement in the percentage of patients meeting a threshold. Other derivations on these models could be to reward only the pharmacies that are in the top two deciles of current performance or improvement.

The advent of pharmacy P4P is near. A small number of drug plans are beginning to implement simple models of P4P to drive improvements in selected measures of efficiency or quality. These models may be coupled with public reports on pharmacy quality to heighten the stakes for pharmacies and stimulate improvements in areas on which drug plans are being evaluated. Pharmacy owners and managers should become aware of the

TABLE 15-2. Example of Pharmacy P4P Based on Improvement

	Medication Adherence	Medication Safety	Appropriateness: Asthma/Diabetes
No. of patients	200	300	100
Score in 2006	60%	90%	93%
Score in 2007	70%	93%	92%
Improvement	10%	3%	None
Incentive	$1 per patients/ 1% increase	$0.50 per patients/ 1% increase	$2 per patients/ 1% increase
Bonus payment	$1 × 200 × 10 = $2000	$0.5 × 300 × 3 = $ 450	$2 × 100 × 0 = $0

opportunities as well as risks when these models are implemented. A proactive pharmacy may begin efforts now to identify strategies for boosting performance so that the pharmacy will come out "on top" when report cards and P4P systems are implemented.

REFERENCES

1. Institute of Medicine. *Rewarding Provider Performance: Aligning Incentives in Medicare.* Washington, DC: National Academy Press; 2007.
2. Rosenthal MB, Landon BE, Normand ST, Frank RG, Epstein AM. Pay for performance in commercial HMOs. *N Engl J Med.* 2006;355:1895–1902.
3. Gilmore AS, Zhao Y, Kang N, et al. Patient outcomes and evidence-based medicine in a preferred provider organization setting: a six-year evaluation of a physician pay-for-performance system. *Health Serv Res.* 2007;42:2140–2159.
4. IHA. *Advancing Quality through Collaboration: The California Pay for Performance Program.* Available at http://www.iha.org/wp020606.pdf. Accessed September 19, 2009.
5. IHA *The California Pay for Performance Program: The Second Chapter Measurement Years.* Available at http://www.iha.org/FINAL%20White%20Paper%20June%202009.pdf. Accessed September 19, 2009.
6. CMS. *Roadmap for Value-based Purchasing.* Available at http://www.cms.hhs.gov/QualityInitiativesGenInfo/downloads/VBPRoadmap_OEA_1-16_508.pdf. Accessed September 19, 2009.
7. CMS. *Premier Hospital Quality Incentive Program.* Available at http://www.cms.hhs.gov/HospitalQualityInits/35_HospitalPremier.asp#TopOfPage. Accessed September 19, 2009.
8. Lindenauer PK, Remus D, Roman S, et al. Public reporting and pay for performance in hospital quality improvement. *N Engl J Med.* 2007;356:486–496.
9. Institute of Medicine. *Rewarding Provider Performance: Aligning Incentives in Medicare.* Washington, DC: National Academies Press, 2007.

10. NCQA. *State of Health Care Quality 2008*. Available at http://www.ncqa.org/Portals/0/Newsroom/SOHC/SOHC_08.pdf. Accessed September 25, 2009.
11. Werner RM, Dudley RA. Making the "pay" matter in pay-for-performance: implications for payment strategies. *Health Aff.* 2009;28:1498–1508.
12. National Quality Forum. *Measure Evaluation Criteria*. Available at: http://www.qualityforum.org/uploadedFiles/Quality_Forum/Measuring_Performance/tbEvalCriteria2008-08-28Final.pdf. Accessed September 28, 2009.
13. Pilletere DP, Nau DP, McDonough K, Pierre Z. Development and testing of pharmacy performance measures. *J Am Pharm Assoc.* 2009;49:212–219.
14. Lee JK, Grace KA, Taylor AJ. Effect of a pharmacy care program on medication adherence and persistence, blood pressure and low-density lipoprotein cholesterol. *JAMA.* 2006;296:E1–E9.
15. Murray MD, Young J, Hoke S, et al. Pharmacist intervention to improve medication adherence in heart failure. *Ann Intern Med.* 2007;146:714–725.
16. Schectman JM, Schorling JB, Nadkarni MM, Voss JD. Can prescription refill feedback to physicians improve patient adherence? *Am J Med Sci.* 2004;327:19–24.

Part V
Application of Quality Improvement to the Pharmacy Practice Setting

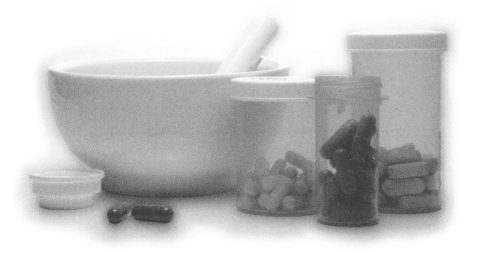

CHAPTER 16

Responding to an Outside Assessment of Pharmacy Quality

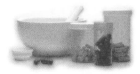

Julie Kuhle and Lynne Schifreen

Learning Objectives

At the end of the chapter, the reader will be able to:

1. Describe how to interpret a pharmacy quality report from an outside assessment.
2. Use the quality improvement process to improve quality as identified by an outside assessment.
3. Apply quality improvement principles to community and hospital pharmacy examples.

> If, and only if, providers have to demonstrate excellent results in addressing specific medical conditions will error decline, unnecessary tests not be performed, unnecessary treatments stop, the use of ineffective treatments cease, and the withholding of effective services come to an end.[1]

The results of quality measurement compiled in a pharmacy performance report can be a valuable tool to assess performance, identify and address quality concerns, and improve patient care. When pharmacy quality performance reports are available to the public, pharmacies can use information about the quality of their services to establish market differences between the health care they provide and service provided by their competition. Pharmacies can use the results in performance reports to differentiate themselves on aspects of patient care or disease management. The reports could also assist consumers in selection of a high-performing pharmacy and could be used by health plans in developing a high-performance pharmacy network. As payment reform leads to incentives based on quality, the mechanism used to give feedback to providers will be performance reports.

Most importantly, quality reports enable pharmacy staff to assess their performance so that patient care quality can be improved and enhanced. The Institute of Medicine defines quality as: *The degree to which health services for individuals and populations increase the likelihood of desired health outcomes and are consistent with current professional knowledge* (http://www.iom.edu/CMS/8089.aspx, accessed August 22).

Quality reports allow the user to determine areas for improvement based on the measure score, impact on patient safety, or stakeholder interest. When a pharmacy quality report is received, the pharmacy should consider the following process for optimizing their response. First, pharmacists should understand who has produced the report, why the report was provided, and what the data source for the report is. A payer such as CMS or a Medicare Part D plan may provide the report, or a chain pharmacy organization may provide quality reports to each of their pharmacies. Quality reports typically are used to provide information or comparison, to stimulate practice improvement, or to base an incentive. The data source for many pharmacy quality measures will be prescription drug claims, but some measures may also include diagnostic, laboratory, or administrative information. Pharmacy survey report cards will use subjective evaluation of the pharmacy's services from patient surveys.

The next step is to interpret the results on the performance report. Pharmacists should develop a good understanding of the measures used and how the score reflects on their practice. Most quality reports will include the measure's name and basic specification. The calculation of the measure uses a specified numerator and denominator. For example, an adherence measure may reflect the percentage of all diabetic patients (denominator) that are adherent to their oral hypoglycemic medications (numerator). In this case a high score is good. Prescription claims data are used to identify diabetic patients and calculate adherence. Another measure will reflect the percentage of all patients over 64 years of age getting a prescription (denominator) who received a potentially inappropriate medication for the elderly (numerator). In this example, a low score reports better performance and the data are derived from a combination of prescription claims data and administrative data to identify the patient's age.

The third step is to select a target for quality improvement activities. Three broad criteria were used by the Institute of Medicine in determining their 20 clinical priority areas[2] (these criteria to can be applied to the pharmacy's practice to determine the focus for quality improvement):

- *Impact*: What is the burden of poor quality on your population?
- *Improvability*: What is the ability to improve the process of care?
- *Inclusiveness*: Will the improvement affect a broad range of the pharmacy's patients considering age, gender, ethnicity, and socioeconomic status?

Compare the pharmacy's score for an individual measure to the report's average score or benchmark for that measure to determine practice variation (improvability). Choosing an area where the pharmacy has low performance will provide a good opportunity to improve care. Consider whether the pharmacy has a specific clinical emphasis where improvement would promote their special services and improve patient care (impact). Priority can be given to measures that include a large proportion of the pharmacy's patients, so that the quality improvement activity will benefit a larger number of people (inclusiveness). Choice of a quality improvement initiative can be based on whether a quality measure reflects either high risk or high cost to patients (impact). Finally, consider the interests and expertise of the pharmacy staff that will be supporting the quality improvement effort.

The following examples illustrate how a pharmacy can use a quality performance report:

● ABC pharmacy receives a performance assessment that includes measures of their patients' adherence to several different medication classes. Compared to the benchmark, this pharmacy's patients are adherent to diabetic medications and ACE inhibitors but are considerably less adherent with hyperlipidemic medications. Based on the measure's low score and variation from practice average, ABC pharmacy vbegins a quality improvement plan to increase patients' adherence to hyperlipidemic medications.

● Jones Pharmacy receives a similar performance assessment with several measure rates below benchmark standards. Instead of choosing the rate that is lowest, they review the low-scored measures to determine which measure may impact patient safety the most. After reviewing their performance scores, Jones Pharmacy sees that they have a high number of patients over 64 years reported in the denominator for the high-risk medications in the elderly measure. The pharmacy staff elects to focus their quality improvement efforts on decreasing their elderly patients' use of high-risk medications.

● Mainstreet Diabetic Center receives a performance assessment from a health care plan that is paying an incentive to pharmacies that provide better care for the health plan's diabetic patients. The quality report shows that Mainstreet Pharmacy scores well on several of the health plan's measures, but falls below goal on the measure of hypertensive diabetic patients receiving an ACE inhibitor. To improve this measure of pharmacy practice and be eligible for the health plan incentive, Mainstreet Pharmacy chooses to focus on the addition of ACE inhibitors for diabetic patients.

Once an area of performance has been selected for improvement, it is important to assess the capability and readiness of staff to implement a change. Several questions should be asked and answered. Is there support from all staff to improve performance? Is there buy-in from management? Who will be the champions of the activity? Are there knowledge deficits that will require additional training? How much time can be dedicated to supporting the quality initiative?

A quality improvement team should be assembled that reflects all areas of the pharmacy including pharmacy leadership, staff pharmacists, and technicians. The QI team is responsible for determining the goal for the quality improvement project, selecting the processes that will be changed to reach the goal, and formulating an action plan that will give structure to the quality improvement activity. A team leader, selected by management or elected by the team, should establish ground rules, facilitate meetings, provide a project timeline, and serve as a spokesperson for the team.[3]

The QI team will start by identifying all the process steps within the focus area to determine which process will be selected for improvement. Each step will be assessed for variability, process failure, or inefficiency. Identify where a system change can be made that will likely improve the desired outcome. Areas of suboptimal performance are listed in Box 16-1. Key factors in the selection are that the process must be

---

BOX 16-1. Areas of Suboptimal Performance

Ineffective or inefficient process
Variation in process
Communication gaps
Staffing limitations
Deficient, incomplete, or ineffective policy
Equipment failure or need
Knowledge gaps

---

observable, measurable, and have clearly defined boundaries.[3] Consider if additional steps need be added to the process to improve the outcome.

For example, a pharmacy may want to decrease the number of their elderly patients receiving new prescriptions for propoxyphene products. The QI team begins by listing all the steps associated with receiving the new prescription, determining that another medication should be considered, requesting a change from the prescriber, and providing the new medication to the patient. The team recognizes that the process step most variable in their pharmacy is that of requesting a change from the prescriber. Only a few pharmacists request a medication change for propoxyphene and only if time allows. The QI team decides to focus the quality improvement efforts on developing a fax-back communication tool to the physician that is easily completed and can be uniformly used to request a change in therapy.

There are several methods that can be used to approach quality improvement activities. Examples include the Plan–Test–Act–Check approach, the IMPROVE process, rapid-cycle change, Six Sigma Breakthrough Strategy, and the lean approach. A commonly used method is the Plan–Do–Study–Act (PDSA) cycle. This process includes simple steps that can be repeated to assess the success of the quality improvement intervention[4]:

⬤ *Plan*: Plan a change by studying results of quality measurement, formulate a plan for improvement, determine goals and targets, and determine interventions.

⬤ *Do*: Implement the plan (intervention) on a small scale, educate, and train.

⬤ *Study*: Gather data to evaluate the results of the intervention.

⬤ *Act*: Implement the change on a full scale or restructure the intervention and start the PDSA cycle again.

In the example given, the QI team *plans* a change by studying the steps in the process they want to change and developing a fax-back form to request a different medication whenever a new propoxyphene prescription is received for an elderly patient. The team plans how to implement the new process. They may decide that only two pharmacists will use the form for 2 weeks. The team is interested in how long it takes to complete and send the form, receive a response from the prescriber, and whether propoxyphene prescriptions are decreased. Information is recorded as the fax is used (*do*) during the

---

BOX 16-2. Tips for QI Success

Engage leadership
Select a committed QI team
Identify a single process for improvement
Set a goal relevant to staff and the organization
Research possible solutions
Determine an achievable project timeline
Collaborate with other teams or disciplines
Communicate success

---

test implementation. At the conclusion of the 2-week period, the team meets to *study* the data. The team determines that the fax is uniformly completed, but the fax could also act as an order if it was redesigned, so this *act*ion is taken and the cycle begins again.

Box 16-2 lists a number of tips that will assist teams in their QI efforts.

CASE EXAMPLE: RESPONDING TO PERFORMANCE REPORTS

The Universal Health Plan has recently expanded their Pay-for-performance program for network pharmacies. Since CMS is now rating the plans on drug safety, the plan has extended that rating to the pharmacies in their network. One of these ratings is on the use of high-risk drugs in the elderly. When these pharmacy report cards were sent out, Universal announced a program to reward those pharmacies who could substantially improve their scores.

Master's Excellent Pharmacy was particularly concerned when they reviewed their report card that their rate of filling high-risk drugs for elderly patients was noticeably higher than their peers. Jeff Master, the pharmacist in charge, saw the opportunity to increase reimbursement for his independent pharmacy, and also to improve medication safety for his community, as his pharmacy was adjacent to a large retirement community. Jeff was also thinking ahead to the time when consumers would be able to choose their pharmacy based on performance data. Thinking about these data, Jeff found a journal article on high-risk drugs in the elderly. "Certain drugs cause adverse events in the elderly population. Adverse events may increase falls or confusion. National guidelines identify certain drugs that have limited therapeutic effect and/or potentially serious side effects in the elderly. These drugs can affect a patient's ability to care for themselves independently, thereby decreasing their quality of life. Avoiding certain drugs can prevent hospitalizations or long term care admissions, allowing the elderly to remain at home and independent." (5)

Jeff saw the issue of high-risk drugs as one that could have significant impact on his retired population, due to the potential for avoiding hip fractures and other injuries. He hypothesized that if he could determine which drugs made up 80% of the avoidable prescriptions, then he and his pharmacists might be able to develop an intervention to reduce the number of prescriptions that their pharmacy received for the target drugs and thereby improve their score on this performance measure. Jeff had a staff meeting of his pharmacists and technicians to discuss this project and the impact it could have on their patients. First, he developed a presentation on High-risk Drugs in the Elderly that could be given to his pharmacists as well as the physicians in the area. Jeff also gave the pharmacists the high-risk drug list that was published by the National Committee on Quality Assurance. The pharmacists saw this could be used to screen prescriptions and advise physicians in their daily interactions. The pharmacists were excited to be able to expand their practice by looking at information in a proactive way.

Jeff and his pharmacists developed a comprehensive action plan. Their first action was to evaluate the data on fills for high-risk drugs in their pharmacy based on the data specifications provided by Universal Health Plan. They used their pharmacy data systems to produce a report on the number of fills for each drug on the NCQA high-risk drug list for the last 6 months in order to determine which drugs were filled the most frequently. The data showed that antihistamines, skeletal muscle relaxants, and narcotics made up 98% of the potentially avoidable drugs prescribed. Jeff reran the report for these three drug classes and created a report for each physician. They set up appointments with local physicians to discuss the potential risks of the target drugs and to recommend safer alternatives. The pharmacy technicians then flagged the profiles for each of these patients. The pharmacists developed a sample script for discussing the high-risk drugs with their patients and along with the technicians developed a simple patient information sheet explaining the concern about high-risk drugs.

Jeff was hoping that the program would move forward quickly, but there were numerous barriers. At first, some patients were very upset that their pharmacist was "going over their physician's head" and saying they should not have a medicine that was already prescribed. Likewise, there were physicians who were angry that the pharmacists were upsetting "their" patients. Jeff and his pharmacists went back to their script many times to tweak the language. They also developed a fax flyer they could send to physicians who had questions about the target drugs. Jeff noticed that customer waiting times were increasing at the counter; he found that he needed to bring in relief pharmacist help at key times. Every month when Jeff ran the data, he hoped to see some improvement.

Four months into the program, Jeff began to see improvement. The data noted a 15% decrease in high-risk drugs but with an increase in other prescriptions that could be used in place of the high-risk drugs. The pharmacy staff was elated to see that their work was making a difference. Jeff would continue to run the data and provide the staff with trend charts so that they could see their progress. The high-risk drug program was on the agenda of every staff meeting. Jeff even received an invitation to have a booth at a health fair at the retirement community on the program, and his staff is looking forward to their next project. Masters Excellent Pharmacy's improvements have also been noticed by the Universal Health Plan. Jeff's pharmacy received a quality bonus from the health plan in the quarter following the dramatic improvement in their scores. The shift to safer medications along with the quality bonus made the program a success for their patients while maintaining the revenues for the pharmacy.

REFERENCES

1. Porter ME, Teisberg EO. *Redefining Health Care – Creating Value-based Competition on Results.* Boston, MA: Harvard Business School Press; 2006:102–103.
2. Institute of Medicine. *Performance Measurement – Accelerating Improvement.* Washington, DC: The National Academies Press; 2006.
3. Nau D, Scott V. *Building a Quality Improvement Program for Pharmacy-based Diabetes Management Services.* Chap 3. American Pharmacists Association: Washington, DC: 2001.
4. Deming WE. *Out of the Crisis. Cambridge, MA: Massachusetts Institute of Technology,* Center for Advanced Engineering Study; 1986.
5. QualityNet. *Avoidable Drugs in the Elderly.* Available at: www.qualitynet.org Last accessed: March 19, 2010.

CHAPTER 17

Implementing Your Own Pharmacy Quality Improvement Program

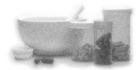

Terri L. Warholak and Mi Chi Song

Learning Objectives

At the end of the chapter, the reader will be able to:

1. Identify the key steps in a quality improvement process.
2. Apply the quality improvement process with real-world examples.
3. Assess the challenges in applying the quality improvement process in pharmacy settings.

INTRODUCTION

Continuous Quality Improvement or CQI is a process improvement technique that focuses on improvement efforts by identifying root causes of problems, intervening to reduce or eliminate these causes, and reassessing the process. The never-ending CQI process recognizes that the majority of problems result from a failure in the process of providing the service (systems issues), as opposed to being attributable to the providers themselves. In this manner, CQI empowers health care providers to improve quality on a daily basis.

Many CQI models exist. Examples of specific models include the PDCA model that stands for plan, do, check, and act, and the FOCUS-PDCA model, which is a nine-step model that incorporates the words find, organize, clarify, understand, select, plan, do, check, and act. The Six Sigma model is also a well-known business management strategy whose use is widespread in many sectors of industry today. Suffice it to say that there are many CQI models and that all include elements that reflect the following core concepts: (1) plan, (2) design, (3) measure, (4) assess, and (5) improve. CQI has been described as a practical application of the scientific method since both processes are similar. With this being said, one can think of the steps in the CQI cycle as parallel to the information found in the sections of a scientific article: background, methods, results, conclusions, and recommendations. A visual representation of the sections of a scientific article can be seen in Figure 17-1.

This chapter will describe the CQI model and explore its use in pharmacy practice. The chapter will review examples of how pharmacists can use CQI to increase quality in pharmacy practice.

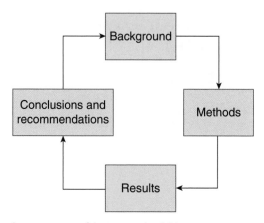

Figure 17-1. A visual representation of the steps in the CQI process.

The following discussion of the CQI process is provided as a review; a more thorough discussion can be found in Chapter 5. A worksheet to guide you through the process is also found in Chapter 5.

BACKGROUND

When doing background work, it is important to investigate the issue to ensure you know and are able to define the following:

1. What is the problem? You need to be sure you are working on the *right* problem.
2. Why is the problem a problem? That is, why is the problem worthy of your attention?
3. What solutions have been tried? This is important and can be derived from the literature. If someone else has tried a solution and it has worked, the same solution may be able to be adapted for your practice setting.
4. State the global goal of the project. The goal should relate to the project stated in #1 above. Some of the options may include: (a) discovery, (b) frequency estimation, (c) measure of a change, or (d) a combination of these.

METHODS

1. Think about the methods that others have used in the past to solve similar QI problems and adapt them for your needs and practice situation.
2. Select the best intervention to accomplish goals.
3. List the process and/or outcome measures necessary to determine if goal(s) were met.
4. Determine what data are already being collected, and what measures exist.
5. Plan data collection methods. You might choose from: (a) inspection points, (b) focus groups, (c) monitoring for markers, (d) chart review, (e) observation, and (f) spontaneous report.

6. Plan statistical analysis – make sure you will collect all information needed.

7. Break the project into steps and detail practical considerations. Focus in on what steps are needed, and determine who–what–where–when–how each will be accomplished.

8. Sketch a preliminary timeline for the project.

9. List challenges to be addressed before the next meeting, and assign a responsible party to address each challenge listed above.

RESULTS

For this portion, you need to put the plan developed in methods into action:

1. Measure your chosen measures.

2. Enter data and analyze them.

CONCLUSIONS AND RECOMMENDATIONS

This is where you can take some time to think about your results and what they mean:

1. What is the bottom line?

2. What worked?

3. What could be done better?

4. What recommendations for further improving the process can you make now? This will help you plan your next QI cycle, as well as rate the success of this one.

Below are some examples of how the quality improvement process can be used in pharmacy practice

---

CASE EXAMPLE 1

Let us use a chain community pharmacy example, focusing on dispensing errors, and go step by step through the CQI cycle. This example is taken from a Doctor of Pharmacy student QI project titled "Implementing Methods for Thorough Demographic Documentation in a Chain Pharmacy: Project PANDA." Each of the sections that follow in this example includes direct quotes (in italics) from Project PANDA as developed by Melissa Badowski, Melanie Cohen, Megan Corrigan, Chantel Hrabe, and Renata Krzyminski.

Background:

1. What is the problem?

> *In the medical field, it is vital to obtain correct patient information to ensure efficient and comprehensive care. To ensure that every patient*

receives the same quality of care, proper demographic information must be routinely collected.

2. Why is the problem a problem?

This is a problem because if the demographic information is either inaccurate or missing, detrimental results may occur. These results may be, but are not limited to, correct medication given to the wrong patient, a medication given to a patient that he/she is allergic to, or inappropriate dosing due not recording or checking date of birth. There is an ample amount of data that supports these issues. For example, in a study done in the Veteran's Healthcare System, out of 82 dispensing errors reported, 24 were medications given to the wrong patient.[1] It has been suggested that "18% of medication errors [are] due to incomplete patient information."[2]

3. What solutions have been tried?

Although there have been attempts made to computerize prescriptions to ensure that the correct patient is given the medication, this has not ameliorated the problem completely.[3] This is extremely significant in the eyes of the patients who receives the wrong medication. The investigators are interested in the topic of demographic errors due to lack of information because it is felt that this is overlooked in many studies. "There is little published evidence related to dispensing errors and near misses occurring in this setting [community pharmacies]."[4] We feel that with a little extra effort at the in window, all necessary demographic information can be obtained in a timely manner.

4. State the global goal of the project.

The overall objective of this project is to decrease the number of demographic errors made in Rx entry and Rx pick-up by implementing a procedure that ensures that the correct information is in the store computer system at one pharmacy. This will include discovery of demographic errors occurring before the implementation of the procedure and measuring the success rate after initiation of the program. The goal is to decrease the number of prescriptions that are entered and sold with the incorrect demographic information.

Methods:

1. Think about the methods that others have used in the past to solve similar QI problems and adapt them for your needs and practice situation.

2. Select best intervention to accomplish goals (listed in #4 above).

After brainstorming, the investigators devised a program to reduce the number of prescriptions entered and dispensed under the wrong profile. The program, entitled PANDA, is a mnemonic device to re-

*mind the pharmacy staff to gather essential information about each
patient. This program enforces standardization among the pharmacy
staff when collecting patient information. The mnemonic stands for:
P – phone number, A – allergies, N – name, D – date of birth, A
– address. In order to execute the idea, the investigators developed a
self-inking stamp of the mnemonic to be utilized at the in-window
and the drive-thru window. They also developed a "Verify PANDA"
stamp to be used by the pharmacist for phoned in prescriptions and
reminded the pharmacy staff to perform a final verification at the out-
window.*

*Procedure: Each member of the pharmacy staff was instructed to
stamp each new prescription with the appropriate PANDA stamp.
They were also trained to fill in each letter with the corresponding information. The pharmacist, while verifying, was then to double-check
the information on the stamp against the information in the computer
to ensure that it was indeed the correct patient. If there was a "Verify
PANDA" stamp placed in the bag, then the out-window staff was
to verify the PANDA information again. There were signs posted in
the pharmacy, pamphlets available for patients, and a letter to the
pharmacy staff explaining the objectives of PANDA. Employees were
also asked to wear pins in support of the program and to encourage
patients to inquire about PANDA.*

3. List process and/or outcome measures necessary to determine if goal(s) were met.

*A baseline count of new prescriptions and a count of errors that left
the pharmacy was documented so that adequate comparison could be
made after the procedure had been implemented. The sample selection
of the program was designed to target the entire store population from
September 21, 2004 until October 18, 2004.*

4. Determine what data are all ready being collected and what measures exist.

None were applicable.

5. Plan data collection methods.

*The investigators collected data prior to the implementation of
PANDA regarding filling and dispensing errors. Throughout the duration of PANDA the investigators collected data involving the number
of stamped prescriptions vs. non-stamped prescriptions, the pharmacist
working and the number of stamped prescriptions, and if the stamp
was filled out in its entirety. The pharmacist documented, over short
spans of time, how many prescriptions he/she returned to the staff during the filling process due to incorrect patient information in one of
the five PANDA fields. A survey was distributed to the pharmacy staff*

to assess their opinions on the PANDA process. The questions were asked with an interval scale (strongly disagree–strongly agree).

6. Plan statistical analysis.

The data were analyzed by counting the number of stamped prescriptions vs. the number of non-stamped prescriptions, looking at the pharmacist on duty vs. the number of stamped prescriptions, evaluating the most and least filled fields of the stamp, and pharmacy staff attitudes regarding PANDA. The data were then compiled into graphs and tables to convey the outcomes of the project.

Results:

For this portion, you need to put the plan developed in the section "Methods" into action.

1. Measure your chosen measures.

Over the four weeks that PANDA was implemented, there were 2158 new prescriptions evaluated. Of the 2158, 1119 were stamped. Although only 51.9% of the new prescriptions were stamped, the program was considered effective because there were no errors that left the pharmacy dealing with incorrect demographic data. The fraction of non-stamped prescriptions increased during a one-week span.

In the 8 weeks prior to the start of the program, there were 3814 new prescriptions and four errors due to incomplete demographic data. The percentage of errors that left the pharmacy in the 8 weeks prior to the start of the program was 0.104%, and after implementation of the program the percentage was 0%.

As can be seen in Figure 17-2, the consistency of new prescriptions stamped varied with the pharmacist on duty. Although there is no

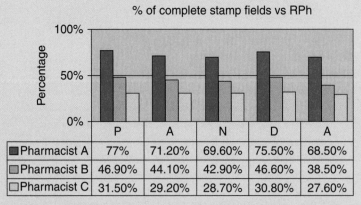

% of complete stamp fields vs RPh

	P	A	N	D	A
■ Pharmacist A	77%	71.20%	69.60%	75.50%	68.50%
▨ Pharmacist B	46.90%	44.10%	42.90%	46.60%	38.50%
☐ Pharmacist C	31.50%	29.20%	28.70%	30.80%	27.60%

Figure 17-2. Consistency of new prescriptions PANDA fields completed by pharmacist.

definite reason for the variation in the percentages, it may be con-
cluded that lack of motivation played a factor; not all fields were filled
out consistently. The "Name" and "Address" sections of the stamp were
not filled out as often than the other fields. The "Phone Number" and
"Date of Birth" sections of the stamp were filled in the most often.
This may have occurred because a search in the store computer system
is performed by inputting the phone number or date of birth first.

After the completion of the program, the pharmacy staff was asked
to complete a survey prepared by the investigators. The survey concluded
that although the program was helpful and did not take an excess
amount of time, they felt that the patients were not aware of the pro-
gram and its usefulness. It is interesting to note that when the pharmacy
staff was surveyed, they conveyed acceptance of the program.

Conclusions and Recommendations:

The limitations of this research program included limits within
the pharmacy and limits dealing with the collection of data. Since
PANDA was not a company mandated program, there was a lack
of motivation; the staff did not always comply with the investigators'
requests involving the stamping of all prescriptions. Also, there was a
lack of complete information due to the fact that controlled prescrip-
tions and refills were not examined. Therefore, there was a large
quantity of prescriptions that were not included in the final data.
One last limitation was that this program was only implemented for a
four-week timeframe. There were not sufficient baseline data collected
and there were only a small amount of actual data collected. One last
limitation was that the investigators did not use the data collected by
the pharmacist over short periods of time to document near-misses.

The implications to the site included improved care, more accu-
rate demographic data collection, an increase assurance of the correct
prescription reaching the correct patient, and ultimately, optimizing
patient outcomes.

The investigators concluded that this research program, if given
enough time to be implemented, would be successful. Even though the
resulting numbers were small and insignificant on the whole, the fact
remains that the project caught potential errors. These errors could
have caused detrimental effects to the one patient who received the
wrong prescription. Also, the research program was well received by
other sectors of the pharmacy field. The district manager, pharmacy
manager, and pharmacists of the store commended the investigators on
their creative solution to the problem at hand.

This PANDA procedure can be modified to encompass refills to
ensure the patient receives continuous quality care. Instead of limiting

*PANDA to only one store in one chain, it can be expanded to mul-
tiple locations across the nation.*

*There needs to be more research in the area of motivation of the
pharmacy staff in order to be more compliant with the stamping. An
emphasis needs to be placed on making sure all fields of PANDA are
filled in completely. Each field is as important as the next and this
needs to be stressed to the staff. Another area of investigation is the
patient's thoughts and feelings about having to constantly give this
demographic information time after time. There needs to be a way to
educate the patient on the importance of consistently retrieving this
information to prevent harm in the long run.*

CASE EXAMPLE 2

Another study was done that looked at improving patient care by performing
a "Comparison of Inventory Accuracy in Pyxis® CUBIE™ and Matrix Systems."
This was also a Pharm.D. student QI project by Arti Patel, Minesh Patel, Thanh
Phan, Kim Tran, Hong Tran, Huong Tran (pharmacy students), and Lisa Mi-
chener (preceptor). Excerpts taken verbatim from the authors are in italics below.
The project and steps are summarized in the interests of brevity.

Background:

   *To further prevent medication errors, the Institute of Medicine
   recommends the implementation of automated dispensing systems
   (ADS).[5] One prospective study reported 34 errors found among 4029
   doses (0.84%) filled manually by technicians versus 25 errors among
   3813 doses (0.66%) filled by ADS devices.[6] Another study concluded
   that the medication error rate was decreased from 16.9% to 10.4%
   after implementation of ADS devices into a nursing unit.[7] With this
   being said, according to the Institute for Safe Medication Practices,
   the use of ADS devices alone, cannot improve patient safety unless a
   cabinet design and use are carefully planned to eliminate opportunities for drug selection and dosing errors.[8]*

   *The Pyxis® brand automated dispensing systems are widely used in
   many health care institutions, and there are different systems/models
   available. The Pyxis® Computerized Unit-Based Inventory Exchange
   (CUBIE) system limits access to one medication at a time, thereby
   reducing risk for medication errors, while the Pyxis® Matrix system
   is an open grid-like system that allows access to multiple medications
   at one time. Pictures of a medication drawer from the Pyxis® CUBIE
   and Pyxis® Matrix systems appear as Figures 17-3 and 17-4 below.
   This study was conducted at a suburban Chicago hospital to compare*

the Pyxis® CUBIE and Pyxis® Matrix systems for the total number of inventory inaccuracies (i.e., wrong inventory count, wrong medication, and expired medications).

Methods:

The inventory accuracy was compared between the Pyxis® CUBIE™ and Matrix systems in the Pyxis® Medstation Rx System 2000, version 4.2. Inventory accuracy was determined by auditing the Pyxis® CUBIE™ and Matrix pocket systems on three consecutive Wednesdays in October 2004. The types of inventory inaccuracies that were audited were for

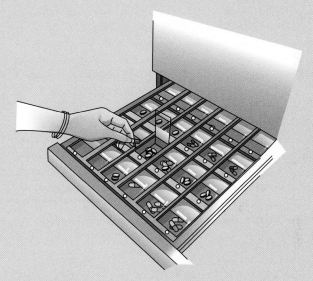

Figure 17-3. The Pyxis® CUBIE™ system.

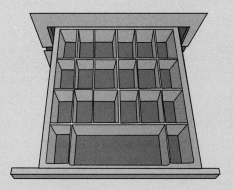

Figure 17-4. The Pyxis® Matrix system.

the wrong count, wrong medication, and expired medications, and chi-squared analyses were performed to determine whether there were statistically significant variances between the two systems.

Results:

As can be seen in Table 17-1 below, the results of the study showed that the total number of inventory inaccuracies as well as total number of inaccuracies for each type of inventory criteria investigated, were significantly lower in the Pyxis® CUBIE™ system compared to the Pyxis® Matrix system. The Pyxis® CUBIE™ system had 93 (19.9%) total inventory inaccuracies compared to 207 (38.6%) total inventory inaccuracies in Pyxis® Matrix system, and all three types of inventory inaccuracies were consistently lower in Pyxis® CUBIE™ system. In the Pyxis® Matrix system, the greatest contributor to inventory inaccuracy was wrong count (70%) followed by wrong medication (17%), then expired medication (13%), while in the Pyxis® CUBIE™ system, the greatest contributor was wrong count (86%), and wrong medication (3%) showed the least contribution to inventory inaccuracies. However, the investigators acknowledge that only three criteria for inventory accuracy were measured, so the findings from this study should not be used to generalize other possible contributing factors in inventory accuracy. Also, due to a short study period, the selection method for Pyxis® Medstation, and the small population of medication pockets audited, the findings from this study cannot be extrapolated to state the overall effect of Pyxis® CUBIE™ system on inventory accuracy is a reduction in medication errors.

Conclusions and Recommendations:

Future studies to investigate other factors influencing inventory accuracy and analysis of the overall cost-effectiveness of implementing the Pyxis® CUBIE™ technology is recommended. Also, since the Pyxis® CUBIE™ system has unique device features, further studies need to

TABLE 17-1. Results from Data Collection and Statistical Analysis

	Pyxis® Matrix	Pyxis® CUBIE™	P-Value (≤.05)
Total pockets audited	536	467	N/A
Total inventory inaccuracies	207	93	<.001
Total wrong count	145	80	<.001
Total expired medications	26	10	<.001
Total wrong medications	36	3	<.001

be done to investigate what errors are specific to the Pyxis® CUBIE™ technology. However, the findings of this study encourage pharmacy and nursing staff to check and update expired medications regularly, make sure that the right drug is in the right pocket, increase the frequency of inventory audits, and report any medication errors for further improvements in medication distribution.

SUMMARY

The examples above, while not perfect, do demonstrate many of the important lessons of using the CQI process. That is, the CQI process:

- is applicable to varied pharmacy practice settings;
- can be used for a variety of reasons (the examples in this chapter show how the process can be used to measure the impact of a system change as well as to assess which dispensing machine might produce less errors);
- often requires only the use of descriptive statistics;
- can be used effectively by pharmacists and pharmacy students with a little training;
- can help little changes have a big impact.

Remember, all pharmacists and pharmacy students have the potential to increase the quality in their practice setting if they use the CQI process.

REFERENCES

1. Rolland P. Occurrence of dispensing errors and efforts to reduce medication errors at the Central Arkansas Veteran's Healthcare System. *Drug Saf.* 2004;27:271–282.
2. Leape L, Bates DW, Cullen DJ, et al. Systems analysis of adverse drug events. *J Am Med Assoc.* 1995;274:35–43.
3. Kennedy AG, Littenberg B. A modified outpatient prescription form to reduce prescription errors. *Jt Comm J Qual Saf.* 2004;30:480–487.
4. Ashcroft DM, Quinlan P, Blenkinsopp A. Prospective study of the incidence, nature and causes of dispensing errors in community pharmacies. *Pharmacoepidemiol Drug Saf.* 2004. 14:327–332
5. Institute of Medicine (IOM) Committee on Quality Health Care in America. *Crossing the Quality Chasm: A New Health System for the 21st Century.* Washington: National Academy of Sciences; 1999.
6. Klein EG, Santora JA, Pascala PM, et al. Medication cart-filling time, accuracy, and cost with an automated dispensing system. *Am J Hosp Pharm.* 1994;52:1193–1196.
7. Borel JM. Effect of an automated nursing unit-based dispensing device on medication errors. *Am J Hosp Pharm.* 1995;52:1875–1679.
8. Institute for Safe Medication Practices (ISMP). *Survey of automated dispensing shows need for practice improvements and safer system design.* June 15, issue 1999.

Index

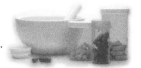